Mobilizing against AIDS

Mobilizing against AIDS

REVISED AND ENLARGED EDITION

Institute of Medicine
National Academy of Sciences

EVE K. NICHOLS

HARVARD UNIVERSITY PRESS
Cambridge, Massachusetts
London, England
1989

Library of Congress Cataloging-in-Publication Data

Mobilizing against AIDS, revised and enlarged ed.
  Bibliography: p.
  Includes index.
  1. AIDS (Disease) I. Nichols, Eve K. II. Institute
of Medicine (U.S.)
RC607.A26M63 1989   616.97'92   88-30100
ISBN 674-57763-9 (alk. paper)
ISBN 674-57762-0 (pbk. : alk. paper)

Contents

Foreword

AIDS, the acquired immunodeficiency syndrome, is now a serious public health concern in most major U.S. cities and in countries worldwide. Scientific investigation has expanded and intensified as the disease has grown to unquestionably epidemic proportions. The Institute of Medicine organized the scientific session of its 1985 annual meeting around an examination of the disease. The first edition of this book was drawn from that meeting, which also contributed to the convening of a larger body of experts under the auspices of the Institute of Medicine and the National Academy of Sciences. That group's recommendations for actions against the epidemic, issued in late 1986 as the report *Confronting AIDS*, attracted wide official and public attention to the directions in policy and size of investment needed.

Since 1986 there have been impressive advances in understanding of the AIDS virus, its mechanisms, and its routes of transmission. Researchers are creating virtually a new generation of tools to probe the virus in the laboratory and to screen for its presence in the population. But these hard-won discoveries have not yet led to a drug that can cure infection with the virus or to a vaccine that can prevent it, nor is either breakthrough expected soon. The only way to stem the spread of infection remains the public health approach of educating people about how to avoid infection or, if they are infected, how not to infect others. If these efforts fail, AIDS will exact an increasing toll on its infected victims and an intolerable drain on the health workers and resources employed in combating the disease.

The range and size of this revised edition testify to the pace and volume of efforts in the past few years to understand AIDS: it is more than twice as large as the 1986 version. In the following pages Eve Nichols faithfully recounts the ferment of activities to combat AIDS and presents the rationale for hoping that the epidemic can be quelled.

Samuel O. Thier
President, Institute of Medicine

September 1988

Mobilizing against AIDS

1

The Scope of AIDS

He put his cane down on the table next to his bed and slowly removed his shirt. The bright light coming through the window fell on his chest as he turned reluctantly toward the mirror. For weeks he had been afraid to look at his own reflection. The purplish spots of Kaposi's sarcoma now covered his entire torso. The boyish face crumpled and he cried as he had many times during the past 18 months. He was 24 years old, and he knew that the infections raging through his body would kill him before the spring.

Three years ago, when this account was written for the first edition of *Mobilizing against AIDS,* the American public had just begun to understand the potential impact of acquired immunodeficiency syndrome (AIDS). More than 10,000 people in the United States had died from AIDS, and 9,000 more were battling the disease. The discovery of the human immunodeficiency virus (HIV) had resolved the most basic question about AIDS—what causes it—but had generated many new questions as well. For example, blood tests revealed that a large proportion of apparently healthy people in groups with a high prevalence of AIDS (such as homosexual men and hemophiliacs) were infected with HIV. No one knew how many of them would eventually become sick.

Many scientists now believe that in the absence of a treatment to slow or halt the progression of infection, virtually all of those with evidence of HIV infection in their blood will develop AIDS. This realization, based on several long-term

Table 1.1. (continued)

State	Year ending August 1, 1988		Cumulative total since June 1981	
	Number	(%)	Number	(%)
Delaware	57	0.2	109	0.2
Iowa	35	0.1	85	0.1
Maine	37	0.1	84	0.1
New Hampshire	41	0.1	75	0.1
Nebraska	35	0.1	71	0.1
West Virginia	15	0.1	50	0.1
Alaska	19	0.1	48	0.1
Vermont	20	0.1	34	0.0
Virgin Islands	25	0.1	32	0.0
Idaho	12	0.0	22	0.0
Montana	14	0.0	22	0.0
Wyoming	3	0.0	11	0.0
South Dakota	5	0.0	10	0.0
North Dakota	3	0.0	9	0.0
Guam	4	0.0	5	0.0
Trust Territory			1	0.0
Total	29305	100.0	69366	100.0

Source: U.S. Department of Health and Human Services, Public Health Service, Centers for Disease Control.

blood products before techniques were developed to safeguard the blood supply, heterosexual partners of those at recognized risk of HIV infection (see Figure 1.1), and infants born to infected mothers. Researchers have established that heterosexual transmission occurs from men to women and from women to men, but so far the prevalence of infection among heterosexuals with no known risk factors is low in the United States. (This fact suggests that an opportunity exists for prevention strategies designed to stop the spread of HIV infection.) Repeated studies in both the United States and Africa have found no evidence for HIV transmission by casual contact or by biting or bloodsucking insects.

Those most familiar with the devastating consequences of HIV infection continue to be the nation's homosexual men. In cities across the United States they describe the anguish of

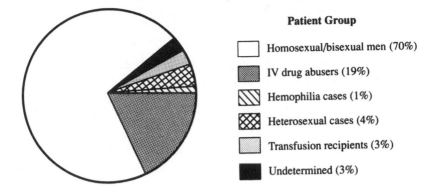

Patient Group

☐ Homosexual/bisexual men (70%)

▨ IV drug abusers (19%)

◪ Hemophilia cases (1%)

▧ Heterosexual cases (4%)

▦ Transfusion recipients (3%)

■ Undetermined (3%)

FIGURE 1.1. Reported adult cases of AIDS (total = 68,258) in the United States: percentage by patient group, 1981 to August 1, 1988. (Seven percent of the homosexual/bisexual men reported having used intravenous drugs.) Source: U.S. Department of Health and Human Services, Public Health Service, Centers for Disease Control.

watching one friend after another weaken and die. The loss of a dozen friends in less than 6 months is not uncommon in cities hardest hit by the epidemic. Most of the dead have been young men; almost 90 percent of AIDS patients are between the ages of 20 and 49.

The geographic variation in HIV infection among homosexuals is relatively low. In contrast, the prevalence of HIV infection among intravenous (IV) drug abusers varies widely, ranging from 5 percent or less in cities such as Denver, San Antonio, and Tampa to more than 60 percent in New York City. Historical studies indicate that once HIV enters a drug-abusing population it can spread very rapidly. For example, the prevalence of HIV infection in Manhattan increased to more than 40 percent within 3 years after collection of the first HIV-seropositive blood sample.[2] Researchers are attempting to identify the factors responsible for the rapid spread (beyond sharing of needles and syringes within friendship groups) and to determine whether local efforts can prevent it.

Areas with the greatest number of HIV-infected IV drug abusers also have the greatest number of infected women and children. A 1987 study by the CDC showed that the two major risk factors among women with AIDS are intravenous drug abuse and heterosexual contact with an intravenous drug abuser.

One consequence of the strong link between drug abuse and heterosexual transmission of HIV infection in the United States is the disproportionate impact of the epidemic on racial and ethnic minorities. The socioeconomic factors associated with high rates of intravenous drug abuse among minority populations, including poverty, unemployment, and inadequate education, are also associated with higher rates of HIV infection. More than 70 percent of all women with AIDS are black or Hispanic, as are about 75 percent of all children with AIDS.

Greater recognition of the magnitude of HIV-related problems among urban minorities is essential to the development of effective measures to limit the spread of HIV infection. Risk-reduction education has reduced high-risk sexual behavior among homosexual men and has had a limited impact on needle sharing among intravenous drug abusers. There is little evidence, however, that AIDS education has had any effect on those at greatest risk of heterosexual transmission of HIV. In fact, over the past 4 years public health officials have witnessed a dramatic resurgence in syphilis and other sexually transmitted diseases among heterosexuals in the United States. The problem has been most severe among young men and women in inner-city neighborhoods.

Researchers need to learn more about the factors that motivate behavior change. Studies in other fields indicate that effective education programs must be highly specific and must create a supportive social environment for those willing to change.

An important element of current prevention programs is to encourage as many potentially infected people as possible to seek counseling and voluntary testing. (The National AIDS Hotline provides confidential information and referrals to HIV testing and counseling centers; see Appendix A.) Such programs will be most successful if federal, state, and local authorities strengthen measures to ensure confidentiality and to protect records from unauthorized disclosure. Several states have reexamined protections afforded to all types of health records. Federal and state lawmakers also are evaluating legislation to prevent discrimination against those who are infected or thought to be at risk of HIV infection.

Public health officials support voluntary use of the HIV test by individuals whose behavior places them at high risk of infection because the test is believed to foster individual behavior change and slow the spread of the epidemic. The assumption is that people who test positive will use condoms regularly and adopt other safer-sex practices to avoid passing the infection to their sexual partners.

People seeking voluntary testing benefit in several different ways. A negative test result is reassuring. In addition, the counseling session that accompanies the test should provide those who are HIV-seronegative with practical information about how to avoid future infection.

Receiving news about a positive HIV test is an extremely stressful experience. At first patients may be so distraught that they are unable to absorb educational or referral information. But early diagnosis can prolong the life of a person infected with HIV. It allows the physician to be on the lookout for life-threatening opportunistic infections that may be the first clinical signs of immune suppression. As discussed in Chapter 3, therapies for *Pneumocystis carinii* pneumonia and some of the other opportunistic infections common in HIV-infected patients have improved dramatically since the beginning of the epidemic. In 1981 only 18 percent of HIV-infected patients diagnosed with *P. carinii* pneumonia in New York City survived more than a year; by 1985 the one-year survival rate had increased to 48 percent.[3] Researchers now are exploring the benefits of various prophylactic treatments to prevent episodes of *P. carinii* pneumonia in high-risk patients.

Despite progress in treating the opportunistic infections associated with HIV infection, long-term survival of AIDS patients will depend on strategies that attack the virus itself. The euphoria that followed the discovery of AZT (azidothymidine or zidovudine; the trade name is Retrovir), the first

anti-HIV drug licensed by the U.S. Food and Drug Administration, has faded. AZT prolongs the lives of some patients
but is too toxic for others. Many different drugs will be
needed to combat the diverse effects of the very complex virus
reponsible for AIDS. Chapter 7 explores the requirements for
potential drug candidates: they must be suitable for oral
administration, inexpensive, safe enough for lifelong use, and
able to cross the physiologic barrier between the bloodstream
and the central nervous system.

The design of possible future drugs will be based on greater
understanding of the structure of HIV, its life cycle, and its
interactions with various cells in the body. Initially, researchers
believed that HIV infected only one population of white blood
cells, the T4 or "helper" cells. (Loss of the T4 cells prevents the
body from responding effectively to many external challenges.)
Further studies have revealed, however, that the virus also
infects monocyte/macrophages (another class of white blood
cells), certain cells in the brain, Langerhans cells in the skin,
endothelial cells (cells that line blood vessels), epithelial cells in
the small intestine and rectum, cervical cells, cells in the retina,
and blood-forming cells in the bone marrow. This array of
targets makes the virus a formidable opponent indeed.

Increased knowledge about HIV has made scientists less
sanguine about the prospects for an AIDS vaccine. In early 1984,
Margaret M. Heckler, then secretary of the U.S. Department of
Health and Human Services, predicted that a vaccine might be
ready for clinical trials in 2 years. Seventeen months later, a
long-range plan developed by the Public Health Service (PHS)
to control AIDS acknowledged that it was unlikely that a
vaccine would be generally available before 1990. Today the
PHS assessment also is viewed as overly optimistic.

Recent attempts to develop a vaccine have been discouraging. Scientists have tried all the "obvious" solutions—
solutions based on experience with other types of viral
infections—and none of them has worked. Potential vaccines
have failed to protect laboratory animals from viral challenges.
Despite these results, several vaccine candidates have been
approved for human safety trials in the United States and

elsewhere. Chapter 7 discusses the rationale behind these trials and the concerns of those who believe that human trials should wait until protection against infection has been demonstrated in an animal model.

The road to an HIV vaccine will be long and arduous. Efficacy trials will require thousands of willing, thoroughly informed volunteers who are at high risk of infection but still uninfected. Follow-up for years after immunization will be necessary to detect signs of HIV-related disease or adverse reactions to a vaccine. The logistics and expense of such trials present enormous obstacles. The Institute of Medicine has recommended that planning begin now for large-scale human efficacy trials even though suitable vaccine candidates have not yet been identified.

For now, the only way to slow the spread of HIV is through education and other public health measures. Considerable controversy exists, however, about what these other measures should be. For example, public health experts have very different views about the reporting of HIV test results. Some believe that mandatory reporting and partner notification are necessary to slow the spread of the epidemic; they say that identifying and counseling the sexual partners of people infected with HIV may be especially beneficial in populations with a low prevalence of disease. Others express concern that mandatory reporting might discourage some people who practice high-risk behavior from taking the test. Disagreements grow even sharper over the ethical and moral implications of mandatory testing and the possibility of quarantining HIV-infected people who continue to engage in high-risk behavior without concern for the health of others. Maintaining an appropriate balance between the health needs of the community and the civil rights of those infected with HIV will continue to challenge policymakers as the epidemic grows.

Another extremely important challenge is the provision of adequate health care for HIV-infected patients. The relatively sudden appearance of large numbers of patients with complex HIV-related diseases has highlighted inadequacies in both the organization and the financing of health care in the

period (for example, 6 or 7 years after infection), they would be unlikely to get it at all. However, data from long-term studies of HIV-infected patients indicate that the risk for disease progression does not decrease with time; rather, it appears to increase. Thus, without effective therapy the great majority of people infected with HIV will eventually progress to AIDS.

Development of the Epidemic

When the first cases of AIDS were reported in 1981, epidemiologists at the Centers for Disease Control immediately began tracking the disease backward in time as well as forward. They determined that the first cases of AIDS in the United States probably occurred in 1977.[1]

By early 1982, AIDS had been reported in 15 states, the District of Columbia, and 2 foreign countries, but the total remained low: 158 men and 1 woman. More than 90 percent of the men were homosexual or bisexual. Interviews with patients did not provide any definite clues about the origin of the disease.

Then in July 1982 the CDC published a report from the University of Miami describing unusual infections and Kaposi's sarcoma in 34 recent Haitian immigrants (including 4 women) in 5 states. The authors of the report noted the similarities between this new phenomenon and the pattern of disease previously described in homosexual men and intravenous drug abusers. None of the Haitian men reported homosexual activity, however, and only one had a history of intravenous drug abuse.

The puzzling report about the Haitian patients was followed immediately by news that 3 heterosexual men with hemophilia had developed AIDS. Together, these reports provided strong support for the theory that the syndrome was caused by an infectious agent that could cause disease in anyone, homosexual or heterosexual.

The potential magnitude of the AIDS problem became

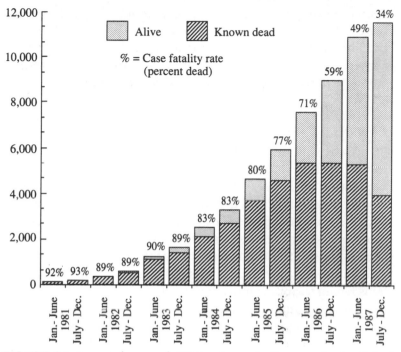

FIGURE 2.1 Reported cases of AIDS and case-fatality rates in the United States, by date of first report to the Centers for Disease Control, 1981 through 1987. Bottom (hatched portion of bar) indicates number of cases in each half-year group known dead as of July 18, 1988. (A recent assessment of reporting delays suggests that additional cases will be reported for the second half of 1987.) Source: U.S. Department of Health and Human Services, Public Health Service, Centers for Disease Control.

clear in 1983 (see Figure 2.1). By December of that year, 3,000 cases of AIDS had been reported in adults from 42 states, the District of Columbia, and Puerto Rico, and the disease had been recognized in 20 other countries. Researchers had identified cases suggesting transmission from mother to baby, either during pregnancy or at the time of delivery, and through blood transfusions. The risk group pattern in the United States began to take on many of the characteristics still observed today: 71 percent of cases involved homosexual or bisexual men, and 17 percent involved men and women who abused intravenous drugs. Of the remaining patients, 5 percent were Haitian immigrants, 1 percent were hemophiliacs, 1 percent were heterosexual partners of men or women in high-risk groups, and 1 percent were transfusion recipients. About 4 percent did not fit any known risk category.

Recognizing the Extent of Infection

Soon after the epidemic became manifest, scientists began to take a closer look at the health of the general homosexual population in the areas with the largest number of cases of the new disease. Physicians had known for many years that homosexual men who reported large numbers of sexual partners had more episodes of venereal disease and were at higher risk of hepatitis B virus infection than the rest of the population, but coincidentally with the appearance of AIDS, other debilitating problems began to appear more frequently. The most common was chronic generalized lymphadenopathy (swollen glands), often accompanied by extreme fatigue, weight loss, fever, chronic diarrhea, mild immune system abnormalities, decreased levels of blood platelets (cells that prevent excessive bleeding), and fungal infections in the mouth. This condition was labeled AIDS-related complex, or ARC. Some ARC patients appeared to remain stable indefinitely. Others developed AIDS.

Researchers suspected that AIDS, ARC, and a range of milder aberrations of the immune system probably represented different responses to the same infectious agent. The possibility that some people without symptoms might be capable of transmitting the infection was suggested by several cases of transfusion-associated AIDS, in which the donors had appeared healthy at the time of blood donation but later developed signs of ARC or AIDS.

The isolation of HIV in 1983 and 1984 and the development of techniques to produce large quantities of the virus paved the way for a battery of tests to determine the relationship between AIDS and ARC and the magnitude of the carrier problem.

Antibody Tests

Using several different laboratory tests, scientists looked for antibodies (proteins produced by the immune system in response to infection) against HIV in the blood of AIDS and ARC patients. They found that almost 100 percent of those with AIDS or ARC had the antibodies—they were seropositive. In contrast, less than 1 percent of persons with no known risk factors were seropositive.

The next step was to look for antibodies in people from groups at recognized risk for AIDS. Researchers were surprised by the large numbers of risk-group members who tested positive. Early studies showed that the rates of seropositivity were between 10 percent and 70 percent for homosexual men (men who lived in cities with the highest prevalence of AIDS and those who had more sexual partners were more likely to be positive); between 50 and 60 percent for intravenous drug abusers in New York City and northern New Jersey; between 15 percent and 90 percent for patients with hemophilia (depending on the type and severity of the hemophilia); and between 10 and 60 percent for women who were sexual partners of HIV-infected men.

What did these high seropositivity rates mean? How many of those who were HIV-seropositive were capable of transmitting the disease to others? How many would eventually become ill?

The presence of specific antibodies in the blood against viruses that cause acute diseases, such as measles, shows that a previous infection has registered on the body's immune system or that a vaccine has elicited an appropriate antibody response. The antibody molecules that remain in the bloodstream are like scouts; if the virus appears again, the scouts recognize it immediately and prevent it from gaining a foothold. Thus, people rarely develop measles a second time, although they may encounter the measles virus hundreds of times after initial exposure. In the case of many infectious diseases, such as polio, a person can develop protective antibodies against the causative agent without showing any signs of disease.

HIV produces a chronic viral infection. Researchers quickly discovered that the presence of antibodies to HIV did not correlate with elimination of the virus. Harold Jaffe of the Centers for Disease Control and his colleagues were able to isolate active virus from the blood of 12 out of 20 homosexual men who had antibodies but had shown no symptoms for between 2 and 6 years. In 1985 Robert C. Gallo of the National Cancer Institute and his coworkers reported that they could isolate virus from the blood of more than 80 percent of people with detectable antibodies.

These findings mean that most, if not all, people who have antibodies against HIV carry active virus. Thus, every person who is HIV seropositive should be considered infectious. Like people with HIV-related diseases, however, asymptomatic seropositive individuals can spread the virus only through sexual practices that involve an exchange of body fluids, through sharing of contaminated needles and syringes, through contamination of blood or blood products, through transplantation of organs or tissue, and, for women, through transmission to their unborn or, very rarely, breastfed children.

Progression to AIDS: The Long Incubation Period

Questions about the outcome of infection took longer to answer because of the very long period that elapses between infection with HIV and the development of AIDS.[2] James Curran, director of the AIDS Program at the CDC's Center for Infectious Diseases, explains that in 1984 the observed average incubation periods for transfusion-associated AIDS were 21 months in children and 31 months in adults. But these figures underestimated the true incubation periods, because those with longer incubation periods had not yet become ill. A mathematical model developed in 1987 suggests that the mean incubation period for persons aged 5 to 59 with transfusion-associated HIV infection will be 8.2 years.

Efforts to determine the mean incubation periods for HIV infections acquired in other ways are more difficult because scientists rarely know exactly when infection occurred. The data suggest, however, that homosexual men and adults with hemophilia progress to AIDS at about the same rate as adults with transfusion-associated infections.[3] In contrast, hemophiliac patients infected with HIV as children or teenagers appear to develop symptoms of AIDS more slowly (see below). The reasons for this difference are under investigation.

Information about the proportion of HIV-infected patients who will develop AIDS comes primarily from long-term studies of homosexual men in San Francisco. In the San Francisco City Clinic Cohort Study, 36 percent of HIV-infected participants progressed to AIDS within 88 months, and more than 40 percent had other signs or symptoms of infection. Only 20 percent remained symptom free.

Projections by Andrew Moss of San Francisco General Hospital and his coworkers are equally grim. In a study of a cohort of homosexual men recruited in 1983 and 1984, they found that progression to clinical AIDS after infection with HIV was the norm rather than the exception. On the basis of observations and laboratory test results, they predict that half of their HIV-seropositive subjects will progress to AIDS within 6 years (assumed to be about 9 years after infection) and that three-quarters will have either AIDS or an AIDS-related condition.[4]

Revision of the CDC Case Definition of AIDS

When epidemiologists at the Centers for Disease Control developed a definition for acquired immunodeficiency syndrome in 1982, they placed clear constraints on the types of cases that would be included:

CDC defines a case of AIDS as a disease, at least moderately predictive of a defect in cell-mediated immunity, occurring in a person with no known cause for diminished resistance to that disease. Such diseases include KS [Kaposi's sarcoma], PCP [*Pneumocystis carinii* pneumonia], and serious OOI [other opportunistic

further leap of faith is required since we must also assume that the relative size of the (self-reported) homosexual population is the same in the 1980s as it was in the 1940s."[18] Despite this problem, most public health experts consider the estimates developed by the CDC to be reasonable for general planning purposes.

HIV Antibody Surveys

Planning at the local and state levels requires more specific information about the prevalence of HIV infection in recognized risk groups, in heterosexually active persons, and in accessible segments of the general population. To meet these needs, U.S. Public Health Service officials announced in December 1987 that they would support a "comprehensive family of HIV surveys" in 30 metropolitan areas: 20 with a large number of reported AIDS cases and 10 with a moderate to low prevalence of AIDS.

Antibody tests are being conducted on blood samples from persons treated at selected hospitals and at family planning clinics, sexually transmitted disease clinics, drug addiction treatment centers, and tuberculosis clinics. (Antibody studies in "sentinel" hospitals are conducted on blinded samples, that is, samples from which identifying information has been removed. In other settings, tests may be conducted on nonblinded samples, but only with informed consent and appropriate pre- and post-test counseling.) In addition, the Public Health Service has entered a cooperative agreement with 15 private and public colleges to perform blinded tests on 1,000 blood specimens drawn for other purposes at college health clinics, and has contracted with a major university to conduct a serosurvey of 10,000 inmates in ten state prisons.

HIV infection among childbearing women. A very important element in this nationwide survey project is the testing of blood from newborn babies. The presence of HIV antibodies in the blood of a newborn indicates that the newborn's mother is infected with the virus (scientists estimate that 25 to 50 percent of such babies are actually infected with HIV; see Chapter 3).

In 1987 researchers at the State Laboratory Institute of the Massachusetts Department of Public Health pioneered a technique for detecting HIV antibodies in neonatal blood specimens routinely collected for other purposes, such as screening for the metabolic disease phenylketonuria (PKU).[19] A punched disk from the absorbent paper used to collect the infant's blood is soaked overnight in a special saline solution. The tiny amount of serum eluted from the disk produces accurate results on primary HIV screening tests and on a miniaturized version of the Western blot (see Appendix C). Samples are processed in batches, without personal identifiers, to prevent accidental decoding of the identities of babies or mothers.

The system of studying blood from newborns to assess the prevalence of HIV infection in the general population of childbearing women provides an unusually unbiased sample. Current estimates of the prevalence of HIV infection in the general population are based primarily on data obtained from screening blood donors and military recruits, but in both cases the samples may be biased by self-selection (for example, women who know they are at high risk for HIV infection are discouraged from donating blood). In Massachusetts, researchers found that estimates of the prevalence of HIV infection in women obtained through newborn screening tests were considerably higher than those obtained by screening of blood donors and military recruits.[20]

Blinded serologic testing of blood samples collected from newborns is under way in the 30 cities selected for the comprehensive family of surveys. In addition, several states are using the newborn testing system to follow statewide trends in HIV infection.

National household seroprevalence survey. To obtain a more complete picture of the prevalence of HIV infection in the United States, public health officials would like to conduct a nationwide household-based sample survey. Data from an

AIDS information questionnaire administered as part of the National Health Interview Survey in 1987 indicated that 71 percent of the 3,097 adults questioned were willing to have their blood tested with assurances that the test results would remain private.[21] However, a pilot study in Washington, D.C., to evaluate the feasibility of a household-based survey was canceled in August 1988 because of strong community opposition. Federal officials are working with community leaders in other regions to develop alternative sites for the pilot study.

Trends in HIV Infection

Long-term projections of the course of the AIDS epidemic require data on the incidence of HIV infection (the number of new infections over time), but these data are extremely difficult to gather.

The information that is available suggests that the incidence of HIV infection has dropped dramatically among homosexual and bisexual men in the United States but remains high among intravenous drug abusers in some cities. The rate of new infections among transfusion recipients and hemophiliacs has been very low since 1985, when blood banks instituted serologic screening of blood and plasma donors and other protective measures.

The decline in new HIV infections among homosexual and bisexual men has been demonstrated in 8 different studies.[22] For example, Warren Winkelstein, Jr., of the University of California at Berkeley and his coworkers report that the annual HIV infection rate among participants in the San Francisco Men's Health Study decreased from an estimated 18.4 percent per year from 1982 to 1984, to 5.4 percent and 3.1 percent respectively during the first and second halves of 1985, to 4.2 percent during the first six months of 1986. (During the last 3 periods the prevalence of HIV infection remained stable at about 50 percent.) These declines were associated with reductions of 60 percent or more in high-risk sexual practices.[23]

The incidence of HIV infections among intravenous drug abusers has declined in some cities, such as New York and San

Francisco, but is still increasing rapidly in others. Don C. Des Jarlais of the New York State Division of Substance Abuse Services warns that even in cities that appear to have a constant overall infection rate, the spread of HIV continues. For example, in New York City the prevalence of HIV infection among IV drug abusers has stabilized at between 55 and 63 percent; but the drug-using population is constantly changing as some users seek treatment, others die, and new people enter the population. Studies indicate that each year about 6 percent of IV drug abusers who were not formerly infected acquire the virus.[24]

In June 1988 Des Jarlais told participants at the Fourth International Conference on AIDS in Stockholm that "efforts to reduce sharing of dirty needles by addicts have been more successful than efforts to encourage addicts to use condoms and limit their sexual partners."[25] This is particularly worrisome because IV drug abusers represent the main conduit of HIV infection to women and children. The proportion of AIDS cases attributable to heterosexual transmission (most involving a partner who uses IV drugs) is increasing more rapidly than the proportion of cases in any other risk category, but the data are insufficient to identify trends of HIV infection in this population.

The CDC reports that in the two general population groups tested over time, applicants for military service and first-time blood donors, HIV antibody prevalence rates have remained relatively stable for two years (although the prevalence among blood donors has fluctuated seasonally).[26] The overall prevalence among first-time donors in the period 1985–1987 was 0.043 percent; the prevalence among military applicants, adjusted for the age, sex, and racial and ethnic composition of the U.S. adult population, was 0.14 percent. New infections may be masked, however, by increasing rates of self-deferral by those who believe themselves to be at risk. Preliminary results from a CDC survey of four sentinel hospitals in the United States indicate that 3 of every 1,000 patients hospitalized for conditions not associated with AIDS or related conditions are infected with HIV. This figure is

Heterosexual activity. In an excellent review of the modes of transmission of HIV, Gerald Friedland and Robert Klein of the Albert Einstein College of Medicine recall that the first evidence for heterosexual transmission of the virus was reported in 1983.[32] Since then, numerous studies from the United States, Haiti, and Africa have documented both male-to-female and female-to-male transmission. These studies indicate that most heterosexual transmission of HIV occurs during unprotected vaginal intercourse.

The proportion of U.S. AIDS patients infected through heterosexual intercourse with a person at risk for AIDS is increasing faster than the proportion of cases in any other risk category. In 1985, 1.7 percent of the adult cases of AIDS reported to the CDC were acquired through heterosexual activity; projections suggest that by 1991 the proportion will rise to 5 percent (3,700).[33] Friedland and Klein estimate that if these cases are combined with cases among people born outside the United States in countries where heterosexual transmission is thought to predominate, and with cases among people with no identifiable risk factor (most of whom are thought to have become infected through heterosexual intercourse), the proportion of cases resulting from heterosexual transmission could approach 10 percent by 1991.[34]

Heterosexual contact is the only transmission category in which women with AIDS outnumber men with AIDS. Heterosexual contact accounts for 29 percent of AIDS cases among women in the United States, but for only 2 percent of cases among men. Mary Guinan and Ann Hardy of the CDC suggest that the larger number of heterosexually acquired AIDS cases among women in this country may be the result of two factors: "(1) a greater proportion of men are infected, and therefore a woman is more likely than a man to encounter an infected partner; and (2) the efficiency of transmission of HIV from man to woman may be greater than from woman to man."[35]

For now, the pool of infected women appears to be too small to sustain an HIV epidemic in people who do not belong to one of the known risk groups. Sustaining the spread of disease requires a "chain of transmission" from individuals practicing high-risk behavior to their partners, and then to individuals with no known risk. This chain of transmission would have to include a sufficient number of infected women interacting with men who would not otherwise be at high risk. Researchers are worried that IV drug abuse could create such a reservoir of infected women. About 30 percent of IV drug abusers are women, and between 30 and 50 percent of these women report that they have engaged in prostitution to obtain funds for illicit drugs. HIV antibody prevalence is three to four times higher among prostitutes who acknowledge IV drug use than among those who do not.

There have been no studies in the United States exploring the risk of HIV infection from prostitutes. The number of male AIDS patients reporting contact with prostitutes as their only risk factor has been quite small. In New York City, only 22 AIDS cases involving sexual contact with prostitutes were reported through January 1987, despite the fact that about half of the city's drug-abusing prostitutes are believed to be infected with HIV. Des Jarlais suggests that the apparently limited transmission from prostitutes may be a result of safer sex practices—more than 90 percent of street prostitutes in New York report that they regularly require customers to use condoms.[36]

One approach to monitoring for heterosexually acquired infection is to measure the prevalence of HIV infection among people seeking treatment in sexually transmitted disease clinics. Physicians in these clinics see patients whose behavior puts them at highest risk of infection with HIV and other sexually transmitted diseases. In December 1987 the CDC reported that in nine surveys of STD clinics in six major cities, the prevalence of HIV infection among heterosexuals with no known risk factors ranged from 0 to 2.6 percent. In studies conducted in clinics in which data were collected during personal interviews (not through self-administered questionnaires), and in which seropositive men and women were interviewed a second time to obtain better data on their risk status, the prevalence of HIV infection among persons with no in Belgium and his coworkers say that in one study of men who acquired a sexually transmitted disease from a group of prostitutes with a high prevalence of HIV infection, "a single sexual exposure was apparently associated with a female-to-male transmission risk of 5 to 10 percent provided particular cofactors were present."[39] This rate is considerably higher than any estimates of heterosexual infection rates in the United States.

Two other factors that have been associated with increased risk of HIV infection in Africa are the use of oral contraceptives in women and noncircumcision in men. Both factors require further study.

In 1988 Norman Hearst and Stephen Hulley of the University of California at San Francisco developed estimates of the risk to heterosexuals of sexual encounters with partners in different risk categories.[40] Their estimates of the risk of HIV transmission in unprotected intercourse with a person known to be infected with HIV are 1 in 500 for a single sexual encounter and 2 in 3 for 500 sexual encounters. The use of a condom reduces these odds to 1 in 5,000 for a single encounter and to 1 in 11 for 500 encounters. (They assume a condom failure rate of 10 percent.) In contrast, they estimate the risk of unprotected intercourse with a person who does not have a history of high-risk behavior and who has had a negative AIDS test to be 1 in 500 million, with condom use reducing the risk to 1 in 5 billion.

Hearst and Hulley also address the risk of sexual encounters with a partner whose infection status is unknown. For partners not in any high-risk group,[41] they estimate the risk of a single protected encounter to be 1 in 50 million. The risk rises to 1 in 1,000 for a single unprotected sexual encounter with a member of a high-risk group in a metropolitan area with a high prevalence of AIDS. Five hundred unprotected sexual encounters with such a partner increases the risk to 1 in 3.

The California researchers conclude that careful choice of partners provides greater protection against HIV transmission than using a condom, avoiding anal intercourse,[42] reducing the number of sexual partners, or requiring that one's partner have a negative HIV antibody test. They acknowledge, however, that it may be difficult to assess the risk status of a potential partner. They encourage gradual courtships and asking potential partners directly about any history of high-risk activities. They advise against casual sex or sex with prostitutes. Other scientists warn that the estimates developed by Hearst and Hulley are group averages and do not reflect potential variations in the infectivity of a seropositive partner or the susceptibility of a seronegative partner.[43] Moreover, a recent California study suggests that both men and women often lie to prospective partners about past sexual experiences. Thus, the recommended precautions involving condom use, avoidance of anal intercourse, and limiting the number of sexual partners are still warranted.

Transmission by Intravenous Drug Abuse

The prevalence of HIV infection among intravenous drug abusers shows enormous geographic variation. In April 1988, W. Robert Lange of the National Institute on Drug Abuse and his coworkers described the results of a study to monitor HIV seroprevalence trends among IV drug abusers in six geographic regions.[44] Study subjects were enrolled in drug treatment programs, and all had a history of at least 12 months of IV drug abuse. In the New York City area, 61 percent of blood samples obtained in late 1986 were HIV seropositive (up from 50 percent of samples obtained in the same area in early 1985). The seroprevalence rate in Baltimore was 29 percent. In contrast, samples from programs outside the northeastern United States had much lower rates: 5 percent in Denver, 2 percent in San Antonio, 1.5 percent in southern California, and 0 in Tampa.

The geographic variation in HIV seroprevalence among intravenous drug abusers is much greater than that observed for homosexual and bisexual men. The probable explanation for this difference is that the IV drug abuse population is less mobile than the homosexual population. Regions with close cultural connections to New York City and northern New Jersey (including Puerto Rico) have high seroprevalence rates; other regions have much lower rates.

Lange and his colleagues expected that the geographic variation also might be associated with differences in lifetime needle-sharing practices. (Sharing of unsterilized needles and syringes and the common practice in "shooting galleries" of drawing blood back into the syringe before injecting a drug are the likely sources of HIV transmission among IV drug abusers.) They found, however, that needle sharing was very common in all geographic regions; in fact 99 percent of subjects questioned in San Antonio reported needle-sharing experiences. This finding is disturbing because it highlights the extreme vulnerability of areas where the HIV seroprevalence rate is still relatively low.

Historical studies in the United States and Europe indicate that the introduction of HIV into a drug-abusing population may be followed by a period of very rapid spread. For example, historically collected sera (sera collected in the past for other reasons) from IV drug abusers in Manhattan show that seroprevalence rates rose to more than 40 percent within three years after the first seropositive sample was collected.[45] In Edinburgh, Scotland, HIV seroprevalence rose to almost 50 percent within two years after the first seropositive sample.[46] Researchers are attempting to identify the factors responsible for the rapid spread (beyond sharing of injection equipment within friendship groups) and to determine whether local efforts can prevent it.

Recent data from New York City indicate that the impact of HIV infection on the IV-drug-using population has been much greater than previously recognized. Stephen Joseph, commissioner of health for New York City, reports that a study of all drug-related deaths in the city from 1982 through 1986 revealed 2,500 deaths that could be attributed to HIV in addition to those meeting the CDC definition of AIDS. Among these were deaths caused by endocarditis, nonpneumocystis pneumonia, and tuberculosis in people who had symptoms compatible with HIV infection, such as oral thrush.

The large increase in deaths from "non-AIDS" infections began at the same time as the introduction of HIV into the drug-using population and has taken a greater toll than AIDS itself. When HIV mortality is adjusted to account for these excess deaths among addicts, the AIDS-related deaths involving IV drug abusers in New York City surpasses AIDS-related deaths among homosexual men by more than 15 percent.[47]

The rate of progression to AIDS among IV drug abusers may be influenced by the frequency of drug injection. In a study by Des Jarlais and his coworkers, high frequencies of drug injection in seropositive subjects were associated with an increased loss of T4 cells. This finding is compatible with the results of laboratory studies in which immunologic stimulation of HIV-infected T4 cells led to increased viral replication and cell death. Sources of immunologic stimulation associated with the act of injecting drugs include nonsterile drug preparation, nonsterile injection procedures, and exposure to blood in a shared needle and syringe.[48] Thus, reducing the frequency of drug injection may protect the health of an HIV seropositive drug abuser, as well as diminish the possibility of HIV transmission to an uninfected needlesharing acquaintance.

Controlling HIV infection among IV drug abusers is essential to limiting the scope of the AIDS epidemic. CDC epidemiologist Martha Rogers reported in April 1987 that more than half (65 percent) of reported AIDS cases in women, 69 percent of cases in heterosexual men, and 73 percent of cases in children infected at or before birth were related to IV drug abuse or sexual contact with an IV drug abuser.[49]

Transmission by Blood or Blood Products

People who have acquired HIV infection through blood or blood products can be grouped into three categories: transfusion recipients, hemophiliacs, and health care workers with occupational exposures.

Transfusion recipients. By August 1, 1988, the CDC had reported 1,863 cases of AIDS (1,721 in adults and 142 in children) associated with blood transfusions. All but a handful resulted from transfusions received before March 1985, when blood service organizations began testing donated blood for HIV antibodies and discarding all positive units. The blood products associated with HIV infection have included whole blood, blood cellular components (red cells and platelets), plasma (the liquid part of blood), and clotting factors (used in the treatment of hemophilia). Other products prepared from blood—immunoglobulin, albumin, plasma protein fraction, and hepatitis B virus vaccine—have not been implicated in HIV transmission.

Scientists estimate that between 66 and 100 percent of people who receive a transfusion from an HIV-infected donor will become infected.[50] Recipients are more likely to become infected if the transfusion occurs close to the time that the donor develops symptoms. In one study, all recipients became infected if the donors developed AIDS within 23 months of the donation.[51]

Researchers believe that about 12,000 people now living in the United States may have acquired a transfusion-associated HIV infection between 1978 and 1984.[52] The risk was probably greatest the year before the initiation of blood-bank screening of donated blood; as many as 7,200 persons may have been infected in 1984. (Scientists estimate that about 60 percent of these recipients would have died from the disease for which they were originally hospitalized; this would leave about 2,900 living recipients who acquired a transfusion-related HIV infection in 1984.)

In June 1986 the American Red Cross and other blood-banking organizations launched a "look-back" program to identify patients who had received blood before 1985 from donors who later tested positive for HIV antibody. In one region, 70 percent of recipients identified through such a program were seropositive.[53] The CDC recommends that other pre-1985 transfusion recipients who are concerned about the possibility of HIV infection should discuss HIV testing with their physicians. In general, the risk of infection was very small. Public health officials are most concerned about people who received multiple transfusions in an area with a high prevalence of AIDS.

Many patients with transfusion-related HIV infections probably have not yet developed symptoms. A mathematical model developed by G. F. Medley and his coworkers suggests that the mean incubation period for transfusion-associated AIDS in people aged 5 to 59 will be 8.2 years. For children under age 5, the model places the mean incubation period at 1.97 years.[54] (Recent studies indicate that young children may do better than was previously expected. Thomas Mundy of the Cedars-Sinai Medical Center in Los Angeles describes the status of 20 children who were infected with HIV through pre-1985 transfusions. One-third of the children have remained healthy, one-third are in good general health but have more than the usual number of childhood infections, and one-third have developed AIDS. This rate of progression to AIDS is comparable to that seen in adults.[55])

The risk of acquiring a transfusion-related HIV infection has fallen dramatically since the adoption of antibody screening tests for donated blood. Existing screening tests for HIV antibodies are extremely sensitive. Experts estimate that the test's false negative rate is in the range of 4 to 5 per million (that is, 4 to 5 of every 1 million donors screened as negative may actually be positive). The potential for HIV transmission through blood transfusions may be slightly higher than this figure indicates, however, because of the problem created by new infections in donors who have not yet developed antibodies. Studies have shown that most people infected with HIV develop antibodies within 6 to 14 weeks, but some may remain seronegative for more than a year.[56]

John W. Ward of the CDC and his coworkers recently studied 13 transfusion recipients who became HIV seropositive after receiving blood from donors who were screened as negative for HIV antibody at the time of donation.[57] They found that all the donors had subsequently seroconverted. Six of the 7 donors had identifiable risk factors for HIV infection and should have refrained from donating blood.

The researchers conclude that there is a small but identifiable risk of HIV infection for recipients of screened blood. Calculations that include worst-case estimates of the number of HIV-infected but seronegative donors suggest that between 72 and 460 of the nation's almost 4 million blood recipients could be infected with HIV each year.

Measures to minimize the very small risk of transfusion-associated AIDS include communicating more effectively to potential high-risk donors the reasons for not donating blood (Figure 2.2 illustrates the type of information provided to prospective blood donors); employing new assays that detect HIV infection earlier; improving physician education to minimize the number of unnecessary blood transfusions; and promoting the use of autologous transfusions (in which patients receive their own blood donated several weeks before an elective surgical procedure).[58] The decision to adopt new tests for HIV in blood-bank screening programs must involve a careful assessment of both benefits and costs (the latter includes the cost of blood donations discarded because of false positive results).

PATIENT SAFETY

Some people must not give because their blood might spread an infection to the people who receive it.

Do not give blood if you are at risk for getting and spreading the AIDS virus. You are at risk if . . .

- You are a man who has had sex with another man since 1977, *even one time.*
- You have ever taken ("shot up") illegal drugs by needle, *even one time.*
- You are a native of Haiti, Sub-Saharan Africa, or any island close to Sub-Saharan Africa and came to the United States after 1977.
- You are a hemophiliac who has taken clotting factor concentrates since 1977.

- You have ever had a positive test for AIDS or the AIDS virus.
- You have AIDS or one of its symptoms, which include—
  —Weight loss (10 pounds or more in less than 2 months) that you can't explain.
  —Night sweats.
  —Blue or purple spots on or under your skin.
  —White spots or unusual sores in your mouth that last a long time.
  —Lumps in your neck, armpits, or groin that last more than a month.
  —Fever higher than 99 degrees that lasts more than 10 days.
  —Diarrhea that lasts more than one month.

- You have, since 1977, had sex with any person described above.
- You are a woman or man who has been a prostitute at any time since 1977.
- You are a man who has had sex with a female prostitute or a woman who has had sex with a male prostitute in the last six months.

Do not give blood to find out whether you have a positive AIDS test. The tests we use are very good, but they are not perfect. A person may be infected and have a negative test result. That's why you must not give blood if you are at risk for getting AIDS. A Red Cross nurse can tell you where you can get an AIDS test without giving blood and without giving your name.

Do not give blood if you . . .
- Have ever had hepatitis (liver disease caused by a virus).

- Have had malaria or have taken drugs to prevent malaria in the past three years.
- Have syphilis.

If you decide that you should not give blood, you may leave now. If you're not sure, ask to talk privately with a Red Cross nurse.

If you decide to give blood today, you will be given a form to let us know whether your blood is safe to be given to another person. You will be told how to use the form so that no one at the blood drive will know what you have said. If your blood should not be given to another person, you *must* let us know with this form.

If you give blood today, but decide later that your blood may not be safe for another person, call the telephone number on the back of this pamphlet *as soon as possible* and state that your blood should not be give to another person.

FIGURE 2.2. Warning to prospective blood donors in the American Red Cross brochure *What You Must Know before Giving Blood* (Washington, D.C., June 1988).

Hemophiliacs. More than 5 percent of people with severe hemophilia A in the United States have been diagnosed with AIDS (722 cases reported among all hemophiliacs as of August 1, 1988), and more than 80 percent have antibodies against HIV. A bright note is that new procedures for inactivating the virus in the blood products used to treat hemophilia, combined with donor screening for HIV antibody, have virtually eliminated the risk of HIV infection for hemophiliacs diagnosed in the future.

Hemophiliacs lack one of several blood proteins required

for normal clotting. The most common form of the disease is hemophilia A, caused by an inability to manufacture the antihemophilia factor, or factor VIII; patients with hemophilia B lack another clotting factor, called factor IX. Before the development of techniques to extract factor VIII and factor IX concentrates from human plasma, these patients endured frequent bleeding, and some were in danger of fatal bleeding episodes.

Former methods of manufacturing these concentrates placed the hemophiliac population at high risk of infection with HIV. The concentrates are extracted from pooled plasma obtained from thousands of donors. Unlike some other blood products, such as albumin, the concentrates could not be pasteurized because heat inactivated the clotting factors. Plasma from one infected donor could contaminate the entire pool and thereby transmit the virus to many hemophiliacs.

In the fall of 1984 several laboratories announced new methods of protecting the clotting factors from high temperatures. With these techniques, manufacturers can heat the pooled blood fractions sufficiently to inactivate HIV and still retain the clotting function. In addition, the FDA recently approved a solvent-detergent method for inactivation of virus in factor VIII concentrates and an immunologic technique for purifying factor VIII. All hemophiliacs in the United States now use either the heat-treated or solvent-detergent-treated products.[59]

Overall, about 70 percent of tested persons with hemophilia A and 35 percent with hemophilia B in the United States have been HIV seropositive. (Hemophilia B tends to be less severe than hemophilia A, so patients with hemophilia B generally have had fewer exposures to HIV-contaminated factor concentrates.) These figures may overstate the true prevalence of HIV seropositivity among hemophiliacs, however, because most of the serologic surveys have been done at hemophilia treatment centers, where patients are more likely to have severe hemophilia than a mild form of the disease.[60]

For several years it appeared that hemophiliacs might be less likely to progress to AIDS or might have a longer incubation period than other people infected with HIV. Recently, however, scientists have determined that seropositive adults with hemophilia progress to AIDS at the same rate as seropositive homosexual men. In one study, 30 to 35 percent of HIV-infected adults with hemophilia had symptoms of AIDS within six to seven years. In contrast, only 10 percent of hemophiliacs who were infected as children or teen-agers had AIDS.[61] Thus, age appears to be an important cofactor in the development of HIV-related disease.

Numerous studies are under way to determine why children and teenagers with hemophilia fare better than adults. Some researchers believe that hormonal differences may explain the disparity. Better understanding of the impact of age could lead to new measures for prolonging the well-being of all people infected with HIV.

Health care workers.   The occupational risk of acquiring HIV infection in health care settings is low and is most often associated with the accidental injection of blood from an HIV-infected patient. There is no evidence that the virus spreads either through the air or through casual contact. In studies by the CDC, the National Institutes of Health, and the University of California, less than 1 percent of health care workers reporting needlestick injuries or other puncture wounds involving HIV-contaminated equipment have become infected with the virus.

As of December 31, 1987, the CDC had tested 1,070 workers at least 90 days following exposure to HIV-infected blood or other body fluids. The workers were grouped into three categories: 870 had experienced needlestick or other puncture wounds involving contaminated blood; 104 had reported blood splashed onto mucous membranes (such as the inside of the mouth) or open skin lesions; and 96 had been exposed to other body fluids (saliva or urine). Four of the 870 workers (0.5 percent) in the first category were seropositive for HIV antibody (in one case, however, heterosexual transmission from an HIV-seropositive partner could not be ruled out); none of the other workers was infected.[62]

Transmission through non-needlestick injuries is extremely rare (the precise level of risk cannot be determined because no one knows how often such events occur). In May 1987 the CDC described 3 isolated cases in which health care workers apparently became infected with HIV after substantial exposure of either mucous membranes or inflamed skin to HIV-infected blood. The exact routes of transmission in these cases are not known. One worker had blood splattered into her mouth when the top flew off a blood collection tube; the second had chapped hands and was not wearing gloves when she helped care for an emergency room patient later found to be infected with HIV.

In their review of HIV transmission, Friedland and Klein say that 40 percent of reported needlestick injuries and 2 of the 3 non-needlestick injuries described above could have been prevented if workers had followed existing infection control guidelines (see Appendix D).

Adherence to biosafety recommendations for HIV also is essential for workers in research and virus-production laboratories. In 1988 the director of the National Institutes of Health convened an expert team to investigate HIV infections in two workers employed in laboratories producing large quantities of highly concentrated virus. The experts concluded that there was a need "for more proficiency and discipline in laboratory safety practices."[63]

Mother-Infant Transmission

In the United States more than 1,100 children under age 13 have been diagnosed with AIDS, and more than half of them have died. As shown in Figure 2.3, three-quarters of these children come from families in which one or both parents have AIDS or are at increased risk of developing AIDS; the virus is transmitted from mother to child during pregnancy, at the time of delivery, or shortly after birth. Most of the remaining pediatric patients are hemophiliacs or recipients of multiple transfusions. About 4 percent of AIDS cases in children are unexplained; most of these are awaiting further

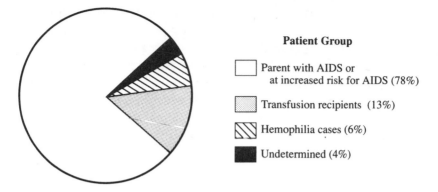

FIGURE 2.3. Distribution of pediatric AIDS cases (total = 1,108) in the United States: percentage by patient group, 1981 through August 1, 1988. Source: U.S. Department of Health and Human Services, Public Health Service, Centers for Disease Control.

information about the antibody and risk behavior status of the parents.

The geographic and racial distribution of AIDS cases in children closely parallels that in women. Most cases have been reported in New York, New Jersey, and Florida—the states with the highest numbers of women with AIDS. Seventy-six percent of all children with AIDS are black or Hispanic, as are 71 percent of all women with AIDS. The source of most cases of perinatal transmission is intravenous drug abuse by the mother or her sexual partner.

Most children with maternally transmitted HIV infections develop symptoms within the first two years of life, but some have remained well for six years or more. Infants who become ill before their first birthday tend to do poorly, especially if they develop *Pneumocystis carinii* pneumonia.

Even women who appear completely healthy can transmit HIV to their offspring. In a study by Gwendolyn Scott and her colleagues at the University of Miami School of Medicine, 15 of 16 mothers whose infants developed AIDS shortly after birth were clinically well at the time of delivery, although all had some abnormal immune functions. Five of these women later developed AIDS, and 7 developed milder symptoms of HIV infection.

Several recent studies indicate that the overall rate of perinatal transmission is between 25 and 50 percent.[64] Some women have borne one or more uninfected children after giving birth to an infected child. Researchers in Zaire report that mothers whose own immune systems are failing are more likely to transmit HIV to their offspring.

The frequency and efficiency of the different modes of transmission of HIV from mother to child remain unclear. Support for transmission in the womb comes from a case described by Canadian physicians who found evidence of HIV infection in an infant delivered by caesarean section from a mother with AIDS who died 2 hours later. In addition, the virus has been isolated from the central nervous system of a 13-week fetus and from a 15-week fetus.[65]

The discovery of HIV-infected cells in cervical tissue suggests that some infants might be infected when they come into direct contact with infected cells during vaginal delivery. Some researchers believe that infants who are infected with HIV during the perinatal period may have a longer incubation period—remain healthy longer—than infants infected early in pregnancy (see Chapter 6).

A report from Australia and two reports from Rwanda indicate that infants also can be infected after birth, probably through breast milk; the researchers describe AIDS in infants whose mothers developed antibodies to HIV following post-partum transfusions.[66]

On the basis of data from other viral diseases, researchers had feared that pregnancy might accelerate the progression of HIV-related disease in the mother. Preliminary data from several studies indicate, however, that the number of T4 cells and other measures of immune function in HIV-infected women do not change significantly during pregnancy. The incidence of opportunistic infections also remains the same.

Disease progression may accelerate in the postpartum period, but this has not been established with certainty. Scientists tracing the natural history of HIV infection in women who were identified because their infants developed AIDS-related symptoms found that between 45 percent and 75 percent of the mothers became ill within 28 to 30 months of delivery.[67] This is a much higher rate of disease progression than that seen in homosexual men, IV drug abusers, or hemophiliacs. It is possible, however, that women who transmit HIV infection to their offspring may represent a unique subset of women with a higher burden of virus and a greater likelihood of disease progression.

Recent surveys of HIV seroprevalence among childbearing women (performed by testing samples of blood from newborns) indicate that the number of HIV infected infants in the United States will grow rapidly during the next few years. The New York State Health Department estimates that 700 infected babies will be born in that state alone in 1988. Other regions on the East Coast with a high prevalence of HIV infection among IV drug abusers face similar problems.

The CDC recommends that women of childbearing age with identifiable risks for HIV infection be routinely counseled and tested for HIV antibody, regardless of the health-care setting (see Appendix E). This includes all women living in communities where there is a known or suspected high prevalence of HIV infection among women. The identification of seropositive women before they become pregnant allows them to avoid pregnancy and the risk of transmitting HIV to their infants. Early diagnosis of HIV infection during pregnancy enables women to make an informed choice about continuation of the pregnancy; in cases in which the pregnancy is continued, early diagnosis affords physicians time to plan for appropriate medical care for the mother and child.

Patients with No Recognized Risk Factors

AIDS cases of undetermined origin are those not immediately traced to homosexual activity, intravenous drug abuse, receipt of contaminated blood or blood products, or heterosexual intercourse with someone in one of the main transmission categories. In March 1988, Kenneth Castro and his coworkers reviewed the origins of the 2,059 AIDS cases with no recognized risk factors reported to the CDC through September 30, 1987.[68] In 921 cases, risk history was incomplete or unobtainable (because of death, refusal to be interviewed, or loss to follow-up). Further investigation allowed researchers to place almost three-quarters of the remaining 1,138 cases in one of the conventional risk categories. In addition, 32 cases were found to involve incorrect diagnoses —the patients did not have AIDS.

Risk factors could not be identified for the remaining 281 cases despite additional information. The researchers found, however, that a relatively high proportion of these patients had a history of other sexually transmitted diseases. Also, 34 percent of the men interviewed reported sexual contact with prostitutes. These facts suggest a possible association between a small number of AIDS cases in the United States and heterosexual promiscuity.

The CDC researchers concluded that modes of transmission of HIV in this country have remained unchanged. They found no evidence for new modes of transmission among AIDS cases of undetermined origin.

Routes *Not* Involved in Transmission of HIV

Education about the known routes of transmission of HIV is the principal tool available for slowing the spread of the AIDS epidemic. It is equally important that the general public understand how HIV is *not* transmitted.

Household or Casual Contact

Long-term studies of more than 400 family members of adult and pediatric AIDS patients demonstrate that the virus is not transmitted by any daily activity related to living with or caring for an AIDS patient.[69] Siblings of children with AIDS have remained free of infection even after sharing beds and toothbrushes with a sick child. Personal interactions typical in family relationships, such as hugging, kissing on the cheek, and kissing on the lips, have not resulted in transmission of the virus among household members who did not have additional exposure to HIV infection through sexual activity or perinatal transmission.[70]

The only documented case of a family member acquiring HIV infection through nonsexual contact involved the mother of a congenitally ill infant with transfusion-associated AIDS. The mother was a registered nurse; she provided intensive nursing care to her child and was frequently exposed to the infant's blood and bloody feces. She did not wear gloves. Family members who perform medical procedures that involve regular exposure to infected blood should follow infection control guidelines established for health care workers (see Appendix D). Such activities are not considered casual contact.

After reviewing all existing information on the lack of HIV transmission through household and casual contact, AIDS researcher Alan Lifson of the San Francisco Department of Public Health wrote:

If HIV is not transmitted between persons in households (where exposures are repeated and may be prolonged), it would be even less likely to occur in the workplace or school. No known risk of transmission to coworkers, clients, or consumers exists from HIV-infected workers in such settings as offices, schools, and factories. Evidence also indicates that blood-borne and sexually transmitted infections such as HIV are not transmitted during the preparation or serving of food or beverages, and no instances of HIV transmission have been documented in this setting.[71]

Guidelines from the U.S. Public Health Service say that workers known to be infected with HIV should not be restricted from work solely because they are infected, nor should they be restricted from using telephones, office equipment, toilets, showers, eating facilities, or water fountains.

Body Fluids Other than Blood or Semen

Fears about the possibility of catching AIDS through casual contact were most intense among the general public

The International Prevalence of AIDS

The United States has reported more cases of AIDS than any other country, but the AIDS epidemic is clearly a global problem. By mid-March 1988, 136 countries had reported a total of 84,256 cases of AIDS to the World Health Organization (WHO). Taking into account underrecognition and underreporting of AIDS cases (especially in countries where large segments of the population do not have access to modern diagnostic and treatment facilities), WHO scientists estimate that the actual world total probably exceeds 150,000 cases.[76]

The current distribution of AIDS cases reflects the spread of HIV infection in the late 1970s and early 1980s. Surveys to determine the number of currently asymptomatic people who are infected with HIV (and thus at high risk of developing AIDS or a related disease) present a grim picture for the future. WHO estimates that between 5 and 10 million people are infected worldwide.

The basic modes of HIV transmission are the same throughout the world. But the relative importance of these transmission mechanisms varies. WHO epidemiologists recognize three broad geographic patterns of transmission.[77]

Pattern One

The first pattern is characteristic of industrialized nations with large numbers of reported AIDS cases, such as the United States, Canada, countries in Western Europe, Australia, New Zealand, and parts of Latin America. In these areas most AIDS cases have been attributed to homosexual or bisexual activity and intravenous drug abuse (primarily in urban centers). Heterosexual and perinatal transmission are responsible for only a small percentage of cases, though the proportion is growing. Transmission through exposure to contaminated blood and blood products occurred between the late 1970s and 1985 but has been reduced to extremely low levels by the self-deferral of blood donors at increased risk of HIV infection and by routine blood screening. The ratio of male to female AIDS patients in countries with this pattern ranges from 10:1 to 15:1. The prevalence of HIV infection in the overall population is estimated to be less than 1 percent but has been reported to exceed 50 percent in some groups practicing high-risk behavior (for example, intravenous drug abusers and men with multiple male sexual partners).

As of March 21, 1988, 7 countries in this category had more than 1,000 reported AIDS cases: the United States, France (3,073), Brazil (2,325), the Federal Republic of Germany (1,669), Canada, (1,517), Italy (1,411), and the United Kingdom (1,227).[78]

Pattern Two

The second pattern is observed in areas of central, eastern, and southern Africa and in some Caribbean countries. Most AIDS cases in these areas occur among heterosexuals, and the male-to-female ratio approaches 1 to 1; perinatal transmission is relatively common. The principal risk factors associated with HIV infection include number of heterosexual partners, sex with prostitutes, and being a sexual partner of an HIV-infected person. Intravenous drug abuse and homosexual transmission are either nonexistent or rare. WHO researchers report that the overall level of HIV infection in many of these countries is estimated to exceed 1 percent, and, "in a few urban areas, up to 25 percent of the sexually active age group is infected."[79]

Transmission through contaminated blood and blood products remains a significant problem in these countries. A study reported in January 1988 suggests that almost 1 in 15 children in central Africa receiving a blood transfusion to treat malaria-related anemia may become infected with HIV.[80] NIH researcher Thomas Quinn estimates that 1,000 children in central Africa may have been infected with HIV in this way in each of the last 5 years. The use of unsterilized needles or other skin-piercing instruments for medical or ritual purposes (such as scarification) has also been implicated in AIDS transmission in "pattern two" countries.[81]

One of the most puzzling features of the international

AIDS epidemic has been the different roles played by heterosexual transmission in the United States (pattern one) and Africa (pattern two). The relatively low frequency of HIV infection among the regular sex partners of seropositive transfusion recipients and hemophiliacs in the United States does not seem consistent with the rapid spread of HIV infection among heterosexuals in parts of central Africa. Over the past several years, researchers have begun to examine various biological and social factors that could account for this phenomenon.

The discovery that genital ulcers and other sexually transmitted diseases greatly increase the risk of HIV infection —perhaps because they provide a more direct portal of entry for the virus—has been an important starting point. Genital ulcers are more prevalent among certain sexually active populations in Africa than they are among heterosexuals in the United States.

Another possibility is that African heterosexuals are more susceptible to HIV infection because of chronic exposure to other viral or parasitic infections. Laboratory studies have shown that activated T cells are more susceptible than resting T cells to productive infection with HIV. Quinn and his coworkers explored the role of other infectious agents in HIV infection in a study of the immune systems of African and U.S. AIDS patients, healthy heterosexual men and women, and homosexual American men. They found that heterosexuals from the United States had a much lower prevalence of antibodies (evidence of previous infection) to cytomegalovirus, Epstein-Barr virus, hepatitis A and B viruses, herpes simplex virus, syphilis, and toxoplasmosis than the African heterosexuals. The prevalence of infection among the African heterosexuals was comparable to that found among the AIDS patients and the homosexual men. The researchers concluded: "These data demonstrate that the immune systems of African heterosexuals, similar to those of U.S. homosexual men, are in a chronically activated state associated with chronic viral and parasitic antigenic exposure, which may cause them to be particularly susceptible to HIV infection or disease progression."[82]

There is an urgent need for more information about possible cofactors that increase the risk of HIV infection and the risk of disease progression among those infected with the virus. New HIV and AIDS surveillance systems in many African countries may help provide this information.

Thirty-eight countries in Africa have reported 13 percent of the world's total AIDS cases. As of March 21, 1988, Zaire and Zimbabwe had each reported 300 to 500 cases; and Burundi, Congo, Kenya, Malawi, Rwanda, Tanzania, Uganda, and Zambia had each reported more than 500 cases.[83] The principal cause of AIDS in these countries is believed to be HIV-1 (the original AIDS virus). A second virus associated with AIDS, HIV-2 (see Chapter 4), is more common in West Africa (countries such as Guinea, Guinea-Bissau, and Senegal).

Pattern Three

The third pattern of transmission occurs in regions of Eastern Europe, the Middle East, Asia, and most of the Pacific. Scientists believe that HIV was introduced into these areas in the early to mid-1980s. Few AIDS cases have been reported. Most involve people who have traveled to areas with a high prevalence of HIV infection or who have had sexual contact with someone from such an area. Some cases have been attributed to the use of imported blood or blood products.

In recent testimony before the U.S. presidential commission on HIV infection, Jonathan Mann, director of WHO's Global Programme on AIDS, expressed concern about the potential for rapid spread of HIV infection in areas that until now have been relatively unaffected by the AIDS epidemic. The recent increase in HIV seropositivity among IV drug abusers in Bangkok, Thailand, may be an important warning signal. In 1987, 1 percent of tested IV drug abusers in Bangkok were seropositive; during the first three months of 1988 the figure rose to 16 percent. Mann says, "This Thai experience shows very clearly that Asia is just as vulnerable to an explosion of HIV infection as any other part of the world."[84]

Global Strategies to Control AIDS

The WHO Global Programme on AIDS (GPA) is coordinating the international effort to stop the spread of HIV infection. More than 150 countries have now established national AIDS committees; WHO has provided technical assistance to at least 115 of them. These committees are overseeing efforts to establish HIV and AIDS surveillance systems; educate health workers; ensure adequate laboratory support; develop, implement, and evaluate prevention programs; and strengthen health care and social services for AIDS patients and their families.[85] The GPA helps developing nations elicit support for these programs and also provides a substantial amount of direct financial assistance. In addition, GPA officials are working with the United Nations Development Program (UNDP) and other international agencies to help Third World countries incorporate AIDS-prevention measures into their development plans.

WHO also has launched a global blood safety initiative to reduce the risk of transfusion-related HIV infection. It has drawn together the International Society for Blood Transfusion, the International League of Red Cross and Red Crescent Societies, UNDP, and other organizations to increase the availability of low-cost, reliable blood screening techniques.

As HIV infection spreads throughout the world, the need for international collaboration in the fields of biomedicine, epidemiology, behavioral research, and public health becomes more apparent. The United States has an important role to play in this collaboration because of its strong foundation in scientific research, its experience with AIDS, and its relative affluence.

Conclusion

AIDS and other disease processes associated with HIV infection will continue to be a serious problem in the United States for the foreseeable future. Over the next decade, the vast majority of cases will occur among groups that have already experienced heavy losses as a result of HIV infection:

homosexual and bisexual men, intravenous drug abusers, recipients of blood and blood products, heterosexual partners of those at recognized risk of HIV infection, and infants born to infected mothers. The annual incidence of new HIV infections has decreased among homosexual men but remains high among intravenous drug abusers in the Northeast. HIV transmission through blood and blood products in the United States has been virtually eliminated as a result of donor-exclusion measures, systemwide testing for HIV antibodies, and procedures to inactivate the virus in clotting concentrates. Although heterosexual transmission occurs both from men to women and from women to men, so far the prevalence of infection among heterosexuals with no known risk factors is low in the United States. This fact suggests that an opportunity exists to stop the spread of HIV infection through education and other public health measures. But the task will not be easy; high-risk sexual behavior resulted in a major increase in syphilis among U.S. heterosexuals in 1987.

3
The Spectrum of Disease

The man and woman seemed to have nothing in common except their deaths. Both succumbed to respiratory failure and deteriorating brain function.

He was a 40-year-old homosexual with a history of more than 900 anonymous sexual encounters. He had been well until July 1982, when he began to tire easily and was sometimes too weak to leave the house. Later he developed persistently swollen glands and daily fevers. When he entered the hospital he had pneumonia, two kinds of cancer, and a viral infection that was destroying the retina in both eyes. The cancers and pneumonia initially responded to treatment, but symptoms recurred when therapy was stopped. Meanwhile, he developed signs of brain disease: his memory failed, he appeared drowsy, and his handwriting changed. Four months after diagnosis he died.

The woman was 22 years old and a recent immigrant from Haiti. For nine months before being hospitalized she had suffered frequent fevers, watery diarrhea, and excessive weight loss. Her left arm and leg had grown progressively weaker until she was unable to walk. Diagnostic tests showed four different intestinal parasites and a large tubercular lesion in the brain. Antituberculous drugs produced some improvement, but her overall condition worsened. When she died after more than 3 months in the hospital, an autopsy revealed viral pneumonia and a brain infection with the protozoan *Toxoplasma gondii*, in addition to the tubercular lesion.

Both of these patients had AIDS. Their conditions,

described in a 1985 issue of the *Journal of the American Medical Association*,[1] were typical of the first AIDS cases. Most patients had multiple problems and failed to respond to standard therapies; when they did respond, symptoms often returned as soon as a treatment course ended. Coping with such treatment failures was very difficult for a society with enormous confidence in the power of medical science.

Seven years of experience with the AIDS epidemic has reduced but not eliminated the shock. Scientists have begun to sort out the effects of human immunodeficiency virus type 1 (HIV-1) from those of the opportunistic infections that often herald its presence (see Table 3.1). They have learned to anticipate treatment problems and, in some cases, to overcome them. Although AIDS remains incurable, more than 15 percent of patients now survive at least 5 years after diagnosis (most long-term survivors are homosexual men with an initial diagnosis of Kaposi's sarcoma).

Classifying HIV-1 Infections

Any discussion of the clinical findings associated with AIDS must begin with the understanding that AIDS is only one outcome of infection with HIV-1. People infected with the virus may be completely asymptomatic; they may have mildly debilitating constitutional symptoms; or they may have life-threatening conditions caused by progressive destruction of the immune system, the brain, or both.

Several different terms, including AIDS-related complex (ARC) and lymphadenopathy syndrome, have been used by physicians and researchers to describe the less severe signs and symptoms of HIV infection. The inconsistent use of these terms has created problems for scientists attempting to track the natural history of HIV infection and has made it difficult to compare different patient populations. The CDC's revised surveillance case definition (Appendix B) has in effect rendered the term *ARC* obsolete.

To improve communication about the broad spectrum of HIV-related illnesses, the Centers for Disease Control has

Table 3.1.   Microorganisms causing opportunistic infections in patients
with AIDS

Microorganisms	Syndromes
Viruses	
Cytomegalovirus	Encephalitis, chorioretinitis, pneumonia, hepatitis, colitis, adrenalitis, disseminated infection
Herpes simplex virus	Persistent, recurrent, or disseminated skin ulcers
Varicella-zoster	Local, severe, or disseminated infection
Epstein-Barr virus	Lymphoma
Papovavirus-JC	Central nervous system infection
Adenoviruses	Colonization, disseminated infection
Bacteria	
Mycobacterium avium-intracellulare[a]	Disseminated infection, severe gastrointestinal disease, massive intraabdominal lymphadenopathy
Mycobacterium tuberculosis[a]	Adenitis, pulmonary infection, meningitis
Mycobacterium species[a]	Disseminated infection
Nocardia asteroides[a]	Pulmonary-pericardial infection, brain abscess
Salmonella species[a]	Typhoidal syndrome, severe gastroenteritis with bacteremia
Listeria monocytogenes[a]	Bacteremia
Legionella species[a]	Pneumonias, cellulitis
Streptococcus pneumoniae[b]	Pneumonia, bacteremia
Haemophilus influenzae[b]	Pneumonia, bacteremia
Staphylococcus aureus[c]	Bacteremia, skin infections, pneumonia
Clostridium perfringens[c]	Bacteremia
Shigella species[c]	Diarrhea, bacteremia
Parasites	
Pneumocystis carinii	Pneumonia
Toxoplasma gondii	Encephalitis, brain abscess
Cryptosporidium species	Gastroenteritis
Fungi	
Candida species	Oropharyngitis, esophagitis, vaginitis
Cryptococcus neoformans	Meningitis, disseminated infection, pneumonia
Histoplasma capsulatum	Disseminated infection
Aspergillus species	Pneumonia

Source: Adapted, with permission, from D. Armstrong et al., "Treatment of
Infections in Patients with the Acquired Immunodeficiency Syndrome," *Annals of
Internal Medicine,* 103 (November 1985), p. 739, table 1.
   a. Commonly take advantage of T-cell defects. (See Chapter 5 for discussion of
specific cell defects.)
   b. Commonly take advantage of B-cell defects. (See Chapter 5.)
   c. Not associated with identified cell defect.

developed 2 hierarchical classification systems—one for adults and the other for children with HIV infection. The system for adults is summarized in Table 3.2. It is important to note that classification in Group IV does not provide specific information about the severity of symptoms. For example, HIV-infected patients whose only clinical symptom is thrush (candidiasis infection limited to the mouth) would be included in Group IV even though they are not sick enough to fit the CDC case definition of AIDS (see Chapter 2).

The following pages use the CDC classification systems as guides to examine the incidence and characteristics of some of the more common findings in adults and children infected with HIV-1. New treatment alternatives for specific disorders are described briefly; Chapter 7 examines the effects of antiviral agents, such as azidothymidine (AZT, also called zidovudine), which could have a major impact on the course of all HIV-related illnesses.

Acute Infection with HIV-1

One of the first signs of HIV-1 infection in some patients is an acute mononucleosislike or flulike disease. The condition

Table 3.2. Summary of the CDC classification system for human immunodeficiency virus (HIV) infection in adults

Group I	Acute infection
Group II	Asymptomatic infection[a]
Group III	Persistent generalized lymphadenopathy[a]
Group IV	Other disease
Subgroup A	Constitutional disease
Subgroup B	Neurologic disease
Subgroup C	Secondary infectious diseases
Subgroup D	Secondary cancers[b]
Subgroup E	Other conditions

Source: Centers for Disease Control, "Classification System for Human T-Lymphotropic Virus Type III/Lymphadenopathy-Associated Virus Infections," Morbidity and Mortality Weekly Report, 35 (1986), 334–339.

a. Patients in Groups II and III may be subclassified on the basis of a laboratory evaluation.

b. Includes patients whose clinical presentation fulfills the CDC surveillance case definition of AIDS.

lasts from a few days to several weeks and is associated with fever, sweats, exhaustion, loss of appetite, nausea, headaches, sore throat, diarrhea, swollen glands, and a rash on the trunk. The acute syndrome was first described by physicians monitoring the health of almost 1,000 homosexual and bisexual men in Sydney, Australia.[2]

In one patient in the Australian study, the illness developed 6 days after probable exposure. Three other patients developed antibodies against the virus 19, 32, and 56 days after onset of the illness. (The length of time between infection and antibody production is discussed further in Chapter 5.) Laboratory studies showed that all the patients had some immunologic abnormalities, but not the extreme changes seen in AIDS patients.

Some of the symptoms of the acute illness may result from HIV-1 invasion of the central nervous system. In a recent article in *Annals of Internal Medicine*, Dana Gabuzda and Martin Hirsch of the Massachusetts General Hospital described retrospective studies suggesting that 5 to 10 percent of patients with HIV-related conditions have clinically apparent aseptic meningitis early in the course of their disease. (Typical signs include fever, headache, neck stiffness, and partial paralysis of some of the facial nerves.) In some cases the clinical findings have correlated with the presence of HIV-1 in the cerebrospinal fluid. The meningitis usually is self-limited; symptoms disappear along with the rash and other signs of acute viral disease.[3]

The significance of this acute illness is not known. It is relatively rare. Physicians are conducting long-term studies to determine if there is a relationship between the initial response to the virus and subsequent development of AIDS or other problems.

Asymptomatic Infection and Persistent Generalized Lymphadenopathy

Soon after AIDS was identified as a new disease, physicians noticed that a large group of previously healthy homosexual men were seeking treatment for persistent swollen glands not explained by specific illnesses or drug use. The epidemiologic characteristics (age, racial composition, and residential patterns) of this population were identical with those of the population of AIDS patients. As the epidemic progressed, similar findings were reported among intravenous drug abusers, hemophiliacs, and the heterosexual partners of some AIDS patients.

When the blood test for HIV-1 antibodies became available, researchers demonstrated that lymphadenopathy was a frequent consequence of infection with the virus. Initially it was believed that people who developed persistent lymphadenopathy were more likely to progress to AIDS than infected patients whose glands remained normal. The results of a recent prospective study of almost 5,000 homosexual and bisexual men in 4 American cities challenges this theory.

Richard Kaslow of the National Institute of Allergy and Infectious Diseases (NIAID) and his coworkers studied the relationship between persistent generalized lymphadenopathy and the level of T-helper lymphocytes in the blood. The researchers found that, in the absence of other symptoms, persistently swollen glands are not indicative of a declining immune system.[4]

Clinical and laboratory findings that did correlate strongly with T-helper cell depletion in the Kaslow study were fever, thrush, anemia, and neutropenia (loss of neutrophils—white blood cells that engulf and destroy bacteria). Fatigue and thrombocytopenia (a decrease in the number of platelets, or blood clotting cells) were more weakly correlated with low T-helper cell counts.

These findings underscore the need for careful follow-up of HIV-infected patients with and without lymphadenopathy. Useful markers of disease progression include the appearance of viral core proteins in the blood (see Chapter 5) and elevated serum levels of a small immune molecule called $beta_2$-microglobulin.[5] If specific immunologic tests are not available, standard blood tests combined with careful clinical assessments may provide clues about the status of the patient's underlying immune disease.

Constitutional Disease: HIV Wasting Syndrome

During the early years of the AIDS epidemic, patients without opportunistic infections or cancers known to be associated with HIV infection often received less attention than others with HIV-related conditions. Their symptoms were deceptively simple: persistent fever and diarrhea, involuntary weight loss, and chronic weakness. Such patients often were not eligible for the benefits and services designed for those with the most "serious" consequences of HIV infection. Yet many were severely disabled. Some died without ever meeting the CDC case definition of AIDS.

An increase in reports of a condition known as "slim disease" among HIV-infected patients in Africa led to gradual recognition that the wasting syndrome was a direct effect of the newly discovered virus. In August 1987 the CDC added HIV wasting syndrome to the official surveillance definition of AIDS. Physicians were instructed to look for

profound involuntary weight loss greater than 10 percent of baseline body weight plus either chronic diarrhea (at least two loose stools per day for more than or equal to 30 days) or chronic weakness and documented fever (for more than or equal to 30 days, intermittent or constant) in the absence of a concurrent illness or condition other than HIV infection that could explain the findings (e.g., cancer, tuberculosis, cryptosporidiosis, or other specific enteritis).[6]

Scientists do not know what causes the wasting syndrome, but some experts speculate that it might result from the abnormal regulation of proteins called monokines. Monokines are produced by monocytes, white blood cells known to be susceptible to infection with HIV-1. In the late 1960s, scientists showed that one of the monokines, IL-1, acts on the part of the brain called the hypothalamus to induce fever. Elevated levels of another monokine, tumor necrosis factor, are associated with tissue wasting in certain parasitic diseases. Researchers in several laboratories are exploring the relationship between HIV-1 infection and monokine production.

AIDS-related gastrointestinal symptoms also may be

caused directly by HIV infection of intestinal cells. In February 1988, California scientists confirmed the presence of HIV in biopsy specimens taken from the small intestine and rectum of AIDS patients with a history of chronic diarrhea.[7]

Neurologic Disease

The neurologic manifestations of HIV infection also are receiving increasing attention. As noted earlier, between 5 and 10 percent of patients with AIDS and HIV-related conditions have bouts of acute aseptic meningitis. A much bigger problem, however, is the degenerative brain disease called subacute encephalitis (or AIDS dementia complex). About two-thirds of AIDS patients have clinical evidence of this disorder.

In adults with AIDS, the first symptoms of subacute encephalitis may be diminished concentration or mild memory loss. Many patients also report motor abnormalities, such as loss of balance or leg weakness. Behavioral problems, including apathy, social withdrawal, depression, and personality changes, may precede or follow other symptoms. (In one study, behavioral changes were the first signs of neurologic disease in 20 percent of patients.)

The rate of progression of HIV encephalopathy varies from several months to more than a year in untreated patients. In the latter stages of disease, loss of cognitive and motor functions may be accompanied by seizures, incontinence, partial paralysis, and extreme psychiatric disturbances. Death usually occurs from 1 to 6 months after the onset of severe dementia.

HIV infection also has been associated with degeneration of the spinal cord (vacuolar myelopathy) and abnormalities of the peripheral nervous system. Symptoms of the former include progressive loss of coordination and weakness. Involvement of the peripheral nervous system may result in shooting pains in the limbs or in numbness and partial paralysis.

Autopsies reveal signs of neurologic disease in 80 to 90 percent of people who die from AIDS. Clearly, the nervous system is a primary target of HIV. These findings underscore the need for drugs that can suppress the effects of the virus in the brain as well as in the immune system.

Treatment. In a preliminary study by Robert Yarchoan and his coworkers, the drug azidothymidine produced some improvement of symptoms in 6 of 7 patients with AIDS-associated dementia, peripheral neuropathy, or both. Additional studies will be required to determine the long-term effects of AZT. Chapter 7 describes other drug candidates that may be useful in HIV-related neurologic diseases.

Functional impairment. In December 1987 the U.S. military services announced that military personnel infected with HIV but otherwise healthy would be removed from sensitive, stressful jobs "because of new evidence that the virus could impair mental function, even in people who show no overt symptoms of the disease."[8] The decision was based in part on a study by Igor Grant and his coworkers at the University of California at San Diego and the San Diego Veterans Administration Medical Center. They administered neurological and psychological tests to 55 homosexual men in four groups: 15 had AIDS, 13 had less serious HIV-related clinical symptoms, 16 were infected with HIV but did not have symptoms, and 11 were seronegative. The researchers reported neuropsychological abnormalities in 13 (87 percent) of the AIDS patients, 7 (54 percent) of the less seriously ill patients, 7 (44 percent) of the asymptomatic individuals, and 1 (9 percent) of the uninfected men.[9]

Grant and his colleagues were surprised at the number of men with asymptomatic HIV infections who showed deficits, but cautioned that confirmation of their results would require more extensive cross-sectional studies, as well as long-term observations of asymptomatic seropositive and seronegative people at risk. In an interview with *Science News*, Grant said: "HIV may affect brain function early on in infection, but it's premature to make any conclusions from this study."[10]

Public health officials and civil rights advocates have

criticized the ruling by the military services because it limits job opportunities for an entire group, rather than focusing only on individuals who actually show signs of impairment. (The Department of Defense is now reviewing the policy.) Some critics have worried that civilian employers might view the military's action as justification for HIV testing of their employees.

In March 1988 the World Health Organization brought together 48 neurologists, psychiatrists, neuropsychologists, clinical researchers, health policy experts, and others from 17 countries to review and evaluate the data on HIV-related functional impairment. They found no evidence that people with asymptomatic HIV infection are more likely than uninfected people to have clinically significant neurological or neuropsychological abnormalities. The group concluded: "Therefore, there is no justification for HIV-1 serologic screening as a strategy for detecting such functional impairment in asymptomatic persons."[11]

Secondary Infectious Diseases (Opportunistic Infections)

HIV destroys the body's defensive capabilities, opening the door to whatever disease-producing agents are present in the environment. In populations that have a high incidence of tuberculosis (such as intravenous drug abusers and immigrants from some developing countries), AIDS is associated with extremely aggressive tubercular lesions in sites not usually affected by the bacterium. Africans with AIDS are prone to cryptococcal meningitis, an infection caused by a yeastlike organism. The parasitic disease toxoplasmosis occurs frequently among AIDS patients born in Haiti. Homosexuals with AIDS often develop persistent herpes infections because the immune cells that previously kept the virus in check have been destroyed.

The diagnosis of secondary infections in AIDS patients and others with HIV infection is complicated because some of the standard diagnostic tests may not work. Often such tests detect the immune response to a disease-producing microorganism rather than the organism itself. For example, the standard tests for syphilis measure antibodies produced by the body in response to infection with the spirochete *Treponema pallidum*. Patients with an impaired immune system may not make such antibodies.[12] Similarly, some AIDS patients with tuberculosis may not be able to mount the type of immune response (a cell-mediated immune response) required for a positive reaction on the Mantoux skin test.[13] Physicians caring for patients with HIV-associated diseases must rely heavily on their own clinical judgment—if laboratory test results fail to confirm a diagnosis based on a patient's clinical symptoms, the physician may have to use more invasive diagnostic procedures (such as tissue biopsies) or develop new approaches to the diagnosis. Rapid diagnosis is extremely important because infectious diseases tend to be much more aggressive in HIV-infected patients than in other people.

Pneumocystis carinii *Pneumonia.*   The most common life-threatening opportunistic infection in AIDS patients is *Pneumocystis carinii* pneumonia, a parasitic infection previously seen almost exclusively in cancer and transplant patients receiving immunosuppressive drugs. The first signs of this disorder are moderate to severe difficulty in breathing, dry cough, and fever.

A recent study of AIDS patients in New York City indicates that the short-term survival of patients with *P. carinii* pneumonia has improved signficantly since the early days of the epidemic. In 1981 only 18 percent of New York patients who were diagnosed with this form of pneumonia survived more than a year; by 1985 the one-year survival rate had increased to 48 percent.

With early diagnosis and appropriate drug therapy, 85 to 90 percent of AIDS patients survive their first episode of *P. carinii* pneumonia, but many require longer treatment regimens than transplant or cancer patients with the same symptoms. In one study, almost 75 percent of AIDS patients continued to have high concentrations of *P. carinii* in their lungs after two to three weeks of therapy. In contrast, most other patients treated for this infection have no detectable parasites within 3 to 14 days after treatment begins.

Another problem in caring for AIDS patients with *P. carinii* pneumonia is that an unexpectedly large number—up to 55 percent—have adverse reactions to the sulfa drugs commonly used to treat the disorder. The reasons for this phenomenon are unknown, although a similar intolerance has been reported in patients with other immune system defects. Researchers have developed several new forms of therapy to help AIDS patients who cannot tolerate or who fail to respond to conventional drugs.

One new treatment regimen combines a metabolic inhibitor called trimetrexate with a vitaminlike substance called leucovorin. Trimetrexate interferes with the metabolism of all living cells. Leucovorin rescues human cells from the toxic effects of trimetrexate but does not protect the *P. carinii* organisms. In October 1987, researchers from the National Institutes of Health and George Washington University Medical Center reported that the trimetrexate-leucovorin combination was safe and effective and was tolerated well by AIDS patients.[14] In the first clinical trial only 1 of 49 patients had an adverse reaction severe enough to require withdrawal of the trimetrexate.

Other physicians have tried new ways of delivering conventional medications. For example, San Francisco researchers report a marked decrease in side effects when the drug pentamidine, usually administered through the veins, is delivered instead in an aerosolized spray. (Conventional therapy with pentamidine frequently causes low white blood cell counts, liver damage, and rashes.) In a study described in *Lancet*, 13 of 15 AIDS patients with mild *P. carinii* pneumonia were successfully treated with three weeks of inhaled pentamidine; the only adverse reaction was coughing.[15] A second pilot study also produced favorable results, although 3 of 10 patients appeared to have had early relapses.[16]

Perhaps the most exciting development related to *P. carinii* pneumonia is the advent of prophylactic treatment. Margaret Fischl and her coworkers at the University of Miami

School of Medicine recently described the results of a study involving 60 patients with newly diagnosed Kaposi's sarcoma. Thirty of the patients received antibiotics commonly administered to treat *P. carinii* pneumonia (sulfamethoxazole and trimethoprim), and 30 received no preventive therapy. Between the beginning of the study in June 1984 and June 1987, none of the 30 patients receiving suppressive therapy developed *P. carinii* pneumonia, compared with 16 of 30 patients in the control group. The antibiotics did not prevent death from other opportunistic infections and cancers, but overall survival was markedly better in the treatment group. Eighteen patients in the treatment group died during the course of the study, compared with 28 in the control group. The authors conclude that prophylactic treatment for *P. carinii* pneumonia should be considered for any patient with an HIV-related disease. They add that further studies are needed to determine whether HIV-infected patients without symptoms should receive antibiotic therapy.[17]

Several other agents also are being evaluated for the prevention of *P. carinii* pneumonia. For example, at the Fourth International Conference on AIDS in Stockholm, 9 groups presented preliminary evidence that inhaled pentamidine could reduce but not completely prevent *P. carinii* pneumonia in high-risk patients (including those who had already experienced one episode of the disease).[18] Large-scale clinical trials are needed to compare the benefits and risks of the different treatment alternatives for this very widespread AIDS-related problem.

Candida albicans.   Infection with *Candida albicans*, a yeastlike fungus, may be one of the first signs of an immune system weakened by HIV. In patients with early HIV-related symptoms, the whitish mouth sores characteristic of candidiasis (commonly called thrush) indicate a high risk of developing full-blown AIDS. AIDS patients often have candidiasis lesions that extend into the esophagus, and a few patients have been reported with candidiasis lesions in the brain.

Infections with *C. albicans* usually respond to antifungal

therapy, but in patients with AIDS the disease often reappears as soon as therapy has been completed.

Cryptosporidium. This protozoan parasite causes severe, protracted diarrhea. Scientists had been interested in the organism for many years because of its effect on calves and other domestic animals; the first recognized case of human cryptosporidiosis occurred in 1976.

In people with normal immune systems, *Cryptosporidium* causes a self-limited disease that lasts 1 to 2 weeks. In AIDS patients, the diarrhea often becomes chronic and may lead to severe malnutrition. Treatment of this disorder remains experimental, but several drugs have shown promise in a few patients.

Cytomegalovirus (CMV). The majority of patients with full-blown AIDS have active CMV infections. This virus is a member of the herpesvirus family. The most common sign of its presence in AIDS patients is spots on the retina, which may lead to blindness. The virus also causes pneumonia and inflammation of the esophagus (esophagitis) and colon (colitis). It may be the principal cause of death in some AIDS cases.

CMV infection rarely produces clinical symptoms in healthy adults, although it does cause some cases of a mono-nucleosislike syndrome. Before the appearance of AIDS, the populations most at risk from CMV were newborns with congenital infections and transplant and cancer patients receiving immunosuppressive drugs.

Infections with this virus generally respond poorly to antiviral chemotherapy, but several new drugs have shown promise in clinical trials. One of these drugs is ganciclovir. Martin Hirsch of Massachusetts General Hospital in Boston says that ganciclovir has a response rate of more than 80 percent in patients with CMV retinitis. Unfortunately, lesions on the retina usually return as soon as treatment is stopped. Prevention of blindness requires intravenous injection of the drug about 5 times a week for life. Hirsch notes that some patients with CMV retinitis have been able to maintain full-time jobs with the aid of home health services that administer intravenous ganciclovir in the evenings.

The major drawback of ganciclovir is that it has the same serious side effect as AZT. Both drugs suppress the blood-forming activities of the bone marrow; thus, they cannot be taken at the same time. Patients may have to choose between a drug that prevents blindness and a drug that could prolong their lives.

Laboratory studies described in Chapter 5 suggest that CMV and some other DNA viruses may accelerate the course of HIV infections. If this relationship is documented in vivo, the control of CMV infections will become even more important.

Herpes zoster.   One of the first signs of a declining immune system following HIV infection may be the development of shingles. Shingles is caused by the herpes zoster virus, which is indistinguishable from the varicella virus that causes chicken-pox in children. After the childhood illness, the virus may establish a latent infection in the bodies of sensory nerve cells. The latent virus produces no symptoms.

Activation of the latent virus frequently occurs in older adults, in patients with certain types of cancer, and in those receiving immunosuppressive drugs. The virus travels down sensory nerve fibers, causing sudden pain and tenderness, a mild fever, and a rash of small blisters along the path of the nerve fibers.

A recent study by American and Danish scientists showed that shingles is part of the clinical spectrum of HIV infection and often precedes a diagnosis of AIDS.[19] The researchers followed 109 homosexual men treated for shingles by physi-cians in an internal medicine practice. They found that more than 70 percent of the men developed AIDS within 6 years of the shingles diagnosis. Shingles involving the head and neck, severe pain, and repeated episodes of the disorder were associated with a greater likelihood of progressing to AIDS.

Patients with shingles involving multiple nerve systems are classified in Group IV of the CDC classfication system for HIV-related disorders.

Syphilis. Syphilis is not included in the CDC classification system for HIV-related infections, but physicians and public health specialists have expressed growing concern about the way in which the two diseases interact.

In 1987 the incidence of syphilis in the United States increased by more than 25 percent. This dramatic rise, concentrated mainly among the urban poor in a few major metropolitan centers, is disturbing for many reasons. First, it occurred at a time when public health experts were urging people to reduce unsafe sexual practices. The increase in syphilis indicates that an important segment of the population—the segment most likely to be at risk of hetero-sexually transmitted HIV infection—has not been responding.

The second reason for concern is the apparent relationship between genital ulcers and HIV transmission. Studies in Africa have shown that people with genital sores caused by chan-croid, syphilis, and other sexually transmitted diseases are more likely to become infected with HIV than those without such sores. The rise in syphilis cases may mean that certain segments of the population are more vulnerable to HIV infection than they were in the past.

Finally, numerous reports in the medical literature indicate that coinfection with HIV has a major impact on the course of syphilis in both treated and untreated cases. Since the introduction of penicillin half a century ago, the severe consequences of syphilis—neurologic disease and death—have been very rare. Most patients have responded well to standard courses of therapy. Recently, however, physicians from several major medical centers have described cases in which standard regimens have not been sufficient to prevent life-threatening progression of the disease. These have been cases complicated by HIV infection. In one patient, neurosyphilis (characterized by blurred vision, weakness, dizziness, head-ache, and paralysis) developed just 5 months after what appeared to be an appropriate response to penicillin therapy for secondary syphilis. The normal incubation period for neurosyphilis, even in untreated cases, is a decade or longer.

In an editorial in the *New England Journal of Medicine*,

Edmund C. Tramont of Walter Reed Army Medical Center recommended that "all HIV-infected patients should be screened for syphilis, and vice versa."[20] Although such screening may not always be possible, physicians need to be aware of potential interactions between the two diseases. (Paul Volberding, director of AIDS Activities at San Francisco General Hospital, says that the presence of any sexually transmitted disease can be regarded as evidence that a patient is engaging in unsafe sexual practices. Thus, HIV counseling and voluntary testing are warranted each time a sexually transmitted disease is diagnosed.) HIV-infected patients may require higher doses of penicillin and more prolonged therapy than others with syphilis.

Toxoplasma gondii.   The protozoan parasite *Toxoplasma gondii* is a frequent cause of neurologic disease in AIDS patients. Most patients improve clinically within 2 to 3 weeks of the start of appropriate therapy, but relapses are common even after 6 months of treatment. Patients who appear to recover need careful follow-up; many medical centers continue therapy indefinitely.

Tuberculosis and other mycobacterial infections.   A 30-year pattern of decline in the incidence of tuberculosis in the United States ended in 1985, when the number of new tuberculosis cases reported to the CDC failed to drop below 1984 levels. In 1986 the number of new cases actually increased by 2.5 percent. Most researchers attribute this increase to the occurrence of tuberculosis among persons with HIV infection.

Tuberculosis is caused by bacteria from the genus *Mycobacterium*. The agent responsible for most cases of tuberculosis in human beings is *Mycobacterium tuberculosis*. However, people with HIV infection are also susceptible to other mycobacterial species, including *M. avium* complex (which causes an illness called MAC disease) and *M. kansasii*. MAC disease is most common in AIDS patients from populations with a low incidence of tuberculosis. AIDS patients from low-income areas in major cities and from developing countries are more likely to be infected with M. *tuberculosis* than with the other mycobacterial species.

In one Connecticut study, the 3-year incidence of tuberculosis among AIDS patients was more than 100 times the incidence of tuberculosis in the general population (adjusted for sex, race, city size, and age). Researchers believe that most of these cases represent reactivation of old infections. People who have been exposed to M. *tuberculosis* often carry a small number of bacteria deep within their lungs. The organism does not spread because it is held in check by the immune system. Infection with HIV destroys the cells that provide this protection and allows the mycobacteria to multiply and infiltrate new areas.

Patients with HIV infection and tuberculosis or MAC disease usually respond relatively well to standard antituberculosis drugs, but they often need a longer course of treatment than other patients. Also, the disease is more likely to spread beyond the lungs to other tissues. Common sites include the lymph nodes, brain, blood, bone marrow, genitourinary tract, liver, and peritoneum (the smooth membrane that lines the abdominal cavity and covers the visceral organs). Almost one-third of AIDS patients treated at the National Institutes of Health before 1986 had M. *avium* complex infections in the brain or other locations outside the lung.

Controlling M. *tuberculosis* infection in AIDS patients and others with HIV-related disease is extremely important, both for the patient and for family members and health care workers. Unlike MAC disease, P. *carinii* pneumonia, and other opportunistic infections that occur in AIDS, tuberculosis can be transmitted to people with a normal immune system. To minimize this potential problem (HIV-related tuberculosis transmission has never been reported in a health care worker) and to improve the treatment of AIDS patients, the CDC published extensive guidelines on the diagnosis and management of mycobacterial diseases and HIV infection.[21]

These guidelines emphasize that all patients who have tested positive for HIV should be given a tuberculin skin test. Anyone who has a significant tuberculin reaction but no other signs of tuberculosis should receive preventive therapy. Moreover, patients with severe HIV-related diseases should receive a chest x-ray as well as a skin test, because of the high probability of a false-negative tuberculin test in patients with an impaired immune system. Conversely, the CDC physicians and their collaborators recommend that the identification of risk factors for HIV infection should be a standard part of the evaluation of patients with tuberculosis. Voluntary testing for HIV is recommended for all tuberculosis patients who have such risk factors and for those who have unusual manifestations of the disease.

Cancers

The association between AIDS and cancer has been clear from the early days of the epidemic when physicians in several cities began reporting numerous cases of a previously rare form of cancer called Kaposi's sarcoma. The increase in Kaposi's sarcoma was concentrated among young, male homosexuals. Later studies showed that the same population also was experiencing a dramatic rise in cancers called non-Hodgkin's lymphomas.

The discovery of HIV and its deleterious effects on the immune system helped explain the source of these new cancers. Scientists knew that suppression of the immune system could trigger malignancies in transplant patients. They were not surprised, therefore, that the damage inflicted by HIV on the immune system could also cause cancer.

Kaposi's sarcoma.   The signs of Kaposi's sarcoma are blue-violet to brownish skin blotches or bumps. When the first blotch appears, it may be mistaken for a bruise, but unlike a bruise it does not go away after a week or 10 days. Kaposi's sarcoma is usually described as a cancer or tumor of the blood vessel walls. Before the appearance of AIDS, it was rare in the United States and Europe, where it occurred primarily in men over age 55 or 60, usually of Mediterranean origin.

More than 95 percent of AIDS patients who have Kaposi's sarcoma are homosexual or bisexual men. For those in whom Kaposi's sarcoma is the first sign of AIDS, the average survival time is slightly more than 1.5 years. Studies of the immune systems of these patients indicate that they generally are less depleted than those of patients whose AIDS diagnosis is based on an opportunistic infection.

Kaposi's sarcoma is rarely life-threatening for the middle-aged and elderly men who develop the disease in the absence of AIDS. Their lesions usually occur on the legs, grow very slowly, and do not invade other tissues. But the epidemic form of the disease is quite different. More than 75 percent of AIDS patients with Kaposi's sarcoma have disseminated disease, usually involving the lymph nodes, the lungs, or the gastrointestinal tract. Physicians treating AIDS patients in San Francisco have found several cases of Kaposi's sarcoma in the brain, a phenomenon that had been reported only once before in the medical literature.

Many different therapeutic approaches have been employed in AIDS-related Kaposi's sarcoma. Between 30 and 40 percent of patients respond initially to alpha interferon, a natural substance that stimulates the immune cells most affected by HIV. Radiation therapy sometimes produces temporary reductions in superficial lesions, and aggressive chemotherapy in the late stages of disease may produce sufficient improvement to allow a hospitalized patient to return home. Kaposi's sarcoma rarely is the principal cause of death in these patients, but it may be extremely debilitating, and it further weakens patients who eventually succumb to opportunistic infections.

Three aspects of Kaposi's sarcoma in AIDS have puzzled scientists: its tendency to behave like an opportunistic infection; its predominance in homosexual men; and the gradual decline in the proportion of AIDS patients with this form of cancer. Before 1984 it accounted for 21 percent of reported AIDS diagnoses; by August 1988 it accounted for only 9 percent of diagnoses overall.

Some scientists believe that answers to the first two puzzles may be related in part to the apparent connection between Kaposi's sarcoma and CMV. Researchers in central Africa, where classic Kaposi's sarcoma is more prevalent than in the United States, have found several types of evidence linking the virus to this form of cancer. Moreover, blood samples from homosexual men in the United States indicate that more than 90 percent have been exposed to CMV, a much higher proportion than among other groups at risk of AIDS. Epidemiologic studies, however, have failed to confirm the link between HIV-associated Kaposi's sarcoma and CMV. Some researchers suggest that a different, as yet unidentified, infectious agent may be involved.

The existence of cofactors associated with life-style also has been suggested as a possible explanation for the unique distribution of Kaposi's sarcoma. In several early studies, the development of Kaposi's sarcoma among HIV-infected homosexual men was linked to the use of nitrite inhalants. In a more recent study by James Goedert and his colleagues, cofactors associated with the disease included receptive fellatio, enemas, methaqualone use, and high levels of antibody to hepatitis B virus.[22] If such cofactors do play a role in Kaposi's sarcoma, reductions in high-risk behavior might be one reason for the apparent decrease in the proportion of people with HIV infection who develop this form of cancer.

In June 1988, Robert C. Gallo of the National Cancer Institute and his coworkers proposed a new explanation for the association between Kaposi's sarcoma and HIV infection. At the Fourth International Conference on AIDS, Gallo and his colleagues reported that HIV-infected cells appear to secrete a substance that triggers a massive increase in the growth of blood vessels. Administration of the partially purified growth factor to laboratory mice produced purplish lesions similar to those seen in AIDS patients.[23] The growth factor hypothesis, however, does not explain the decline in the incidence of Kaposi's sarcoma or why it occurs primarily among HIV-infected homosexual men in the United States.

Lymphomas.   From 1980 to 1983 cancer registry data in the San Francisco Bay area and Los Angeles County showed a threefold increase in the number of young, never-married men with high-grade lymphomas, which are aggressive cancers characterized by unregulated proliferation of certain white blood cells. Most of the affected men were homosexuals; many had generalized lymphadenopathy when their cancers were diagnosed, and some had full-blown AIDS.

Clinical researchers now believe that non-Hodgkin's lymphomas in patients at high risk of AIDS are another sign of infection with HIV. These lymphomas resemble cancers that develop in children with congenital immune defects. The tumors often appear outside the lymph nodes, and most respond poorly to treatment.

In one study of 90 homosexual patients with lymphomas from four major cities, 42 percent had tumors in the central nervous system (23 percent directly in the brain), and 33 percent had bone marrow involvement. The frequency of lymphoma of the brain in other patients with similar types of lymphoma is about 2 percent. Kaposi's sarcoma or severe opportunistic infections characteristic of AIDS developed in almost half of those who had generalized lymphadenopathy at diagnosis and in 3 of 12 who initially had no AIDS-related conditions. Patients who had evidence of ARC or AIDS were less likely to respond to treatment, relapsed more frequently, and had a higher mortality rate.

HIV does not appear to cause the lymphomas on its own, but it may depress immune functions sufficiently to allow other viruses to act. For example, many homosexual men have evidence of exposure to the herpesvirus Epstein-Barr virus (EBV). EBV has been implicated as a causal factor in the development of Burkitt lymphoma in Africa (Burkitt lymphoma is very difficult to distinguish microscopically from the lymphomas most common in AIDS patients) and of nasopharyngeal carcinoma in the Far East. Abnormalities of immune regulation caused by infection with HIV may allow EBV to initiate the processes that eventually lead to cancer.

Non-Hodgkin's lymphoma is included in the surveillance case definition of AIDS only if it is limited to the brain or if it occurs in association with a positive test for HIV (see Appendix

B). Other cases are not included because lymphomas may cause, as well as result from, damage to the immune system. (Paul Volberding says that all cases of non-Hodgkin's lymphoma, especially in young adults, should prompt an immediate test for HIV antibodies, because the prognosis and approach to therapy in HIV-infected patients are quite different from those in HIV-seronegative patients.)[24]

Miscellaneous cancers. The full extent of the relationship between HIV and cancer remains unclear. In a 1987 report in the *American Journal of Epidemiology*, Robert Biggar and his co-workers at the National Cancer Institute examined cancer rates through 1984 in a group known to be at high risk of AIDS—never-married men in San Francisco between the ages of 20 and 49. They found that statistically significant increases in cancer were confined to Kaposi's sarcoma and non-Hodgkin's lymphoma. The researchers recommended, however, that increases in other malignancies, including Hodgkin's disease and hepatoma (liver cancer), be monitored carefully in the future.[25]

Individual case reports also have linked HIV infection to oral cancers, testicular cancers, and leukemias, but scientists do not have sufficient data to establish that such cases are anything more than coincidental. Biggar and his colleagues explain that the length of time between the start of immunosuppression and the appearance of particular tumors varies. For example, transplant patients exhibit an increased risk for lymphoma within the first year after surgery, but do not show an increased risk for other tumors until 2 years later. Some physicians are concerned that people who survive the early years of HIV infection will develop a broad range of cancers as they age.

Oral Signs of HIV Infection

Many of the infections and cancers common in HIV-infected patients cause unusual lesions in the mouth. Oral candidiasis is described above. Oral lesions of Kaposi's sarcoma have been found in AIDS patients with and without skin lesions. Herpes simplex ulcers on the tongue and other oral mucosa of HIV-infected patients are larger and more variable than herpes infections in HIV-seronegative patients.[26]

The most distinctive oral lesion associated with HIV infection is hairy leukoplakia, which usually appears as white raised patches on the sides of the tongue. The term *hairy* refers to the hairy or corrugated texture of the lesion. In one study, 99 percent of patients diagnosed with hairy leukoplakia were found to be HIV-seropositive.[27]

Researchers believe that hairy leukoplakia may be caused by simultaneous infection with Epstein-Barr virus and papillomavirus.[28] The lesion is considered to be an important predictor of progression to AIDS.

Other Conditions

The descriptions above cover just a few of the diagnostic and treatment challenges associated with HIV infection. Physicians in every specialty report increases in previously rare conditions and unusual presentations of familiar disorders. For example, physicians have reported hundreds of new cases of a rare form of arthritis called Reiter's syndrome; almost all the new patients test positive for HIV.[29] Similarly, dermatologists describe an extremely aggressive form of psoriasis associated with HIV infection. Ophthalmologists report "cotton wool spots" (small white areas of retinal thickening) and bacterial infections of the retina in HIV-infected patients with no other symptoms, as well as in those with ARC and AIDS. A new syndrome called AIDS-associated nephropathy (deterioration of the kidney) produces kidney failure in just a few weeks. And cardiologists have identified an AIDS-associated cardiomyopathy (destruction of the heart muscle).

Treatment of these conditions can be extremely complex; standard therapies are often either ineffective or unsafe for patients with HIV infection. For example, patients with AIDS-associated nephropathy respond poorly to kidney dialysis, even with intensive nutritional supplementation. Physicians treating Reiter's syndrome and psoriasis in HIV-infected patients cannot use the broad-spectrum immunosuppressive drugs that often help others with the disease, because the drugs might lead to further progression of AIDS-related symptoms. The potential impact on the health care system of a large patient population with multiple problems of this type is discussed in Chapter 9. It underscores the importance of developing new techniques to rebuild dismantled immune systems and to block the primary culprit, HIV.

AIDS in Children

Pediatric AIDS is a very different disease from AIDS in adults, especially when it occurs in young babies (see Table 3.3). These infants get the opportunistic infections often seen in adult patients, but they also develop a wide range of other problems. Some of the more common signs of HIV infection in young children include frequent bacterial infections, lymphoid interstitial pneumonitis (LIP), failure to thrive (failure to follow growth curves for height and weight), and loss of

Table 3.3.   Differences between pediatric and adult AIDS

---

1. Kaposi's sarcoma and B cell lymphoma are rare in children.
2. Hepatitis B virus infection is less frequent than in adults.
3. Hypergammaglobulinema is more pronounced in children.
4. Peripheral lymphopenia is uncommon in children.
5. Lymphoid interstitial pneumonitis (LIP) is much more common in children.
6. Some children will have normal ratio of helper to suppressor T cells (although quantitatively T helper cells are diminished).
7. Serious bacterial sepsis is a major problem in children.
8. Dysmorphic features may be found in some children.
9. Acute mononucleosislike presentation is rare in children.
10. Progressive neurologic disease secondary to primary HIV infection of the central nervous system is more pronounced in children.

Source: James Oleske, "Natural History of HIV Infection II," in *Report of the Surgeon General's Workshop on Children with HIV Infection and Their Families*, DHHS Publication no. HRS-D-MC 87-1 (Washington, D.C.: U.S. Department of Health and Human Services, 1987), p. 25.

developmental milestones (for example, a baby who had been able to sit or to talk becomes unable to do so).

As noted in Chapter 2, those at risk of pediatric AIDS include infants born into families in which one or both parents have AIDS or are at high risk of developing AIDS, children who received blood transfusions from donors with risk factors, and children with hemophilia. The development of antibody screening tests and of procedures to inactivate HIV in clotting factor concentrates has substantially reduced the risk of AIDS and related disorders among new recipients of blood or blood products. However, AIDS will continue to appear in children who were infected through contaminated blood products before 1985.

A recent European study of children born to HIV-seropositive mothers indicates that about 40 percent of infants with congenital HIV infection develop AIDS or a related illness within 10 months.[30] In contrast, it takes about nine years for a similar proportion of HIV-infected adults to develop severe disease.[31] Stephen Chanock and Kenneth McIntosh of Children's Hospital in Boston say that some of the differences between the adult and congenital forms of HIV infection may be explained by the timing of the infection, especially as it relates to the development of the immune system.[32]

The immune system in an adult consists of many different cell populations working together to recognize and destroy disease-producing microorganisms (see Chapter 5). Although this system cannot rid the body of an HIV infection, it does appear capable of suppressing viral activity for many years. But the situation is quite different when the target of HIV infection is the immature immune system. Maturation of the immune system is a complex process in which substances produced by one cell population stimulate the growth and development of other cell populations. If certain key cells are disabled by HIV infection, entire populations of immune cells may fail to develop normally. Thus, babies with congenital HIV infection may begin life with severely impaired immune responses.

Physicians who care for HIV-infected children often divide their patients into three groups. The first group consists of children who develop severe opportunistic infections, including *P. carinii* pneumonia or HIV encephalopathy, during the first year of life. These children often have very poor immune responses, and many die in infancy. The second group consists of children with lymphoid interstitial pneumonitis. Patients in this group show a variety of clinical and laboratory abnormalities (described below), but they often respond well to treatment. The third group consists of HIV-infected children whose immune functions appear normal and who have few or no signs of disease. Several infected children have passed their seventh and eighth birthdays with only the normal spectrum of childhood illnesses.

Some researchers believe that children in the first group may be those who were infected early in pregnancy. Children in the other 2 groups may fare better because they were infected later in pregnancy or at birth.

Diagnosis of HIV Infection

Two problems complicate the diagnosis of HIV infection in infants. The first is the possibility of confusing HIV-related symptoms with those caused by inherited defects of the immune system, such as severe combined immune deficiency (SCID). Both conditions may cause failure to thrive, chronic diarrhea, and frequent bacterial infections. Specific laboratory tests and a careful family history usually resolve this issue. The second problem is more complex. It involves the interpretation of standard HIV diagnostic tests.

Antibody tests. HIV antibody tests must be interpreted carefully in infants because all young babies have antibodies acquired before birth from their mothers. Commercial techniques for measuring HIV antibodies do not distinguish between these maternal antibodies and antibodies produced by the child in response to infection. A woman infected with HIV may produce a child who is not infected but who carries passively acquired maternal antibodies against the virus. The maternal antibodies usually disappear by about 6 months of age, but in rare cases they may persist for more than a year. Thus, a child under 15 months of age who tests positive for HIV antibodies is not definitely considered to be infected with the virus unless he or she also has immune system abnormalities *and* clinical symptoms associated with HIV (see Table 3.4).

Another problem with using the HIV antibody test in young children is that some HIV-infected infants may not be capable of making antibodies. Early infection with HIV may disrupt the maturation of the immune system to such an extent that antibody-producing cells do not function.

Polymerase chain reaction (PCR) test. For now, the most promising alternative to the antibody test appears to be the poly-

---

Table 3.4.   Summary of the definition of HIV infection in children

---

Infants and children under 15 months of age with perinatal infection

Virus in blood or tissues
    or
HIV antibody
    and
    evidence of both cellular and humoral immune deficiency
    and
    one or more categories in Class P-2ª
    or
Symptoms meeting CDC case definition for AIDS

Older children with perinatal infection and children with HIV infection acquired through other modes of transmission

Virus in blood or tissues
    or
HIV antibody
    or
Symptoms meeting CDC case definition of AIDS

Source: Centers for Disease Control, "Classification System for Human Immunodeficiency Virus (HIV) Infection in Children under 13 Years of Age," *Morbidity and Mortality Weekly Report*, 36 (1987), 225–230, 235.
   a. See Table 3.5 for definition of Class P-2.

merase chain reaction (PCR) test. The PCR test makes it possible to identify minute amounts of viral DNA in infected white blood cells (see Appendix C). Studies are under way to determine whether the test will be a reliable method for early diagnosis of HIV infection in young babies.

HIV embryopathy. The diagnostic problems described above have led some researchers to look for other clues that might help identify children infected with HIV. In July 1986, Robert Marion and his coworkers at the Albert Einstein College of Medicine described a constellation of 10 distinctive physical characteristics that appeared to be more common in infants and children with AIDS or ARC than in other children.[33] The characteristics included growth failure, microcephaly (head circumference less than the third percentile for chronological age), wide-set eyes, prominent box-like appearance of the forehead, a flat nasal bridge, and a well-formed philtrum (the triangular, ridged space directly below the nose). Marion and his associates concluded that these features constituted a new syndrome, HIV embryopathy, caused by infection with HIV early in fetal life. The structural abnormalities tend to be most severe, they said, in patients who develop recurrent infections within the first 6 months of life.

The concept of HIV embryopathy is extremely controversial. Researchers who disagree with Marion's findings suggest that the constellation of features could result from intrauterine exposure to toxic substances, such as alcohol and drugs, rather than from the virus. Some of the features are similar to those associated with fetal alcohol syndrome.

Physicians from New York Medical College, who support the existence of a congenital AIDS-related syndrome but describe it somewhat differently, caution that descriptions of HIV embryopathy must take into account natural variations in bone structure and facial characteristics among different ethnic and racial groups.[34] Further studies will be required to determine the ultimate value of physical appearance as a predictor of HIV infection in infants. Confirmation of the existence of HIV embryopathy would suggest that any future therapy

designed to prevent HIV infection of the fetus might have to
be started very early in pregnancy.

Categories of HIV Infection in Children

The original CDC case definition of pediatric AIDS, like
the early case definition of AIDS in adults, focused exclusively
on some of the most severe consequences of HIV infection.
Physicians in areas with large numbers of affected children
quickly reported that more than half of their patients, including some who were very ill, failed to meet the criteria
established by the CDC. Subsequent revisions have made the
AIDS definition more comprehensive, but the emphasis on
severe consequences has not changed.

In 1987, public health officials at the CDC, acknowledging
the need for a framework that included the entire spectrum of
HIV-related disorders in children, published the classification
system summarized in Table 3.5. Class P-0 includes children

Table 3.5. Summary of the classification system of HIV infection in
children under age 13

Class P-0	Indeterminate infection
Class P-1	Asymptomatic infection
Subclass A	Normal immune function
Subclass B	Abnormal immune function
Subclass C	Immune function not tested
Class P-2	Symptomatic infection
Subclass A	Nonspecific findings
Subclass B	Progressive neurologic disease
Subclass C	Lymphoid interstitial pneumonitis
Subclass D	Secondary infectious diseases
Subclass E	Secondary cancers
Category E-1	Specified secondary cancers listed in CDC surveillance definition for AIDS
Category E-2	Other cancers possibly secondary to HIV infection
Subclass F	Other diseases possibly due to HIV infection

Source: Centers for Disease Control, "Classification System for Human Immunodeficiency Virus (HIV) Infection in Children under 13 Years of Age," *Morbidity and
Mortality Weekly Report,* 36 (1987), 225–230, 235.

family members whose immune systems are not normal. The inactivated polio vaccine offers a safe alternative.

Table 3.6 summarizes recommendations for routine immunization of HIV-infected children; the recommendations also apply to HIV-infected adolescents and adults.

Secondary cancers. AIDS-related cancers, such as Kaposi's sarcoma and B-cell lymphoma, occur very rarely in children. Other tumors associated with HIV infection may be identified as experience with the virus increases.

Other diseases. Laboratory tests and other diagnostic procedures indicate that the direct effects of HIV infection go well beyond suppression of the immune system and destruction of the nervous system. Many children with symptomatic HIV infection have anemia, thrombocytopenia (lack of blood platelets), or both. This fact suggests that the virus may interfere

Table 3.6. Recommendations for routine immunization of HIV-infected children, United States, 1988

| Vaccine | HIV infection | |
	Known asymptomatic	Symptomatic
DTP	yes	yes
OPV	no	no
IPV	yes	yes
MMR	yes	yes[a]
HbCV	yes	yes
Pneumococcal	no	yes
Influenza	no	yes

Source: U.S. Public Health Service, Immunization Practices Advisory Committee, "Immunization of Children Infected with Human Immunodeficiency Virus—Supplementary ACIP Statement," *Morbidity and Mortality Weekly Report,* 37 (1988), 181–183.

Note: DTP = diphtheria and tetanus toxoids and pertussis vaccine. OPV = oral, attenuated poliovirus vaccine; contains poliovirus types 1, 2, and 3. IPV = inactivated poliovirus vaccine; contains poliovirus types 1, 2, and 3. MMR = live measles, mumps, and rubella viruses in a combined vaccine. HbCV = *Haemophilus influenzae* type b conjugate vaccine.

a. Should be considered.

with the blood-forming system (see Chapter 5). Echocardiography, a noninvasive technique for acoustic imaging of the heart, reveals specific cardiac abnormalities in the majority of affected children. In addition, many have abnormal results on standard tests of liver and kidney function. Skin rashes and abnormal reactions to drugs also occur frequently in HIV-infected children.

The relative importance of these different manifestations of HIV infection remains unclear. The one certainty is that pediatricians must be extremely vigilant to manage the multiple problems associated with this devastating and complex disease.

Conclusion

Scientists have made major progress in understanding the consequences of HIV infection, but many questions remain. Studies of large groups of people with HIV infection have shown that patients with lymphadenopathy are no more likely to progress to AIDS than those without lymphadenopathy. Factors more likely to be associated with a depressed immune system in infected patients include thrush, anemia, fever, and depletion of blood neutrophils. The new CDC classification systems for adults and children with HIV infection will help improve communication about the full range of HIV-related problems.

Pediatric AIDS is more difficult to diagnose than adult AIDS, in part because of possibile confusion with inherited defects of the immune system. Also, infants often lack the familiar clinical and laboratory signs of HIV infection. New diagnostic tests that detect viral DNA or viral proteins instead of HIV antibodies should make it easier to identify HIV-infected infants shortly after birth. Early diagnosis is essential to provide these extremely vulnerable children with appropriate care.

Recent evidence indicates that HIV may directly affect the heart, liver, and kidneys, as well as the immune system and the brain. One of the principal goals of future research will be to determine how the virus interacts with tissues throughout the body.

The management of diseases caused by HIV infection is at a crossroads. Scientists have developed better specific therapies for some of the most common AIDS-related disorders, such as *P. carinii* pneumonia and cytomegalovirus infection, but their effects on long-term survival appear limited. The use of multiple drugs may be a problem in itself. Physicians may have difficulty pinpointing a serious adverse reaction to one drug when the patient is taking several powerful medications at the same time.

The new antiviral drugs described in Chapter 6 could change the course of HIV infection and alleviate many of the treatment problems discussed above. Large clinical trials of drugs during the next several years will provide a better indication of the future scope of HIV-related disease.

4

Discovery of
the Virus

The battle against HIV infection illustrates both the power and the limitations of recent advances in molecular biology, virology, and recombinant DNA technology. Less than five years after the disease first attracted attention, researchers had identified the virus that causes it, deciphered its genetic code, and developed a versatile and inexpensive screening test. But these monumental achievements have not produced a solution to the AIDS problem. In fact, each new piece of information has reinforced early impressions that the virus responsible for AIDS represents one of the most complex challenges ever faced by mankind.

This chapter describes the search for and the discovery of the virus now called HIV-1. It also examines the relationship of HIV-1 to other disease-producing microorganisms, including HIV-2 and the monkey virus, SIV.

Searching for a Cause

When the first cases of *Pneumocystis carinii* pneumonia and Kaposi's sarcoma were reported in young, previously healthy homosexual men in the spring of 1981, speculation began immediately about possible causes. What had changed these men from active members of the community to seriously ill invalids in just a few months?

Physicians soon focused on the immune systems of the early AIDS patients. In December 1981 the *New England Journal of Medicine* carried three articles describing immunologic evaluations of 19 male homosexual patients with *P. carinii* pneumonia or an unusually persistent herpes virus infection. All the men had abnormally low numbers of T lymphocytes, white blood cells that play a key role in protecting the body against disease. Subsequent studies showed that one particular subset of T lymphocytes, consisting of cells carrying a T4 (CD4) surface marker, was dramatically reduced in AIDS.

As the epidemic spread through major urban homosexual communities in the United States, theories about the cause of the syndrome multiplied. The possibility of an unknown infectious agent was considered, but early laboratory studies failed to identify a suspect. The life-styles of individual patients were compared with those of healthy homosexuals to highlight any differences that might explain susceptibility to the disease.

Interviews with patients indicated that they tended to be more sexually active than matched populations of healthy homosexuals. Researchers speculated that repeated infections acquired during hundreds of sexual encounters might have overwhelmed the T lymphocytes in these patients, leaving them unable to fight disease. Another theory rested on the immunosuppressive properties of human semen, which could have entered the bloodstream through small tears in the rectum during anal intercourse.

Illicit drug use also was viewed as a potential cause. In February 1982 James Goedert and his colleagues at the National Institutes of Health and the Uniformed Services University of the Health Sciences described immunologic defects associated with the use of amyl nitrite, a drug used by some homosexuals as a sexual stimulant. They speculated that nitrites might be immunosuppressive in the presence of repeated viral infections (laboratory studies later demonstrated that nitrites are not immunosuppressive).

The focus on life-styles continued during the first quarter of 1982, when the disease began appearing in heterosexual men and women who were intravenous drug abusers. This population appeared to have many of the same risk factors as promiscuous homosexuals. The practice of sharing needles and syringes caused a high incidence of multiple infections, and abuse of some illegal drugs had been associated with immunosuppression.

Epidemiologists at the Centers for Disease Control continued to maintain close surveillance of new cases. They documented clusters of disease both in homosexual men and among IV drug abusers. These clusters were analogous to those produced by the spread of hepatitis B virus infection in high-risk populations. Their presence supported the theory that AIDS was transmitted by an infectious agent.

This theory achieved even greater prominence in July 1982, when 3 cases of AIDS were reported in hemophiliacs who had been treated with clotting-factor concentrates to prevent bleeding. Further evidence for the existence of a specific agent transmitted by both sexual contact and blood products accumulated in late 1982 and early 1983.

Laboratories in the United States and in Europe rallied to the search for the AIDS agent. Some investigators believed that the syndrome might represent a new manifestation of a known virus; both cytomegalovirus and Epstein-Barr virus had been shown to suppress the immune system, but neither seemed capable of causing the kind of devastation associated with AIDS. Others suspected that the disease might be caused by a concurrent infection with 2 or more microorganisms. Finally, research teams began searching for an entirely new viral pathogen.

The urgency of the problem and the growth of public concern over it were reflected in frequent newspaper headlines about AIDS. Existing therapies could not stop the progression of the disease, and the number of reported cases was increasing geometrically.

Focusing on the Retroviruses

The idea that a retrovirus might be involved in AIDS crystallized in early 1982 as a result of discussions between Robert C. Gallo of the National Cancer Institute (NCI) and

Myron Essex of the Harvard School of Public Health. The first human retrovirus had been isolated only four years earlier by Gallo and his colleagues in the NCI Laboratory of Tumor Cell Biology.

The basic retrovirus consists of two identical strands of genetic material packaged in a core of viral proteins (see Figure 4.1). The core is surrounded by a protective coat called the envelope, which is derived from the membrane of the previous host cell but modified with glycoproteins (complexes of sugar and protein molecules) contributed by the virus. The molecule carrying the genetic information in a retrovirus is RNA (ribonucleic acid).

In living cells, RNA functions as a messenger between the cell nucleus, which contains the more familiar genetic material DNA, and the rest of the cell. When a new protein is needed

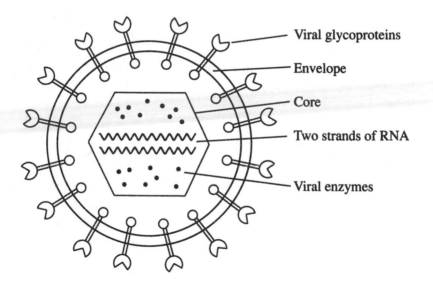

FIGURE 4.1. Schematic diagram of a retrovirus. Two identical strands of RNA and viral enzymes (reverse transcriptase, integrase, and protease) are packaged in a core of viral proteins. The core is surrounded by the envelope, a protective structure derived in part from the membrane of the previous host cell. The envelope is studded with viral glycoproteins.

for a particular function or structure, the portion of the DNA molecule coding for that protein is transcribed into RNA. This RNA molecule then migrates out of the nucleus into the cytoplasm, where it directs the manufacture of the new protein.

A retrovirus reverses this process. Each viral particle carries the enzyme reverse transcriptase, which copies the single-stranded viral RNA into double-stranded DNA (see Figure 4.2). The viral DNA migrates into the cell nucleus and then inserts itself into the host cell DNA. The integrated viral DNA is called a provirus. When the host cell divides, a copy of the provirus is transmitted to each daughter cell. In addition, the viral DNA can coopt the machinery of its host to produce large quantities of viral RNA, some of which is packaged into new viral particles and released by budding through the cell membrane (see Figure 4.3).

The American pathologist Francis Peyton Rous isolated one of the first known retroviruses in 1911. He identified it as the cause of a particular type of cancer, known as a sarcoma, in chickens. Rous sarcoma virus is a member of the subfamily Oncovirinae. Other members of this subfamily cause leukemias and lymphomas in cats, mice, and cows. Before the appearance of AIDS, most research on retroviruses focused on the oncoviruses. There was less emphasis on a second subfamily, Lentivirinae. The only known lentiviruses caused conditions such as encephalitis, anemia, pneumonia, and arthritis in sheep, goats, and horses.

The first human retrovirus, isolated by Gallo and colleagues in 1978, was from the cells of an American man with T-cell leukemia. In published reports of the finding in 1980, Gallo and his coworkers labeled this retrovirus "human T-cell leukemia/lymphoma virus" (HTLV). Additional studies demonstrated that the T4 helper cell was the principal target of this new virus.

Several years later, Japanese and American scientists demonstrated that HTLV was the cause of adult T-cell leukemia syndrome, a disease endemic in certain parts of southwestern Japan. Further studies uncovered many other endemic

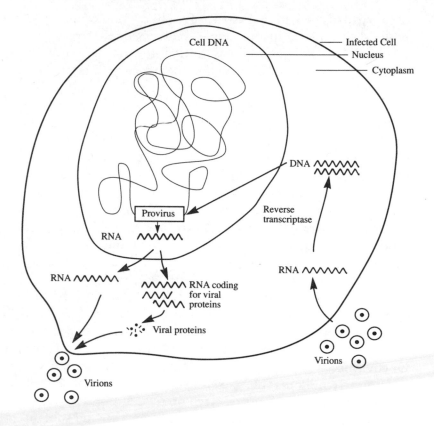

FIGURE 4.2. During the life cycle of a retrovirus, intact viral particles (virions) are taken into the cell via a specific cellular receptor. After uncoating, the single-stranded RNA is reverse transcribed into double-stranded DNA. The DNA enters the cell nucleus, where it integrates itself into the host cell genome. The integrated viral DNA is called a provirus. In some cases the provirus remains dormant or unexpressed. In other cases it is transcribed into viral RNA, leading to the production of viral proteins and the formation of new viral particles. These progeny virions are released by budding from the cell membrane.

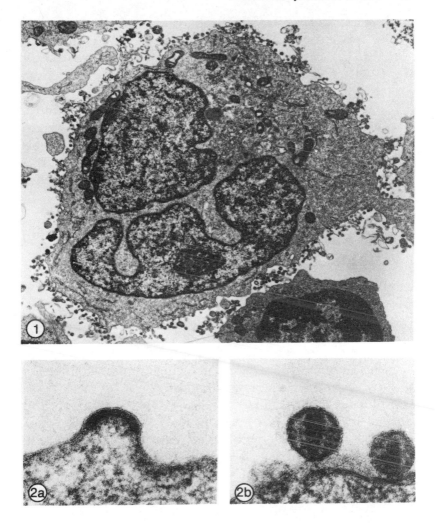

FIGURE 4.3. Electromicrographs of (1) HIV-infected cell (× 15,000) and (2a, b) budding of virus from the cell membrane (× 90,000). Courtesy of Syed Zaki Salahuddin, National Cancer Institute.

areas, including Caribbean islands, the southeastern United States, areas in South America and in southern Italy, and many parts of Africa. Meanwhile, a second but much rarer HTLV (HTLV-II) was isolated from the cells of another American leukemia patient.

The discovery of a virus very similar to HTLV-I—simian T-lymphotropic virus type I (STLV-I)—in African green monkeys and several other primate species provided a possible clue to the ancestry of the human virus. Gallo speculated that HTLV-I originated in Africa, where it infected humans as well as many species of Old World primates.[1]

Isolating the AIDS Virus

Several characteristics of known human and animal retrovirus infections supported the hypothesis that a retrovirus could cause AIDS:

- Some animal retroviruses were known to cause an AIDS-like disease as well as cancer. (The feline leukemia virus actually kills many more cats by inducing immune suppression than by causing leukemia or lymphoma.)
- Like HTLV-I and HTLV-II, the AIDS agent seemed to disrupt the function of T4 cells.
- The suspected modes of transmission of AIDS—through blood products and sexual contact—appeared identical with those implicated in the transmission of HTLV-I. (Leukemias caused by HTLV-I infection are rare in the United States; there is no evidence that other forms of leukemia are transmitted through sexual contact or transfusions.)[2]
- Patients with adult T-cell leukemia also were subject to numerous opportunistic infections, and T cells infected with HTLV-I and HTLV-II showed suppressed immune activity in the laboratory.

Even with this knowledge, efforts to isolate an AIDS agent proved to be extremely frustrating. Scientists could detect transient reverse transcriptase activity in cultured T cells from patients with AIDS or related conditions, but the results were not reproducible. The major problem was that they could not maintain the virus or the T cells in culture. Only later did the scientists learn that the virus was killing the cells before they could complete their analyses.

The first isolation of the virus later shown to be the cause of AIDS was reported in May 1983 by Luc Montagnier, head of the Viral Oncology Unit of the Institut Pasteur in Paris, and his colleagues.[3] They named the virus lymphadenopathy-associated virus (LAV) because they had isolated it from one of the swollen lymph nodes of a patient with lymphadenopathy syndrome (these patients appeared to be at high risk of developing AIDS). Over the next few months, similar retroviruses were isolated from the blood of several AIDS patients, but the researchers continued to have problems with virus propagation.

In May 1984 Mikulas Popovic and his coworkers in Gallo's laboratory reported that they had identified a line of cancerous T cells that had 2 important characteristics: (1) susceptibility to infection with the new virus and (2) the ability to resist the killing effects that had destroyed other infected T-cell cultures.[4] In fact cultures of this cell line could be adapted to produce large quantities of the virus for research and for the development of a much-needed screening test.

The NCI researchers reported that they had isolated the new virus, which they designated HTLV-III, from 48 patients. The meaning of HTLV was changed from "human T-cell leukemia/lymphoma virus" to "human T-cell lymphotropic virus" to reflect the fact that all known human retroviruses shared an attraction to T lymphocytes.[5]

Another virus isolate was described in August 1984 by Jay Levy and his coworkers from the University of California at San Francisco.[6] They named their virus AIDS-associated retrovirus, or ARV.

Molecular analysis of isolates from many different AIDS patients (researchers determined the identity and position of each nucleotide or chemical building block in the viral RNA genome) demonstrated that all were variants of the same virus.

However, much additional work was required to prove that the virus actually caused AIDS and that it was not simply another opportunistic infection attacking a host that was defenseless for some other reason. From mid-1983 to late 1984, researchers on both sides of the Atlantic searched for evidence of infection with the newly discovered virus in the blood of hundreds of healthy volunteers from low-risk groups, genetically immunodeficient patients, healthy individuals from high-risk groups, patients with lymphadenopathy syndrome (persistent swollen glands), and AIDS patients. These studies consistently demonstrated that the acquisition and transmission of the new virus was correlated with AIDS or AIDS-related conditions.

Blood recipients who developed AIDS and their high-risk donors provided an extremely important piece of the puzzle. The detailed records kept by blood banks allowed the researchers to trace the transmission of the disease from one individual to another. Identical virus isolates were obtained from blood recipients with AIDS (who had no other source of infection) and from the high-risk donors who gave the blood.

Competition and Controversy

Three major factors contributed to the rapid pace of efforts to find the cause of AIDS. The first was the sense of urgency created by the epidemic itself—until the cause had been established, researchers could not begin to assess the ultimate scope of the AIDS problem or help those already affected by the disease. The second was the wealth of new techniques in cell biology, virology, and molecular genetics. Without the cell culture techniques and assays for viral proteins developed in the 1970s, it might have taken years longer to identify the new virus. The third factor was intense competition among the research groups working on the problem.

Competition is an integral part of modern science; researchers in every field compete for limited resources and for recognition from their colleagues and the world at large. Unfortunately, the competition to discover the cause of AIDS was so heated that, for a time, it almost overshadowed the major accomplishments of the groups involved. A bitter rivalry between American and French researchers led to a complicated legal dispute and lingering confusion over the correct nomenclature for the AIDS virus.

The legal dispute focused on patent rights for a test to screen blood for antibodies to the AIDS virus. (Viral proteins constitute an integral part of such tests; thus isolation of the AIDS virus was a prerequisite for the patent application.) In December 1983 the Institut Pasteur applied for a U.S. patent for an antibody test-kit based on the work of Montagnier and his coworkers. Five months later the U.S. Department of Health and Human Services (HHS) filed a separate patent application for an assay developed by Gallo and his team. The HHS patent was granted on May 28, 1985; no action was taken on the Institut Pasteur's application.

The Institut Pasteur immediately challenged the HHS patent and, in a separate action, filed suit against the U.S. government for breach of contract. The institute claimed that U.S. scientists had used materials obtained from the French researchers (with the stipulation that they be used only for research purposes) to develop their assay. This claim was strongly denied by Gallo.

The French wanted a share of the millions of dollars in patent royalties generated by use of the AIDS antibody test, but the principal issue underlying the dispute was who should receive recognition for discovering the cause of AIDS. That issue was resolved in the spring of 1987 with the publication of "The Chronology of AIDS Research" (see Appendix F). With the help of Jonas Salk, famous for his development of a polio vaccine, Gallo and Montagnier constructed a chronology of "the main contributions of the two central parties and of some other groups to the determination of the causative agent of AIDS."[7] The chronology became part of a negotiated legal settlement in which Gallo and Montagnier, along with their respective collaborators, were recognized as joint inventors o the AIDS antibody test. HHS and the Institut Pasteur agree to share ownership of the patent and to contribute 80 perce of their royalties (estimated at $4 million each per year) to a new, international AIDS research foundation. Twenty-five percent of the foundation's funds were earmarked for AIDS education and public health programs in developing countries, and the remainder was allocated for AIDS research and studies on other human retroviruses.

Renaming the Virus

One of the consequences of the 3-year conflict over the discovery of the AIDS virus was confusion over the new virus's name. Montagnier and his collaborators named the first AIDS-related virus they isolated LAV, or lymphadenopathy-associated virus. A second isolate identified by the same group was called immunodeficiency-associated virus, or IDAV. Gallo's group called the virus responsible for AIDS HTLV-III, and Levy and his coworkers called it ARV (AIDS-associated retrovirus). Scientific journals in the United States and Europe adopted one of two compound names, HTLV-III/LAV or LAV/HTLV-III.

The compound names afforded recognition to the two principal groups involved in the discovery of the AIDS virus, but they were unwieldy, and they failed to address an issue even more important than who had discovered the virus. This issue was how the new virus related to other known human and animal retroviruses. Early studies showed that although the new human retrovirus resembled HTLV-I and HTLV-II in its preference for T cells, it acted on those cells in a very different way: HTLV-I and HTLV-II caused uncontrolled proliferation of the T cells, whereas the AIDS virus killed them.

The two human T-cell leukemia viruses share many features with the animal oncoviruses (such as bovine leukemia virus), but the structure and function of the AIDS virus are more akin to those of the lentiviruses (such as the visna virus in sheep and the equine infectious anemia virus in horses). The importance of this relationship is that knowledge about the animal lentiviruses may provide clues about disease patterns and preventive approaches to AIDS.

Several events in late 1985 and early 1986 increased the urgency of resolving the name issue. First, researchers identified a monkey virus that appeared very similar to the human AIDS virus. Evidence of the monkey virus was found in both captive macaque monkeys and wild African green monkeys; it was associated with immunodeficiency and lymphomas in the former species but did not appear to cause disease in the latter. Researchers named the virus STLV-III (simian T-lymphotropic virus type III). Several months later, separate research teams led by Essex and Montagnier announced that they had discovered two new human retroviruses in people in West Africa (an area that was relatively free of the original AIDS virus). The Essex group called their virus HTLV-IV, while Montagnier and his coworkers called theirs LAV-2. Subsequent studies showed that the populations studied by Essex and Montagnier were infected with variants of the same virus and that the new virus was more closely related to the monkey virus than to the original AIDS virus in human beings.[8]

Finally, in May 1986 a subcommittee of the International Committee on the Taxonomy of Viruses, chaired by Harold Varmus of the University of California at San Francisco, proposed a new system for naming all AIDS retroviruses in humans and subhuman primates. The human viruses were to be called human immunodeficiency viruses (HIVs). The monkey virus was renamed simian immunodeficiency virus, or SIV. The committee stressed that one of its goals was to pick a name for the AIDS virus that was "sufficiently distinct from the names of other retroviruses to imply an independent virus species."[9]

Table 4.1 shows the new names for the viruses in relation to the old ones. HIV-1 is used to refer to all isolates of HTLV-III, LAV, and ARV. HIV-2 is the official designation for LAV-2 and all related isolates.

The Origin of AIDS

The discovery of HIV-2 has provided a partial answer to a fundamental question raised by the AIDS epidemic: how

Table 4.1.   Appropriate names for the immunodeficiency viruses

Appropriate name	Names used in early descriptions
Human	
Human immunodeficiency virus type 1 (HIV-1)	LAV, HTLV-III, IDAV, ARV, LAV/HTLV-III, HTLV-III/LAV,
Human immunodeficiency virus type 2 (HIV-2)	LAV-2, HTLV-IV[a]
Monkey	
Simian immunodeficiency virus (SIV)	STLV-III

Note: LAV = lymphadenopathy-associated virus; HTLV = human T-cell lymphotropic virus; IDAV = immunodeficiency-associated virus; ARV = AIDS-associated retrovirus; STLV = simian T-lymphotropic virus.

a. The virus isolates originally labeled HTLV-IV have been shown to be identical to an early isolate of SIV (STLV-III$_{mac-251}$). See Chapter 4, note 8.

could AIDS have appeared without warning and then spread so rapidly from one part of the world to another?

Following the isolation of the first monkey immunodeficiency virus, scientists speculated that human AIDS might have resulted from the very recent introduction of a monkey virus into the human population. This speculation seemed consistent with Gallo's theory about the relationship between the human and monkey leukemia viruses (HTLV-I and STLV-I). In addition, biologists had numerous examples of infectious agents that appeared relatively benign in their natural hosts but became highly virulent when introduced into a new species.

When the first member of the HIV-2 group was isolated, it was hailed as a possible missing link between the monkey virus and the original AIDS virus. This concept was reinforced by preliminary data from the Essex laboratory suggesting that HIV-2 might not cause disease in human beings. (The pathogenicity of HIV-2 is discussed further below.) The progression from a benign infectious agent in African green monkeys to a virulent killer in humans seemed a relatively straightforward explanation.

Comprehensive analyses of the genetic sequences of HIV-1, HIV-2, and SIV have produced a very different picture. In 1987 Mireille Guyader and his coworkers from the Institut Pasteur showed that the level of sequence similarity between HIV-1 and HIV-2 (determined by matching the sequence of nucleotide building blocks in the genome of one virus to the sequence of nucleotide building blocks in the other) was well below 50 percent. The researchers suggested that such diversity was not consistent with the speculation that the 2 viruses had a common ancestor just prior to the current AIDS epidemic.

A new computer study of the HIV family tree has reinforced this view. It places the time of divergence between HIV-1 and HIV-2 at roughly 40 to 80 years ago.[11] The same study suggests that the monkey virus could not have been the common ancestor—SIV appears to be an offshoot of the HIV-2 branch of the tree. (Temple Smith of Harvard and the Dana-Farber Cancer Institute in Boston explains that conclusions about the HIV family tree are based on the assumption that SIV has evolved at approximately the same rate as HIV-1 and HIV-2.)

If HIV-1 has existed for decades, why didn't the AIDS epidemic occur sooner? Guyader and his coworkers propose that, until recently, infection with HIV-1 may have been limited to small, relatively isolated populations in rural Africa. The social mores of those populations may not have been conducive to rapid spread of the virus. The few cases of AIDS that did develop could have escaped detection against the backdrop of multiple life threatening infections common in the region.

The major factor responsible for changing this pattern appears to have been urbanization. African cities grew dramatically during and after World War II. As in other parts of the world, urbanization was accompanied by social changes that affected the lives of millions of people. The disruption of families and the anonymity afforded by an urban environment increased the likelihood of behavior that contributes to the spread of sexually transmitted diseases (multiple sexual partners and prostitution). Over time, the prevalence of HIV-1 infection increased sufficiently to make AIDS visible as a new clinical entity in central Africa and elsewhere.

The apparent AIDS-related death of a teenager in St. Louis in 1969 indicates that HIV-1 may have entered the United States several times before the current epidemic. In each case, however, the virus failed to gain a foothold in a large, sexually active population. When the lone carrier died, the chain of infection was broken.

Multiple HIVs

The factors that contributed to the HIV-1 epidemic in central Africa probably also led to the increased incidence of HIV-2 infection in West Africa. Scientists expect to find more members of the HIV group as they investigate AIDS cases around the world. They also expect to encounter new SIVs.

They do not expect, however, that any of these viruses will cause a "new" epidemic. Preliminary evidence indicates that all the viruses are transmitted in the same manner. If this is true, measures taken to reduce the spread of HIV-1, such as using condoms and limiting the number of sexual partners, will also reduce the spread of HIV-2 and other HIVs. A CDC study involving blood samples from more than 20,000 people has not yet found any evidence of HIV-2 infection acquired in the United States.[12]

A major difficulty posed by the presence of mutiple HIVs is how to develop appropriate diagnostic tools. Public health workers need 2 types of tests to reduce the spread of HIV infections: (1) a rapid screening test to determine whether an individual—especially a prospective blood or tissue donor—has been exposed to any of the HIVs, and (2) a more specific diagnostic test to determine which virus is involved in a particular infection. An ELISA (enzyme-linked immunosorbent assay) test using HIV-1 proteins will not reliably detect the presence of antibodies to HIV-2 (see Appendix C). Efforts are under way to develop tests that will meet both types of testing needs.

The importance of determining which virus is responsible for disease in a specific patient or population is underscored by the controversy over HIV-2. The 2 research teams credited with identifying HIV-2 initially expressed very different opinions about whether or not it caused AIDS. The first cases of HIV-2 infection described by Essex and his coworkers all occurred in healthy Sengalese people. In contrast, Montagnier and his collaborators first detected HIV-2 in 2 AIDS patients. Independent follow-up studies by each of the 2 groups led Essex to the conclusion that HIV-2 did not cause disease, and confirmed Montagnier's view that it did. Montagnier and his collaborators suggested that the long incubation period associated with HIV infections might be responsible for the apparent well-being of the subjects in the Essex study. Perhaps HIV-2 had not been in the study area long enough to cause more than a few isolated cases of disease. For his part, Essex questioned the strength of epidemiologic evidence presented by Montagnier and his colleagues to support the link between HIV-2 and AIDS.

Further analysis of the data has produced a tentative compromise between the two groups: the consensus is that HIV-2 clearly causes AIDS but may have a longer incubation period than HIV-1. It is possible that many of those infected with HIV-2 will remain healthy carriers. Epidemiologists caution, however, that more information is needed to make any definite conclusions about the disease-producing capabilities of HIV-2. Long-term studies of healthy carriers of the virus have begun in several West African countries.

Efforts to sort out the natural histories of the different HIV infections will play a crucial role in international public health planning over the next decade. Areas affected by the more aggressive human retroviruses, such as HIV-1, will have to plan differently from areas in which the prevalent human retrovirus is less likely to cause disease. One very important question is what will happen in populations infected with more than one human immunodeficiency virus. HIV-1 has begun spreading into certain parts of West Africa. Researchers do not yet know whether people infected with HIV-2 will be more or less susceptible to HIV-1 infection and disease than those who have never been exposed to a virus in the HIV group.

Comparative studies of the different HIVs and SIVs may lead to important new strategies for the prevention and treatment of HIV infection. Researchers are particularly interested in 2 features of the immunodeficiency viruses: the structure that binds to receptors on host target cells and the regulatory proteins that control the pace of viral replication (see Chapter 5). Scientists also are exploring the different ways in which HIVs and SIVs interact with the host immune system. For example, several laboratories are trying to determine why the prototype SIV causes immunodeficiency in macaques but not in African green monkeys. If researchers could identify an immune response that protected the African green monkey, they might be able to induce a similar response in human beings.

Conclusion

Identification of HIV-1 as the principal cause of AIDS would not have been possible without the molecular biology techniques developed over the past 20 years. Laboratory analysis of the structure and function of this virus already has produced major dividends, including the development of a rapid screening test to limit the spread of infection by way of blood products and to identify those people at greatest risk of disease.

The discovery of additional members of the HIV group has provided a new perspective on the development of the current HIV epidemic. Clearly, the human immunodeficiency viruses have coexisted with human beings for many years. Until recently, however, infections probably were confined to small, isolated communities. The few cases of AIDS that occurred could have gone unnoticed, because patients succumbed to the same infectious agents afflicting others in the population. Many scientists believe that the trend toward urbanization in certain parts of Africa was a major factor responsible for changing this pattern.

HIV-1 may have entered the United States several times before the current epidemic but failed to cause widespread disease. During the 1970s, changing social attitudes led to an increase in the number of people practicing high-risk sexual behavior and IV drug abuse. Such people were particularly vulnerable when the virus reappeared.

Expansion of the HIV family tree has complicated AIDS diagnosis and public health planning, but it also may have a positive impact. Sections of the viral genome that control major biological functions, such as binding to target cells, are more likely to be conserved among the different viruses than other portions of the genome. Thus, comparisons of the genetic sequences of the different viruses may help researchers pinpoint targets for more effective antiviral therapies.

5

HIV and Its Effects on the Body

Confirmation of the role of HIV in the development of AIDS and AIDS-related conditions opened exciting new avenues of research. Experiments were begun to decipher the virus's genetic message and to determine the function of individual viral proteins. Each new discovery has given scientists a better understanding of the kinds of approaches needed to help people infected with HIV and to limit the spread of disease.

To counteract the effects of HIV, scientists also must have information about the types of cells infected by the virus. Initial research has focused primarily on the immune system. Quantitative and qualitative defects in several different populations of immune cells contribute to the AIDS patient's susceptibility to a wide range of infections.

The detection of HIV in cells of the central nervous system offers a partial explanation for the dementia and other neurological problems often associated with AIDS. Scientists still have many questions, however, about the manner in which HIV-related brain disease occurs. Some of these questions are addressed below. The direct infection of nerve cells does not appear to play an important role in the disease process.

Other cells found to be infected with HIV include Langerhans cells in the skin, endothelial cells (cells that line blood vessels), epithelial cells in the small intestine and rectum, cervical cells, cells in the retina, and blood-forming cells in the bone marrow.

The Structure of the Virus

The first pictures of HIV did not reveal any striking differences between the virus and other known retroviruses. The electronmicrographs showed a dense core surrounded by a spherical envelope. As expected, the core was found to contain RNA and the proteins needed for replication of the virus. Scientists were surprised, therefore, when they began studying the virus's full complement of genetic information, its genome. The HIV genome was much more complex than the genome of any previously characterized retrovirus.

Figure 5.1 shows the basic format of a simple retrovirus genome. It consists of 3 structural genes, *gag*, *pol*, and *env*, located between shorter segments called long terminal repeats (LTRs). *Gag* codes for the components of the protein core, *pol* codes for the viral enzymes involved in replication (reverse transcriptase, a protease, and integrase), and *env* codes for the envelope proteins. (The envelope of a retrovirus is derived from the membrane of the host cell that produced the virus, the virus modifies the cell's membrane by inserting the viral envelope proteins.) Adjacent to or within the LTRs are the regulatory signals required for reverse transcription (copying the viral RNA into DNA), insertion of viral DNA into the host cell genome, expression of the virus (the process by which viral genes are transcribed into RNA and then translated into protein), and packaging of the viral RNA.

The HIV genome contains the *gag*, *pol*, and *env* genes, but it also has other sequences that do not correspond to anything

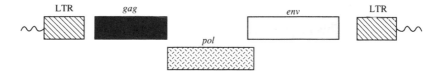

FIGURE 5.1. The basic retroviral genome in the form of the DNA provirus. It consists of the structural genes *gag*, *pol*, and *env* located between sequences called long terminal repeats (LTRs).

genome is reverse transcribed into DNA and then integrated into the host cell genome (see Chapter 4).

A similar mechanism may explain the spread of virus from one cell to another in the absence of free virus. Cells infected with HIV carry envelope proteins lodged in their membrane. These cell-bound proteins can bind to CD4 receptors on uninfected cells. Fusion of the two cell membranes allows partially formed viral particles to move from the infected cell to the uninfected cell. Thus, HIV theoretically could spread through the body without leaving host cells.

Studies of viral mutants lacking small portions of the envelope gene have allowed researchers to identify the segments of gp120 and gp41 that participate in the binding and fusion reactions. These segments of the virus could provide important targets for future vaccines or therapeutic drugs.

Cell death.   HIV infects a variety of cell types, but it preferentially kills the T4 lymphocyte. Some researchers have suggested that T4 cells are more vulnerable to HIV-induced cell death than other cells because they have a higher concentration of CD4 receptors. They speculate that cell death occurs when viral envelope proteins lodged in the membrane of an infected cell bind to CD4 receptors embedded in the same membrane. Multiple self-fusion reactions could destabilize the cell membrane and kill the cell.

Studies of blood samples from people infected with HIV indicate that only about 1 in 100,000 peripheral blood lymphocytes is actively producing virus at any one time, although others may be carrying the viral genome in a latent form. Anthony Fauci, director of NIAID, suggests that if the few T4 lymphocytes with productive infections were the only T4 cells dying, the body probably would be able to replace them without difficulty.[1] Yet AIDS patients and others with HIV-related diseases have dramatic T-cell deficiencies.

One explanation for the massive depletion of T4 cells involves the cell-to-cell fusion reaction described above. In the laboratory, a single infected cell with a high concentration of viral envelope proteins on its surface can bind to hundreds of uninfected T4 cells. The fused cells form giant, multinucleated structures called syncytia, which are extremely unstable and die within a day. One cell with a productive viral infection can cause the deaths of up to 500 normal cells. The fact that syncytia are rarely seen in AIDS patients, however, suggests that other mechanisms probably cause cell death in vivo. For example, cell death might be related to the presence of free-floating viral envelope proteins in the bloodstream. These could bind to uninfected T4 cells, leading to their elimination by the immune system. Other autoimmune mechanisms also may play a role in T-cell depletion; researchers from the Dana-Farber Cancer Institute and New England Medical Center in Boston recently reported that about 10 percent of HIV-infected people produce antibodies against the CD4 receptors on their own cells.[2] The clinical implications of this finding require further study.

In May 1988, Regine Leonard of the Pierre and Marie Curie University in Paris and her coworkers presented evidence that both individual T4 cells and giant syncytia die as a direct result of virus production. They suggest that cell death occurs when intense budding of the virus through the cell membrane results in the formation of tiny holes. The holes disrupt the integrity of the membrane and eventually lead to cell death.[3]

HIV infection also may directly or indirectly suppress the production of new T4 cells. Direct suppression would occur if HIV damaged T4 precursor cells in the bone marrow. Indirect suppression would result if HIV interfered with the production of specific growth factors. Alternatively, infected cells may secrete a toxin that shortens the lifespan of T4 cells or other cells required for their survival.

In some HIV-infected patients the destruction of T4 cells occurs much faster than in others. Robert C. Gallo of the National Cancer Institute and his coworkers suggest that the rapid loss of cells may be caused by a concurrent infection with the recently discovered herpes virus, human herpesvirus-6 (HHV-6; originally called human B-lymphotropic virus, or HBLV).[4] Like HIV, HHV-6 can infect and kill T4 cells. Gallo and his coworkers have shown that infection with HHV-6 is widespread: they reported finding HHV-6 antibodies in 66 percent of a group of patients with AIDS or related diseases, in 47 percent of a group of HIVseronegative homosexual men, and in 24 percent of blood samples from healthy American and European blood donors.[5] The researchers speculate that people may carry latent HHV-6 in their T4 cells. When these cells are subsequently infected with HIV, the HHV-6 virus may be reactivated. Gallo and his associates suspect that the 2 viruses may work together to destroy T4 cells and increase the likelihood of opportunistic infections. Confirmation of the role of HHV-6 in accelerating AIDS-related diseases would suggest that antiherpes drugs might prolong the lives of people infected with HIV.

The envelope and the immune system.   The immune response to HIV infection, described later in the chapter, does not appear to halt the progression of disease. Part of the explanation for this failure probably relates to the structure of the envelope proteins.

The most effective way to stop HIV infection would be to block the binding reaction between gp120 and the CD4 receptor. However, antibodies from infected patients rarely do this. Scientists speculate that the 2 or 3 regions of the gp120 molecule involved in the binding reaction may form a recessed pocket. The inability of antibodies to get inside such a pocket could explain the lack of a protective immune response.

The envelope proteins also are heavily coated with sugar residues. The human immune system does not recognize the sugar residues as foreign because they are products of the host cell rather than of the virus. (The sugar residues added to the viral envelope proteins are identical with those found on normal membrane proteins in uninfected cells.) The sugar residues form a protective barrier around sections of gp120 that might otherwise elicit a strong immune response.

Vaccine researchers are particularly concerned about one other feature of gp120: it contains some regions that are highly variable. Early studies of HIV isolates from different people showed a surprising amount of variation in the genetic makeup of the viruses. Subsequent investigations have revealed that many of the genetic differences among HIV isolates occur in portions of the viral genome coding for the envelope proteins.

The high frequency of spontaneous change, or mutation, in the envelope gene raises many questions. Some scientists believe that the high frequency of variation in the envelope gene occurs as a direct result of selective pressure exerted by the immune system. Others believe that the variability is simply a by-product of a very imprecise replication system. The enzyme in HIV that copies RNA into DNA, reverse transcriptase, appears to be much less accurate than enzymes that carry out DNA synthesis in other systems—it is more likely to substitute one chemical building block for another. The replication process may produce mutants with a wide range of mistakes sprinkled throughout the genome, but only certain ones survive. The survivors are variants in which the mutation does not inactivate essential proteins or regulatory sequences. Variability in the envelope gene may be more common among HIV isolates than variability in other genes simply because the envelope gene is more tolerant to change.

Scientists involved in vaccine development are concerned that a vaccine made against the envelope proteins of one viral isolate might not recognize the envelope of another isolate. The impact of the genetic variation among HIV isolates on vaccine prospects will not be known definitely until researchers learn more about the structure of the envelope proteins and their role in eliciting a protective immune response.

Regulatory Genes

Recent evidence indicates that HIV's unusual regulatory genes also contribute to its ability to evade the immune system. In the simplest retroviruses the replication rate is controlled by interactions between the host cell and elements in the viral LTR. The virus itself has no way of regulating when, where, or how much virus is produced.

In contrast, the human immunodeficiency viruses have

elaborate regulatory control mechanisms in the form of specific regulatory genes. Some of the genes permit explosive replication; others appear to inhibit production of virus. Mechanisms that suppress the production of certain viral proteins, such as the envelope proteins, may allow HIV to hide inside infected cells for long periods without eliciting antibodies or other host immune responses. The 6 regulatory genes identified in the HIV-1 genome are called *tat* (transactivator), *rev* (regulator of expression of virion proteins), *vif* (virion infectivity factor), *nef* (negative factor), *vpr* (viral protein r), and *vpu* (viral protein u).[6]

The tat *gene.*   The protein produced by the *tat* gene greatly amplifies (or transactivates) the level of replication of HIV-1. William Haseltine of the Dana–Farber Cancer Institute in Boston likens it to a "fast-forward" switch; it produces more than a 1,000-fold increase in the efficiency of the viral LTR. HIV-1 mutants that lack the *tat* gene do not replicate.

Researchers believe that the *tat* protein acts in 2 different ways: it increases the rate at which viral DNA is transcribed into RNA, and it increases the rate at which viral RNA is translated into protein.[7] Efforts continue to determine the precise mechanisms for these actions. The *tat* protein is found primarily in the nucleus of infected cells.

The rev *gene.*   The *rev* gene, previously called *art* or *trs*, directly or indirectly controls the types of RNA produced by HIV-1. In the absence of the *rev* protein, the virus does not accumulate RNA coding for the structural proteins (*gag*, *pol*, and *env*), but it does accumulate RNA coding for the regulatory proteins. The *rev* gene may play an important role in the transition from a latent to a productive infection; it is essential for viral replication.

The vif *gene.*   The *vif* gene (formerly called *sor*, *A*, *P'*, and *Q* by different research groups) is required for efficient transmission of HIV-1. In cell cultures, viruses with a defective *vif* gene spread poorly and only through cell-to-cell contact.

The nef *gene.* Several research groups have reported that viruses lacking the *nef* gene (formerly called *3' orf, B, E',* and *F* by different groups) replicate more rapidly than normal viruses. If the product of the *nef* gene does act as a brake to viral replication, it may be important in the establishment of controlled infections (infections that do not kill the host cell).

The vpr *gene and the* vpu *gene.* The functions of the *vpr* gene and the *vpu* gene are not known, although some researchers believe that the product of the *vpu* gene also may help the virus slow its growth in infected cells.

The findings described above represent the very early stages of understanding of HIV replication. Discovery of the novel regulatory proteins has increased the number of potential targets for antiviral drugs and also provided a foundation for further studies of interactions between the virus and specific target cell populations.

The Immune System

Knowledge of the human immune system acquired during the 1970s was a primary factor in the rapid scientific response to the AIDS crisis. Physicians recognized abnormalities in the immune function of AIDS patients because researchers in laboratories across the country had made major strides in working out the details of the normal immune response.

Normal Immune Function

The human immune system consists of many different kinds of cells actively seeking out and eliminating germs and other foreign substances from the body. In the blood, the majority of defenders are white blood cells called phagocytes. These cells are generalists; they have a primitive recognition system that allows them to bind to, engulf, and destroy a wide range of bacteria, viruses, damaged or infected host cells, and other materials. This process is called phagocytosis. The system is not very efficient, however, and many microorganisms have physical or chemical characteristics that enable them to escape detection or destruction.

Two different adaptive responses have evolved to supplement phagocytosis. Both involve a group of smaller white blood cells called lymphocytes. Lymphocytes originate in the bone marrow and are divided into two distinct classes, B lymphocytes and T lymphocytes. When a B cell is stimulated with an appropriate antigen (a foreign protein or sugar molecule), it divides rapidly into a large population of identical daughter cells. These daughter cells grow into small factories that produce and secrete antibody molecules.

Antibodies act in many different ways: they coat invading bacteria to make them more palatable for digestion by phagocytes; they neutralize bacterial toxins (poisons); and they destroy virus particles or prevent them from binding to target cells. This antibody, or "humoral," immune response is specific. That is, antibodies made against one microorganism will not react against another microorganism unless the two share a common molecular structure.

The second type of adaptive immune response is called cell-mediated immunity. The principal actor in this type of reaction is the cytotoxic (cell-killing) T lymphocyte. Cell-mediated immunity confers protection against bacteria that live and grow inside host cells (such as the organisms that cause tuberculosis and leprosy) and against certain viruses. Cytotoxic T lymphocytes attack infected cells to prevent the microorganisms inside from replicating and spreading to other cells. Cell-mediated immunity also plays a key role in the rejection of tissue transplants and may be involved in the elimination of some cancer cells.

Recent advances in molecular biology have contributed greatly to our knowledge of these adaptive immune responses. For example, scientists had known for many years that animals without T cells cannot mount an effective antibody response against some antigens, even though T cells do not secrete antibodies themselves. In the late 1970s, researchers established that a specific subclass of T cells (identified by the

T4 or CD4 surface molecule described earlier) was responsible for this activity. Antibody production depended on cooperation between T4 cells and the appropriate B cells.

Subsequent studies have shown that the T4 cell directly or indirectly regulates every aspect of immune function. Fauci refers to this cell as the "conductor of the symphony of the human immune system." Another way to think of the T4 cell is to imagine it as the dispatcher for a communitywide disaster-response network. This dispatcher takes information about impending emergencies from roving patrol cars and sends out specially trained teams to respond. Without the dispatcher, the flow of information would stop. Individual patrols might be able to handle small problems in the field, but any problem large enough to require a coordinated response would quickly overwhelm the community.

T4 cells coordinate the activities of phagocytes, B lymphocytes, cytotoxic T lymphocytes, and several other immune cells. For example, they produce special chemical messengers that control the movements and function of a group of phagocytic cells in the blood called monocytes. These chemical messengers recruit monocytes to the site of an infection, prevent them from leaving, and stimulate them to kill off ingested bacteria or viruses.

As noted above, T4 cells also induce B cells to produce antibodies against some types of antigen. This process actually begins with the monocyte, which predigests the antigen and then presents tiny fragments to an appropriate T4 cell (see Figure 5.3). When the T4 cell recognizes the same antigen bound to the surface of a primed B cell, it produces chemical messengers that induce the B cell to divide and begin producing antibody.

The T4 cell, again assisted by the monocyte, also regulates cell-mediated immunity against diseases such as herpes and tuberculosis. In this case, T4 cells enhance the activity of cytotoxic T lymphocytes, which carry a T8 surface marker (see Figure 5.4). The stimulated T8 lymphocytes multiply and attack infected target cells.

Other elements of the immune system regulated by T4

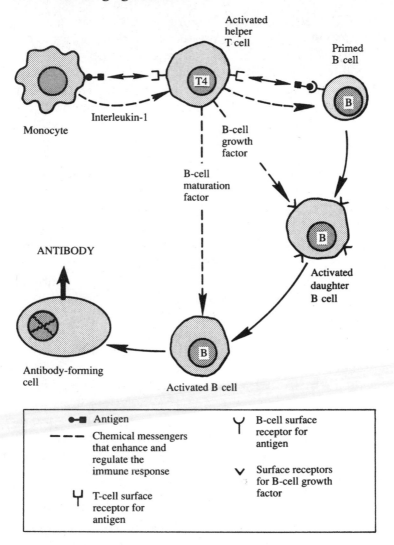

FIGURE 5.3. Simplified view of the cooperation between T4 cells and antigen-specific B cells in the production of antibody. The helper T cell is activated by interleukin-1 produced during interaction with the antigen-presenting monocyte. The activated T cell is further stimulated when it recognizes the same antigen bound to the surface of a primed B cell. (Like the monocyte, the B cell processes antigen and displays a portion of the processed molecule on its surface.) The T cell produces B-cell growth factor,

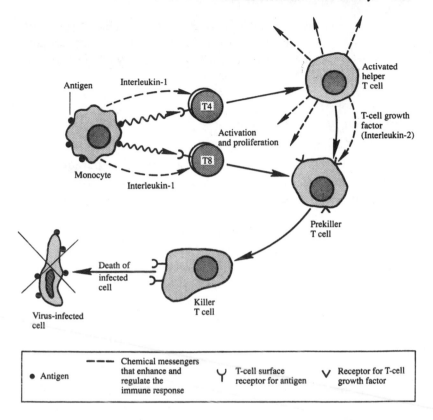

FIGURE 5.4. The cell-mediated immune response. Interaction with the antigen-presenting monocyte results in activation of both the T4 cell and the T8 cell. The activated helper T cell produces T-cell growth factor (interleukin-2) and other chemical messengers that lead to proliferation and maturation of the killer T cell (the cytotoxic T lymphocyte). The killer T cell then attacks and destroys the virus-infected target cell. Source: Adapted, with permission, from Ivan M. Roitt, *Essential Immunology,* 5th ed. (Oxford: Blackwell Scientific Publications, 1984), fig. 3.19 and 3.20, pp. 74, 75.

which stimulates the B cell to divide. B-cell maturation factor, also produced by the helper T cell, stops the cell division and turns the activated B cells into antibody-producing cells. *Source:* Adapted, with permission, from Ivan M. Roitt, *Essential Immunology,* 5th ed. (Oxford: Blackwell Scientific Publications, 1984), fig. 3.16, p. 70.

cells include suppressor cells and natural killer cells. Suppressor cells dampen immune reactions to prevent them from damaging healthy tissues. Natural killer cells destroy some types of tumor cells.

Disruption of Immune Function

The first attempts to assess the effects of AIDS on the human immune system resulted in an apparent paradox: the broad range of clinical signs and symptoms associated with the disease suggested multiple problems crippling many facets of the immune response, but a closer look showed a rather selective defect in one component of the system. The explanation was that HIV was selectively destroying the T4 lymphocyte (see Figure 5.5), the dispatcher cell described above.

In most healthy persons, 60 percent of T lymphocytes in the circulation are T4 cells, and 30 percent are T8 cells, so the T4-to-T8 ratio is 2 to 1. In AIDS patients the number of T4 cells is drastically reduced, so that the T4-to-T8 ratio is much lower and may even be reversed.

Early in the AIDS epidemic, physicians used measurement of the T4-to-T8 ratio in the diagnosis of AIDS. But other viral infections also can alter this ratio, and some of these infections are common in the populations at highest risk of AIDS. This created confusion until researchers showed that the effect of HIV was different from that of the other viruses: the abnormal ratio produced by other viral infections resulted from an increase in T8 cells and not from a decrease in T4 cells. The proliferation of T8 cells was determined to be a normal protective mechanism, and the loss of T4 cells to be a sign of serious disease.

T4 cells from AIDS patients also have a major functional defect: they cannot respond to specific antigen.[8] When normal T cells are challenged in a test tube with a protein such as tetanus toxoid, they immediately begin to divide and multiply. Clifford Lane of the NIAID Laboratory of Immunoregulation and his coworkers have shown that T lymphocytes from patients with AIDS do not proliferate after such a challenge.

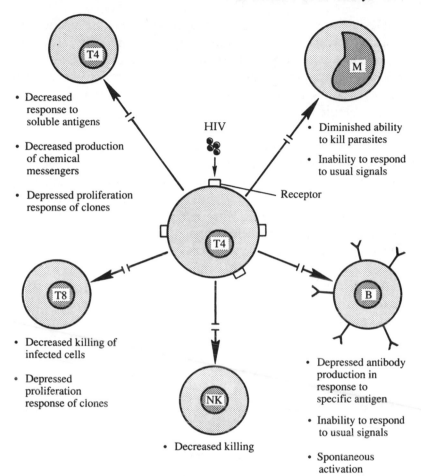

FIGURE 5.5. Some of the many functional defects caused by infection of the T4 helper lymphocyte with HIV. Cells affected include other T cells, B cells, natural killer cells (NK), and monocytes (M). Source: Adapted, with permission, from D. L. Bowen, H. C. Lane, and A. S. Fauci, "Immunopathogenesis of the Acquired Immunodeficiency Syndrome," *Annals of Internal Medicine* (1985), fig. 3, p. 707.

Subsequent experiments have demonstrated that this failure to respond is not caused by an inability to divide; it is caused by an inability to recognize antigen. This defect occurs early in the disease; it was recognized first in cells from patients with early Kaposi's sarcoma who appeared to have only minor immunologic abnormalities.

Monocyte defects. Lane and his coworkers recognized that the failure of T cells to respond might originate in the cells that present antigen to the T lymphocytes, the monocytes, rather than in the T lymphocytes themselves. They explored this possibility by challenging different combinations of lymphocytes and monocytes from twin brothers; one twin had full-blown AIDS and the other was healthy. The researchers found that healthy lymphocytes mixed with healthy monocytes responded normally to antigen stimulation, but that none of the other combinations (healthy monocytes and infected lymphocytes, infected monocytes and healthy lymphocytes, or infected monocytes and infected lymphocytes) produced a similar effect. These experiments showed that monocytes from AIDS patients also have a specific defect, because they cannot respond normally to the chemical signals of healthy T lymphocytes and they are less able to destroy foreign substances.

Subsequent studies have demonstrated that monocytes also can be infected with HIV. The major difference between infected T4 cells and infected monocytes is that the monocytes usually are not destroyed by the virus. They can produce large quantities of viral particles and still remain intact. (Researchers believe that infected monocytes survive because the virus buds into membrane-lined compartments inside the cell instead of budding through the external membrane as it does in lymphocytes.)[9]

The role of the monocyte is to seek out, capture, and destroy viruses and other foreign substances. Therefore, it would not be surprising if monocytes (or macrophages, which are monocyte descendants that have become fixed in certain tissues) were the first cells in the body infected with HIV.

They may transmit the infection to T4 cells. Also, monocytes circulate throughout the body. Scott Koenig and his coworkers at the National Institute of Allergy and Infectious Diseases suggest that circulating monocytes may be responsible for the initiation of HIV infection in the brain.[10] They and others have isolated HIV-infected macrophages from the brains of numerous patients with AIDS encephalopathy.

Interest in the role of monocytes and macrophages in HIV infection increased substantially in mid-1988, when Monte S. Meltzer of the Walter Reed Army Institute of Research in Washington, D.C., and his coworkers reported that they had found the virus in the macrophages of 3 homosexual men who had no other signs of HIV infection. The men were healthy and had no detectable HIV antibodies; tests to find HIV in their T4 cells were negative.[11] Researchers do not yet know how many people who have tested HIV seronegative actually carry HIV in their macrophages or whether patients such as the 3 men described above will have a different pattern of disease progression from others infected with the virus.

At the Fourth International Conference on AIDS in Stockholm, Susan Crowe of the University of California at San Francisco and her coworkers presented evidence that macrophages anchored in the spleen and other parts of the body are a major reservoir of HIV in patients with AIDS-related conditions.[12] They emphasized the importance of testing potential anti-HIV drugs in cell cultures containing monocyte/macrophage populations, as well as in T-cell cultures. A drug that is effective against the virus in T cells may not work in macrophages because the 2 types of cells sometimes metabolize drugs differently.[13]

B-lymphocyte hyperreactivity. Initially, scientists believed that B lymphocytes were not affected by infection with HIV, because patients with AIDS produced normal or higher-than-normal levels of antibodies. Studies have revealed, however, that these high antibody levels do not signify a healthy immune response. Too many B cells are producing antibody for no apparent reason.

The B-cell population in a healthy person contains cells at 3 different stages of activation. Some cells are resting and can be induced to divide and multiply by mitogens, substances that stimulate B-cell proliferation without a T-cell intermediary; a second group is partially activated and ready to respond to T-cell signals; and a third group spontaneously secretes antibody.

An analysis of B-cell populations from 12 patients with AIDS showed that these cells did not follow the pattern described above.[14] Lane and his coworkers reported that the individuals in the study appeared to have no resting B cells; decreased numbers of partially activated cells; and an abnormally high number of fully differentiated, antibody-secreting cells.

The most serious consequence of this hyperreactivity is that the abnormally activated, antibody-secreting B cells are not available to respond to signals that trigger a normal humoral response. When a new antigen enters the body, these B cells cannot be recruited to fight it. The disaster-response analogy mentioned earlier is helpful here, too. If all the specialized response teams were out answering false alarms, they would not be available when an emergency arose that required their unique skills. Similarly, the B cells in HIV-infected patients are busily producing unnecessary antibodies and are not able to respond when a real need arises.

This hyperreactivity diminishes the ability of HIV-infected patients to resist disease and also complicates the diagnosis of many opportunistic infections, because the patient does not make detectable antibodies against invading viruses or bacteria. Also, the presence of large quantities of superfluous antibody increases the likelihood of an autoimmune reaction, in which the body begins to attack itself.

The reasons for the abnormal activation of B lymphocytes in HIV infection remain unclear. Initially, it was thought to result from a concurrent infection with cytomegalovirus or Epstein-Barr virus; both are present in the majority of HIV-infected patients, and both have been shown to cause B-cell hyperreactivity. Further studies have shown, however, that HIV itself can trigger such a response.

The Course of Infection in the Body

Early experiments provided information on the characteristics of cell populations susceptible to HIV infection, but they did not offer a clear picture of how infection progresses in the body. Thomas Folks, Howard Gendelman, Joseph Margolick, and their colleagues at NIAID have developed several laboratory models that help illustrate the chain of events leading to full-blown disease. Their findings may have important implications for carriers of HIV.

In the first model, the NIAID researchers added virus to a previously uninfected culture of T4 cells. The culture grew normally until about the tenth day, when reverse transcriptase activity appeared and cells began to die (as discussed earlier, reverse transcriptase is the enzyme that copies the RNA carried inside each viral particle into the DNA necessary for viral replication). At first it seemed as if the whole culture might succumb, but gradually the reverse transcriptase activity declined and then disappeared. The remaining cells looked and acted healthy, but were they?

Molecular analysis of the surfaces of these cells showed that they were missing the CD4 marker. This was an important clue. Folks and his colleagues suspected that the missing markers might indicate a hidden infection, and indeed when they chemically stimulated the cells to divide, reverse transcriptase activity returned and the cells began secreting viruses. In contrast, cells that were not stimulated continued to grow and were not infectious to other cells.

HIV infection probably follows a similar course in the body. Studies of hemophiliacs and homosexual men indicate that, beginning about 14 days after infection, virus production is high for several weeks. (Patients may or may not have the mononucleosislike symptoms described in Chapter 4.) The early stage usually is followed by a long period—2 months to more than 7 years—during which virus production is very low or undetectable. Patients appear healthy and are symptom-free. Their T lymphocytes, however, respond poorly to new challenges and have a range of subtle surface abnormalities.[15]

In the final stage of HIV infection, virus production increases, the number of T4 cells declines dramatically, and the patient begins the downward spiral toward severe illness and death. The NIAID researchers believe that the "upregulation" of viral genes in immune cells previously harboring a latent viral infection might be a major factor in the conversion of an asymptomatic infection to frank AIDS. They have shown that the HIV genes are switched on when the host cell attempts to respond to a signal that would normally trigger an immune response. The signal might be a noxious chemical, a specific infectious agent, or a growth factor produced by another cell in the immune system.[16] Gendelman and his colleagues also have demonstrated that cells infected with both HIV and another virus (such as cytomegalovirus, Epstein-Barr virus, hepatitis B virus, and herpes simplex virus) produce signficantly more HIV proteins than do cells infected with HIV alone.[17]

The complex interactions between HIV and its target cells will not be worked out completely for many years. These studies suggest, however, that people who know they are infected with HIV may be able to slow the onset of serious disease by avoiding other types of infections.

The Immune System's Response

How does the immune system fight back when it is attacked by HIV? Almost everyone infected with the virus eventually develops both HIV antibodies and a cell-mediated immune response capable of killing HIV-infected cells. Yet neither of these natural defense mechanisms appears to provide permanent protection against severe disease.

Timing of the antibody response.   Researchers believe that most people infected with HIV develop antibodies against the virus within 6 to 14 weeks. Commercially available screening tests for HIV infection, the ELISA and the Western blot (see Appendix C), detect the presence of these antibodies rather than the virus itself. Several new studies indicate, however, that some people may not make antibodies for a year or more after infection; others initially make very low levels of antibodies that do not register on conventional screening tests.

In September 1987, Annamari Ranki of Helsinki University Central Hospital and her Finnish and American coworkers described their analysis of stored serum samples from 9 men who had recently become HIV-seropositive. They found that the men had been infected with HIV for 6 to 14 months before they tested positive on standard antibody tests. Subsequent studies by the researchers revealed that 5 of 25 seronegative sexual partners of known HIV-antibody-positive men (24 men and 1 woman) also were infected with HIV for more than a year without seroconversion.[18] Other laboratories are reevaluating these data.

Steven Wolinsky of Northwestern University Medical School and his coworkers reported similar results at the Fourth International Conference on AIDS. They used a new technique called the polymerase chain reaction (PCR) test to search for small quantities of viral DNA in stored blood samples from 18 homosexual and bisexual men who had recently become HIV-seropositive. They found that 14 of the men had had evidence of the viral genome in their blood for more than a year before they developed detectable antibodies: 6 for 18 months, 2 for 24 months, 2 for 30 months, 1 for 36 months, and 1 for 42 months.[19]

The interpretation of standard antibody tests has been further complicated by evidence that a small fraction of asymptomatic HIV-seropositive people do not remain seropositive. Homayoon Farzadegan of the Johns Hopkins University School of Hygiene and Public Health and his coworkers found that 4 of 1,000 HIV-seropositive men enrolled in a multicenter study gradually lost their HIV antibodies over a period of 2.5 years. At first the researchers believed that these men might have eliminated the virus from their bodies; they could find no evidence of viral replication. But PCR tests revealed that all 4 men had copies of the HIV genome hidden in their blood cells 6 to 18 months after their last positive antibody test.[20] Scientists do not know whether blood from such a person would be capable of transmitting HIV infection to others.

The implications of these findings for members of high-risk groups and for the population as a whole remain unclear. The Wolinsky study was too small to provide an accurate picture of the average time required for antibody production following infection. In addition, most researchers believe that reversion to a seronegative state is quite rare. However, these studies underscore the importance of practicing safer sex and avoiding intravenous drug abuse. A seronegative test result should not be viewed as a guarantee that a partner is free of the virus if the partner has engaged in high-risk behavior in the past.

Public health officials do not believe that the results described here represent a new threat to the blood supply, because there have been very few cases of new transfusion-related HIV infections since the implementation of the anti-body screening tests in 1985. Also, efforts to discourage blood donation by members of groups with a high prevalence of AIDS have been very successful.[21]

Characterizing HIV antibodies. Efforts to characterize the anti-bodies produced during the course of an HIV infection have 2 major goals: (1) to determine whether the presence or absence of certain antibodies in the blood could be used to predict the course of a patient's illness, and (2) to identify antibodies that might be important in vaccine development.

Most HIV-seropositive people make antibodies against all the viral proteins: the envelope proteins (gp120 and gp41), the core proteins (p24 and p17; products of the *gag* gene); the replicative proteins, and the regulatory proteins. The p24 antibody appears to be most useful in predicting the course of disease.

In studies of patients with hemophilia, the appearance of p24 antibody in the blood has been correlated with the disappearance of viral proteins during the first phase of HIV infection. During the months or years of asymptomatic infection, p24 antibody levels remain high. Eventually, however, in patients who are going to become ill, the p24 antibody begins to disappear.

The decline of p24 antibody and the reappearance of viral proteins in the blood of a patient infected with HIV are regarded as signs of impending disease. Patients who fail to develop core protein antibodies altogether generally have a much more severe clinical course than other patients.

Antibody studies directed at vaccine development involve the search for "neutralizing" antibodies. To measure neutralizing antibodies, scientists incubate virus grown in the laboratory in serum taken from an infected patient. (Serum is the clear, yellowish fluid that separates from blood when it is allowed to clot.) Then they add the virus to cell cultures known to be susceptible to HIV infection. Viruses incubated in serum with a high level of neutralizing antibodies will fail to infect the cell culture. (The p24 antibody discussed above is not a neutralizing antibody.)

The presence of neutralizing antibodies against viruses such as measles and polio is associated with suppression of disease symptoms and protection against reinfection. Initially, most scientists thought that HIV did not elicit neutralizing antibodies, because symptoms seemed to progress regardless of antibody production. Studies have shown, however, that most people infected with HIV do make at least some neutralizing antibodies.

Researchers from several laboratories have demonstrated that low blood levels of HIV-neutralizing antibodies are associated with advanced or progressive disease, but no one has established a cause-and-effect relationship. The question remains: do people get sick because they have low or absent neutralizing activity or does the decline in neutralizing activity simply reflect the general deterioration in immune function?

Most of the neutralizing antibodies made in response to HIV infection are directed against the envelope proteins. (The same is true in other retroviral infections.) The goal of current research is to determine whether regions of the envelope proteins that elicit neutralizing antibodies would make good vaccine components. David Ho, then of Massachusetts General Hospital in Boston, and his colleagues described 4 such regions in a 1987 article.[22] Their finding that 3 of the regions were in sections of the envelope common to many different isolates of HIV suggests that the diversity among envelope proteins may not be a major deterrent to vaccine development.

Cell-mediated immunity. Many scientists believe that a vaccine against HIV will be effective only if it elicits a cell-mediated immune response as well as an antibody response. The existence of cytotoxic T lymphocytes specifically armed to kill HIV-infected cells was first reported by researchers in Boston and Paris in July 1987.[23] But the importance of these cells remains unclear. Martin Hirsch, one of the authors of the Boston report, notes that cell-mediated immunity appears to diminish as the disease progresses. Again, it is unclear whether the loss of immune function is a cause or an effect of the disease process.

The French researchers, headed by Fernando Plata of the Institut Pasteur, suggest that interactions between HIV-specific cytotoxic T cells and infected macrophages might be responsible for the lung inflammation seen in some AIDS patients.

HIV in the Brain

Diseases of the central nervous system have been recognized as an important part of the spectrum of AIDS-related problems since the beginning of the epidemic. Some patients had well-defined lesions, such as those caused by tumors and certain parasitic diseases (see Chapter 3). Many others, however, showed signs of a more widespread degeneration of the brain that could not be traced to any specific cause. These patients initially experienced mild memory loss or problems controlling body movements, but the symptoms often progressed to severe dementia or paralysis.

At first the physicians treating these patients thought that they were simply missing or misinterpreting the signs of a familiar viral or bacterial infection, but as the number of cases mounted they became suspicious. If the immune defects associated with AIDS were caused by a new infectious agent, perhaps the same agent was affecting the brain. The discovery of HIV in cells in the brain confirmed this hypothesis.

The dominant cell type infected with HIV in the brain appears to be the monocyte/macrophage. The wandering monocyte probably becomes infected in the bloodstream and then carries the virus across the blood–brain barrier into the central nervous system. The monocyte/macrophage may be the source of infection of brain-derived glial cells and endothelial cells. Glial cells provide structural support to nerve cells, help regulate the transfer of nutrients from blood vessels to nerve tissues, and act like blood phagocytes by removing cellular debris from the brain. Endothelial cells line the blood vessels of the central nervous system.

The degeneration characteristic of AIDS encephalopathy clearly involves the loss of nerve cells in the brain, but direct infection of nerve cells appears to be quite rare. How, then, does the virus inflict such damage? Scientists believe that several different mechanisms may be involved.

Some nerve cells may be destroyed as "innocent bystanders" to an inflammatory reaction triggered by infected monocytes. Activated monocytes secrete a variety of substances that might be toxic to nerve cells in adjacent tissues. Some of these substances specifically attract more immune cells, which might also become infected.

Another mechanism of destruction could involve the infected glial cell. Stephen Dewhurst of Columbia University and his colleagues described the infection of glial cells in December 1987.[24] They showed that glial cells in laboratory cultures do not die as a result of persistent HIV infection; instead, they develop a variety of structural abnormalities. Other virus-induced changes in glial cells could interfere with their ability to maintain an appropriate environment for adjacent nerve cells.

Detrimental changes in the environment of the central nervous system also might result from the infection of endothelial cells. Endothelial cells play a major role in maintaining the blood-brain barrier.

Children infected with HIV frequently develop abnormal mineral deposits in the blood vessels supplying the basal ganglia, large collections of gray matter in the interior of the cerebral hemispheres. Scientists speculate that the deposits result from damage to endothelial cells lining the blood vessels in that part of the brain. No one knows, however, whether such damage is caused directly by the virus or by some secondary process associated with HIV infection, such as a metabolic or hormonal imbalance in the brain.[25]

The presence of the virus in the brain has important therapeutic implications. Various techniques have been proposed to remove virus from the blood and restore the immune system; but if brain cells continue producing virus, any improvements attained with these techniques probably would be temporary. Successful therapy will require a drug that can pass through the physiologic barrier between the bloodstream and the brain and that is nontoxic to brain tissues.

Finally, the association between AIDS and neurological impairment will increase the impact of the disease on the health care system in the United States. The potential needs of a large patient population both with major physical problems and with severe cognitive disabilities could prove overwhelming for some medical facilities.

Other Infected Tissues

HIV infection of the immune system and the brain does not explain all the signs and symptoms associated with AIDS and related diseases. To obtain a more complete understanding of the effects of HIV on the body, researchers have used genetic probes to hunt for the virus in other tissues.

Skin Cells

In 1983 researchers at New York University demonstrated that the outermost layer of skin, the epidermis, in some

AIDS patients was markedly deficient in Langerhans cells.[26] Langerhans cells are part of the body's immune surveillance system: they send out long spindly branches to trap foreign materials entering through the skin and then process them for presentation to nearby T cells. The NYU scientists speculated that the loss of Langerhans cells might play a role in the development of some AIDS-related diseases, but at the time there was not enough information about the cause of AIDS to permit further progress.

The discovery of HIV and the development of powerful assays for the virus reawakened interest in the Langerhans cells. In 1986, researchers from the University of Vienna and the National Cancer Institute detected HIV in very small skin samples from 5 of 25 patients with AIDS or AIDS-related complex.[27] The virus was localized in the Langerhans cells.

Future studies will attempt to determine whether HIV infection impairs the function of Langerhans cells as it does T cells. The results could provide important insights about some of the severe skin disorders that plague HIV-infected patients.

Bone Marrow

Blood cell deficiencies are among the most common laboratory findings in people with HIV-related diseases. Patients often have abnormally low levels of red blood cells and platelets, as well as of white blood cells.

All blood cell production occurs in the bone marrow. Bone marrow progenitor cells are stimulated to grow and mature by a variety of chemical substances, including specific growth factors secreted by T lymphocytes and monocytes.

The most obvious explanation for the cell deficiencies associated with HIV infection was that the virus prevented infected T cells and monocytes from making the factors needed to stimulate normal cell growth and development. But a study by Massachusetts researchers from Genetics Institute, Inc., and the New England Deaconess Hospital suggested another possible explanation: bone marrow progenitor cells also might be infected with the virus.

In a 1987 article the scientists reported that antibodies in the serum of patients with AIDS or ARC could suppress the growth of bone marrow progenitor cells from people infected with HIV, but had no effect on bone marrow cells from uninfected controls.[28] Some of the antibodies involved in this immune-mediated suppression were directed against gp120, the envelope protein of HIV. The researchers speculated that the presence of gp120 on infected bone marrow cells might make them susceptible to damage from antiviral antibodies. In the absence of such antibodies, the cells did not seem grossly affected by the virus.

The Massachusetts scientists suggested that drugs consisting of specific growth factors might be able to overcome some of the bone marrow suppression associated with HIV infection. These drugs are discussed further in Chapter 7.

In June 1988, Thomas M. Folks of the National Institute of Allergy and Infectious Diseases and his colleagues confirmed that normal bone marrow progenitor cells are susceptible to HIV infection.[29] They used a new technique to separate the precursor cells from other components of the bone marrow and then infected them with HIV in the laboratory. Microscopic studies showed that some of the cells became "virtual bags of virus or wall-to-wall virus."[30] (As in monocytes, most virus particles produced in the infected progenitor cells appear to bud into internal compartments rather than through the external membrane.) This finding suggests that bone marrow progenitor cells may be an important reservoir of HIV infection, providing the virus with a safe haven from the immune system.

Tissues Involved in Sexual Transmission

Many of the early reports about homosexual and heterosexual transmission of HIV concluded with the speculation that transmission probably occurred when virus in infected seminal fluid entered the bloodstream through small tears in the lining of the rectum or vagina. But recent evidence indicates that direct access to the bloodstream probably is not necessary for sexual transmission. The virus can infect local tissues in the rectum and the female reproductive tract.

The intestine. In February 1988, Jay Nelson of the Research Institute of Scripps Clinic in La Jolla, California, and his colleagues reported that they had found HIV in bowel biopsy specimens from two AIDS patients.[31] Further studies revealed evidence of HIV infection in the rectum and small intestine of five additional patients.

These findings suggest that rectal tissues should be regarded as a source of HIV transmission between sexual partners practicing anal intercourse. They also indicate that cells in the bowel could be the initial site of virus replication in the receptive partner.

The presence of HIV in intestinal cells may be one cause of the diarrhea and other gastrointestinal problems often seen in AIDS patients. Nelson and his coworkers believe that one of the cell types infected with the virus is the enterochromaffin cell. This cell secretes hormones that control water in the colon. Disruption of the function of enterochromaffin cells could cause severe diarrhea.

The female reproductive tract. HIV was first detected in the cervical secretions of HIV-infected women in 1986. Scientists reported that the virus could be cultured from secretions throughout the menstrual cycle, an indication that the presence of virus was not merely the result of contamination with menstrual blood.

The probable source of HIV in cervical secretions is infected cervical tissue. In March 1988, Roger Pomerantz of Massachusetts General Hospital and his colleagues reported that they had isolated HIV from cervical specimens obtained from 4 seropositive women.[32] The cells most often infected were monocyte/macrophages and endothelial cells.

In male-to-female transmission of HIV, contact with infected semen could lead to local infection of susceptible cervical cells; replication of the virus in those cells might precede systemic infection with HIV. Female-to-male transmission probably results from the sloughing of infected cervical cells into cervical and vaginal fluids.

HIV infection of the uterine cervix also might explain some cases of viral transmission from mother to newborn, although the extent of such transmission is unknown. Researchers have documented transmission before birth (across the placenta) and after birth (probably through breast milk), but no one has demonstrated infection during the birth process. Pediatricians have reported, however, that some infected children have a much better prognosis than others (clinical symptoms appear later and may be less severe); it has been suggested that those who fare better may have been infected later in pregnancy or at birth. If future studies show that direct contact with virus-infected cells during vaginal delivery is a source of transmission, physicians may recommend caesarean delivery for HIV-infected women. So far, researchers have not found an association between method of delivery and newborn infection rates.

Conclusion

Laboratory studies of HIV and the cells it infects are providing important insights into how this virus causes disease. For example, scientists have made major progress in understanding interactions between the virus's envelope proteins and a specific receptor on human target cells, the CD4 molecule. Researchers also have identified a group of novel regulatory proteins that afford the virus an unusual amount of control over its own replication. Each additional piece of information contributes to the development of new antiviral strategies.

HIV infection produces a great variety of immunologic abnormalities, but the principal cause of these abnormalities appears to be the progressive destruction of one subclass of T lymphocytes, the T4 helper cells. These cells play a central role in all the body's major defense mechanisms. Patients who have relatively low T4 levels are more susceptible to opportunistic infections than are those with higher levels.

In addition to this quantitative defect, researchers have discovered a variety of functional defects both in T4 lymphocytes and in other components of the immune system in HIV infection. A T4 cell infected with HIV appears to lose its ability to respond to specific antigens. In addition, the virus serves as a B-cell activator: B cells from HIV-infected patients spontaneously proliferate and secrete antibodies, thus becoming unable to respond to the signals that evoke a normal antibody response.

Monocytes from HIV-infected patients also are defective; they exhibit a diminished ability to respond to chemical signals and to destroy certain parasites. Recent studies indicate that circulating monocytes with productive HIV infections may be responsible for distributing the virus to tissues throughout the body.

Laboratory models of HIV infection suggest that health status may play a role in both susceptibility to infection and the development of serious disease. Scientists believe that a subsequent infection's activation of a lymphocyte harboring an HIV provirus may trigger the production of new viruses and lead to the development of clinical symptoms.

The body's response to HIV remains poorly understood. Almost all infected persons make antibodies against the virus, but these antibodies generally are not protective. More studies are needed to determine the relationship between the type and quantity of antibodies produced and the patient's clinical status. The role of cell-mediated immunity also must be examined more closely.

The presence of HIV-infected cells in the brain helps explain the severe neurological problems and depression seen in some AIDS patients. It also has important therapeutic implications. Successful therapy will require a drug that can pass through the physiologic barrier between the bloodstream and the brain and that is nontoxic to brain tissues.

6

Prevention

In an era in which many young physicians have never seen a case of measles or polio and once-life-threatening bacterial infections can be eradicated with antibiotic therapy, the AIDS epidemic seems almost unreal. At first it was difficult to believe that a vaccine or a miracle drug was not just over the horizon. But public health experts warned that the United States could not wait for a medical solution to the AIDS crisis; the rapid increase in cases necessitated immediate action of a different kind.

More than 90 percent of AIDS cases have been attributed to high-risk sexual behavior or intravenous drug abuse. Control of the epidemic depends on education and other public health strategies to change this behavior. Information alone probably will not be sufficient; sustained change will require constant reinforcement and a social environment supportive of new attitudes about sex and drug use.[1] Preventive measures must be designed to reach such narrowly defined groups as adolescents, non-English-speaking minorities in the cities, and women at risk of having an HIV-infected child.

This emphasis on prevention is not meant to detract from the efforts of hundreds of scientists in the United States and abroad who are hunting for new therapeutic approaches to HIV infection. But this work takes time. Researchers have only begun to understand how to fight chronic viral infections of any kind, much less design a safe and effective agent against the novel HIV. Scientists searching for a vaccine also face many obstacles, and even if they develop a suitable candidate, the logistics of clinical trials and liability issues may delay its use for a decade or longer. Until more effective biological strategies are available, the primary weapon against AIDS is public health education.

Barriers to Education

Risk-reduction education to control HIV infection must be based on the assumption that public health education works, even in areas as sensitive as lifelong sexual behavior, although evidence about the validity of this assumption is mixed. Americans generally do not have a very good record with respect to diseases that require long-term behavioral changes. People of all ages continue to smoke despite the clear connection between smoking and lung cancer. Alcohol problems and dietary habits linked to heart disease are equally resistant to change.

The desire to avoid HIV infection may be stronger, however, because the problem is new and because its most familiar manifestation, AIDS, is uniformly fatal. The dramatic decrease in the incidence of rectal gonorrhea and other sexually transmitted diseases among homosexual men in some parts of the country is one indication that this particular population has responded to local educational campaigns. (The data on gonorrhea do not give a clear picture of the extent or nature of these behavioral changes, however, because the relationship between sexual activity and disease transmission is complicated by many other factors.)

Telephone and written surveys in areas with high and low prevalences of HIV infection indicate that homosexual men generally have fewer sexual partners and are less likely to engage in high-risk activities than they were in the past. But the amount of behavioral change varies widely. Many have not made the major changes in risk-taking behavior required for long-term protection.

Confusion about Risk

The varying responses to the threat of HIV infection among homosexuals have occurred despite consistent information about the need to adopt risk-reduction measures. For heterosexuals, the message has been anything but consistent.

Boston Globe columnist Ellen Goodman complains about a phenomenon she calls "AIDS-information whipsaw."[2] Within a one-month period in 1988, heterosexuals in the United States were confronted with vastly different "expert" opinions about the dangers of unprotected heterosexual intercourse. First, psychiatrist Robert Gould told the readers of *Cosmopolitan* magazine that women engaging in normal vaginal intercourse with men need not worry about HIV infection. Several weeks later, well-known sex experts William H. Masters and Virginia E. Johnson, together with collaborator Robert Kolodny, published a book called *Crisis: Heterosexual Behavior in the Age of AIDS*. In material excerpted in *Newsweek* magazine, the authors declared that "the AIDS virus is now running rampant in the heterosexual community."[3]

Surgeon General C. Everett Koop and scientists who had spent nearly 7 years tracking the AIDS epidemic reacted strongly to both Gould and Masters and Johnson. After the *Cosmopolitan* article, they criticized those who would "lead women to believe they were not at risk from sexual relations with men."[4] In most parts of the country the risk of unprotected heterosexual intercourse is small, but it should not be ignored.

The appearance of the Masters, Johnson, and Kolodny book forced Koop and CDC scientists to tackle the opposite end of the spectrum. Koop labeled the book "irresponsible scare tactics."[5] The 3 authors had not submitted their findings for scientific review or published them in a recognized scientific journal. CDC epidemiologists patiently explained the problems with data used by the authors, but the explanations were often buried by newspaper editors deep inside lengthy articles.

The unfortunate timing of the two incidents exacerbated a situation that has troubled AIDS researchers since the beginning of the epidemic. In the process of responding to unfounded opinions from self-styled "experts," the people who have worked to keep abreast of existing data have had to struggle to maintain their own credibility with the lay public.

The ultimate losers in the push-and-pull of "expert" opinions are the men and women who want to know how to protect themselves against HIV infection. Ellen Goodman concludes: "In the face of all this, the prescription is the same one we heard last month, last year, the year before. Abstinence or a monogamous relationship with an uninfected person is the best protection. The use of a condom and spermicide every time is second best. And while you're at it, be wary of unprotected relationships with untested 'experts.' Misinformation is highly infectious."[6]

Questions of Propriety

Another obstacle to widespread AIDS education has been disagreement about the propriety of some prevention messages. The AIDS crisis sheds light on the ways in which social mores affect our ability to cope with new problems For example, in October 1985 the Los Angeles City Council refused to allow the city health department to put out a flyer on AIDS and drug abuse because the councillors felt that it reflected a permissive attitude toward drug use. (The flyer stated that drug abuse was a problem for many reasons, but that those who used drugs anyway should at least make sure their equipment was clean.)

More recently, the U.S. Congress passed an amendment to the Health and Human Services appropriations bill to limit the scope of federally funded AIDS educational materials. The amendment precludes the use of CDC funds for educational materials "that promote or encourage, directly, homosexual sexual activities." It also requires that any federally funded materials "emphasize abstinence from sexual activity outside a sexually monogamous marriage (including abstinence from homosexual activities)."

These actions reflect the views that government institutions should not be telling people how to conduct illegal activities and that some topics are not appropriate for public discussion. Health experts argue that these attitudes could seriously limit their ability to slow the spread of HIV infection in the population. AIDS is an unusual problem, they say, and it requires unusual and innovative solutions.

Condom Controversy

Much of the controversy about AIDS education has focused on recommendations concerning the use of condoms. In the spring of 1987, network television stations in New York City refused to run 2 of 3 advertisements proposed by the city's health department to reduce the spread of HIV infection.[7] The ads were designed to encourage women to insist on the use of condoms in any encounter outside a long-term monogamous relationship.[8]

Television officials expressed concern that the ads would offend viewers who might interpret them as promoting sexual activity. Indeed, in an interview with the New York Times on May 12, 1987, a spokesman for the Archdiocese of New York, Joseph Zwilling, said: "They [the ads] are an implicit endorsement of promiscuity and seem to promote the notion that if you use a condom you can't get AIDS. They are saying you can fool around, be as promiscuous as you want, and as long as you use a condom you're OK. That isn't the case."

It is important to recognize that the condom debate involves 2 sets of issues, one moral and one scientific. The moral issues concern the impact on premarital and extramarital sexual behavior of promoting condoms. The basic scientific question is whether condoms will reduce transmission of HIV.

Perhaps no one has struggled with these issues more than Surgeon General Koop. In a 1987 editorial addressed to members of the American Medical Association, Koop said:

The emphasis in the media on condoms for protection against HIV infection has diluted an important message: for those who are abstinent or those who have a mutually faithful monogamous sexual relationship, AIDS presents no problem. But for sexually active individuals who are neither abstinent nor have a mutually faithful monogamous relationship, we have little to offer except condoms.

Condoms are not 100 percent effective, but if correctly used they can dramatically reduce one's risk of exposure.

Some of you find it unpleasant to recommend condoms to young people. So do I. Acquired immunodeficiency syndrome is an unpleasant disease and recommending condoms to those who need protection is preferable to treating AIDS.[9]

The challenge in educating people about condoms is to convey the difference between risk reduction and risk elimination. Condoms reduce the risk of infection with HIV and other venereal diseases, but they do not eliminate it. The only way to eliminate risk is to avoid all exposure to the infectious semen, blood, and vaginal fluids of an infected sexual partner.

Measuring the protective effects of condoms is very difficult. In the laboratory, latex condoms completely prevent the passage of HIV. (Natural condoms, usually made from lambs' intestines, may have microscopic holes and are not recommended for prevention of sexually transmitted diseases.) On the other hand, scientists estimate that condoms fail to prevent pregnancy in 1 out of 10 couples who use the method for birth control for one year. Researchers do not know how much of the 10 percent failure rate is caused by condom defects and how much is associated with improper use of condoms. The U.S. Food and Drug Administration has intensified its condom testing program to minimize the sale of defective products.

No condom is effective if it is not used properly. CDC scientist William Darrow reports that a 1971 attempt to stop reinfections with gonorrhea at a Sacramento clinic by offering free samples of condoms failed because patients did not know how to use them.[10] Patients who became reinfected despite regular condom use admitted engaging in sexual foreplay involving contact between the vagina and penis before the male partner put on the condom. Condoms should be placed on the penis after it becomes erect and before it comes in contact with the body of the sexual partner. The condom should be rolled onto the penis, leaving a small space at the end, but allowing no air pockets beyond that point. The penis should be withdrawn from the partner before the erection is

immune system besieged by multiple infections may succumb more quickly to HIV than a resting immune system. Researchers have not yet identified any specific cofactors in vivo. Nonetheless, many physicians recommend that people who have been exposed to HIV should take steps to maintain good general health: eat regularly, exercise, get enough sleep, reduce stress levels, and avoid alcohol and other drugs (including noninjectable drugs). These recommendations will not prevent AIDS, but they may increase the body's ability to fight other infections.

A more direct benefit of early diagnosis through voluntary HIV testing is that physicians can be on the lookout for life-threatening opportunistic infections. As discussed in Chapter 3, therapies for *Pneumocystis carinii* pneumonia and some of the other opportunistic infections common in HIV-infected patients have improved dramatically since the beginning of the epidemic. Early diagnosis may allow outpatient treatment of diseases that previously required long hospitalizations.

Finally, studies in animal models suggest that antiviral drugs such as azidothymidine (AZT) may be most effective if treatment is begun before the onset of symptoms (see Chapter 7). Researchers are conducting large-scale clinical trials of AZT in asymptomatic patients to determine the risks and benefits of such therapy for human beings. If the risk-benefit ratio proves to be acceptable, AZT may be used to prolong the period of well-being between HIV infection and the development of overt clinical symptoms.

Mental Health Consequences

Receiving news about a positive HIV test is an extremely stressful experience. For this reason, public health experts and advocacy groups representing people at high risk of infection emphasize that voluntary testing should be done only in settings that permit adequate pre- and posttest counseling. The pretest counseling should be used to convey information about the purpose of the test and the meaning of both a negative and a positive result. Posttest counseling for a person with a negative result offers a crucial opportunity to provide risk-reduction education (see Appendix E).

Posttest counseling of someone infected with HIV requires an enormous amount of sensitivity. Health care workers have to be ready to answer numerous questions and to make referrals based on the needs of the individual. Some medical centers have found that a single counseling session after a positive test result is inadequate, because people are not able to absorb anything other than the fact that they are seropositive. Educational and referral information are repeated at a second counseling session when the patient has had time to adjust to the diagnosis.

Confidentiality and Antidiscrimination Measures

Public health officials recognize that individuals at high risk of HIV infection are more likely to come forward for voluntary testing if they believe they will not suffer adverse consequences in matters such as employment, school admission, housing, and medical services if they test positive. People must feel assured that their test results will remain confidential and that sanctions are available to prevent unwarranted discrimination.

The confidentiality of health records is governed primarily by state laws. Several states have enacted statutes that firmly restrict the disclosure of HIV antibody test results and severely punish negligent or willful breaches of confidentiality. Other states have used the AIDS issue as a catalyst to reexamine protections afforded to all types of public health and medical records.

The duty to warn. One of the dilemmas in developing the new statutes has been how to handle situations in which a person infected with HIV places an unsuspecting spouse or other sexual partner at risk of infection. People who test positive for HIV are strongly encouraged to notify their sexual partners about the risk of infection and to refer them for counseling and HIV testing. But some seropositive individuals are either afraid, embarrassed, or unwilling to comply with these instructions.

The Council on Ethical and Judicial Affairs of the American Medical Association says that physicians have a responsibility to prevent the spread of infection, as well as an ethical obligation to recognize the rights to privacy and to confidentiality of the person infected with HIV. It recommends that "where there is no statute that mandates or prohibits the reporting of seropositive individuals to public health authorities and a physician knows that a seropositive individual is endangering a third party, the physician should (1) attempt to persuade the infected patient to cease endangering the third party; (2) if persuasion fails, notify authorities; and (3) if the authorities take no action, notify the endangerd third party."[16]

A proposed federal law to provide for the confidentiality of HIV test results would allow physicians the discretion to warn third parties at risk, although it would not create a legal duty to warn.

Partner notification. The direction to "notify authorities" in the AMA statement refers to state or local public health authorities. Many states have voluntary partner notification programs set up to identify and counsel the partners of people infected with venereal diseases such as syphilis and gonorrhea. These programs have an excellent record of preserving the confidentiality of patient information. They are all entirely voluntary—people who refuse to disclose the names of their partners are not penalized. In addition, case counselors never reveal the identity of the index case (the person found to be infected) to those who are contacted.

HIV partner notification has been handled in several different ways. In December 1987 the health commissioner of New York City wrote to all local physicians asking them to inform patients infected with HIV of the "absolute need to tell their sexual partners of the risk of infection." He instructed physicians to provide patients with the telephone numbers of health department counselors, who would carry out notifications for any patients unwilling to do so themselves.[17]

Partner notification is not possible if the index case has had numerous anonymous sexual encounters, and it may not be efficient in populations with a high prevalence of infection. In San Francisco, partner notification has been limited to the heterosexual partners of HIV-infected bisexual men (many of whom are women of childbearing age).[18]

Mandatory reporting of HIV infection. More than a dozen states— most with a relatively low prevalence of HIV infection— base their partner notification programs on information obtained through mandatory reporting of HIV test results. In Colorado, for example, the state board of health requires laboratories to report each confirmed positive test for HIV antibodies with the name and address of the patient and the attending physician. State officials say that the main purpose of the program is individual education—to ensure that all those with positive test results receive skilled follow-up and counseling, either from their own physicians or from health department staff, about the risk of transmitting the disease to others.

Opponents of such a program argue that mandatory reporting of HIV test results is not advisable for several reasons. They are concerned that the potential for abuse of confidentiality rules is too great, especially given the discrimination experienced by many patients with AIDS and less severe symptoms of HIV infection. In addition, they believe that mandatory reporting may discourage voluntary use of the blood test.

Three of the first states to institute mandatory reporting simultaneously strengthened confidentiality provisions. In Colorado, a 1987 statute prevents the release of public health reports under "subpoena, discovery proceedings, search warrants, or otherwise." The statute also prohibits questioning of a public health employee in any hearing in any branch of government concerning personal identifiers and imposes strong penalties on an employee who inappropriately releases identifying information.[19]

Still, some opponents of mandatory testing are wary of any regulation that will establish a list of persons whose high-risk behaviors have resulted in HIV infection. After all, 24 states and the District of Columbia still have so-called sodomy laws, which make homosexual practices illegal even between consenting adults in private. Intravenous drug abuse is illegal in all states, and prostitution is illegal in all jurisdictions except certain counties in Nevada.

Thomas Vernon, executive director of the Colorado Department of Health, says that the number of homosexual and bisexual men being tested in his state has remained stable despite the controversy over reporting requirements. (Proof of identity is not required at testing and counseling sites, and some individuals use pseudonyms.) But the Colorado experience may not be typical. Much more information is needed about the impact of mandatory reporting on the willingness of people to be tested.

Antidiscrimination protections. Public health authorities in several states have recognized that effective voluntary testing programs require strong sanctions against HIV-related discrimination, as well as measures to ensure confidentiality of test results. Legislation in California, Wisconsin, and Michigan prohibits health professionals from discriminating against people having or suspected of having conditions associated with AIDS.[20] California, Florida, Massachusetts, and Wisconsin have enacted laws regulating the use of HIV antibody tests by employers.[21] In addition, ordinances in Austin, Texas, and in several California cities prohibit discrimination in employment, housing, and public accommodations.

Some states have chosen to base their protection of HIV-infected individuals on existing statutes that prohibit discrimination against the handicapped. Questions remain, however, about whether such laws apply to those who are infected with HIV but have no clinical symptoms, or to those who are simply perceived to be infected with HIV. Another problem with many existing antidiscrimination laws is the speed of the review process. If discrimination charges take years to resolve, the HIV-infected patient might die before any wrongs can be redressed.

In recommendations released in 1988, the AIDS Oversight Committee of the Institute of Medicine supported the enactment of a federal statute specifically designed to prevent discrimination on the basis of HIV infection status. One proposed bill reads: "A person may not discriminate against an otherwise qualified individual in employment, housing, public accommodations, or governmental services solely by reason of the fact that such individual is, or is regarded as being, infected with the etiologic agent for acquired immune deficiency syndrome."[22]

Reaching High-Risk Groups

Controlling the spread of the HIV epidemic will depend on broad efforts to change high-risk behavior. The most successful campaigns to change behavior have occurred among homosexuals in San Francisco and New York City. Insights gained from these programs are being used to develop new approaches to risk reduction for homosexuals in areas with a low incidence of HIV infection, for intravenous drug abusers, and for the sexual partners of people at high risk of AIDS.

Homosexual Men

Reports of dramatic changes in behavior among male homosexuals in cities with a high incidence of AIDS have led some observers to conclude that there is no need for further educational efforts among homosexuals. In a study conducted in San Francisco from 1978 to 1985, researchers found a 91 percent reduction in the number of male sexual partners reported by a group of 125 men originally enrolled in a study of hepatitis B virus transmission. The men also reported a 96 percent reduction in unprotected anal receptive intercourse. John Martin of the Columbia University School of Public Health interviewed 745 homosexual men in New York City in 1985. His subjects reported a 78 percent decline in sexual activity (measured in terms of the number of different sexual partners) since first hearing about AIDS.[23]

But such figures can be misleading. Despite the 78 percent decline in sexual activity, men in the Martin study still reported having had anal receptive intercourse with an average of 20 men in the preceding 12 months. Only 14 percent reported being monogamous.

These findings are particularly disturbing in light of a model developed by Harvey Fineberg, dean of the Harvard School of Public Health. He showed that if the prevalence of infection in a population is high, long-term protection from HIV infection requires extreme changes in risk-taking behavior. Moving from 50 partners to 10 partners has very little impact on the probability of acquiring HIV. Only by becoming completely monogamous can a man make a major difference in his chances of becoming infected. Similarly, the benefit from condoms is more substantial in going from halftime to everytime use than in moving from no use to halftime use.[24]

Data from the San Francisco Men's Health Study have allowed researchers to identify certain predictors of high-risk sexual behavior among homosexual men. At the Fourth International Conference on AIDS, Maria L. Ekstrand and Thomas J. Coates of the University of California at San Francisco reported that younger men, men who did not have a friend or lover with AIDS, and men who had thought of themselves as gay from an early age were more likely to engage in high-risk sex than other homosexual men. Alcohol and drug usage also were correlated with unsafe sex practices.[25] This type of information contributes to the development of better educational campaigns for high-risk groups.

Efforts to promote changes in behavior should provide the greatest gains in areas where the prevalence of HIV infection is low. Recent studies indicate, however, that compliance with safer-sex guidelines has been distressingly slight in many such communities. For example, Leonard Calabrese of the Cleveland Clinic Foundation in Ohio and his colleagues found that almost half of the homosexual men they questioned at a 1985 gay-lesbian social gathering in northeastern Ohio were still practicing receptive anal sex without a condom.[26] Clifton C. Jones and his coworkers reported an even higher level of high-risk behavior among men at a sexually-transmit-ted-disease clinic in New Mexico.[27]

The Ohio results are particularly startling because 91 percent of the men believed that they had made changes in their life-styles that would reduce the likelihood of transmit-ting or acquiring HIV. They had decreased both the number of their sexual partners and their use of drugs with sex. But the majority had not taken more meaningful protective measures; only 22 percent reported regular use of condoms.

A comprehensive report on changes in sexual behavior among gay and bisexual men, prepared by researchers at the University of California at San Francisco for the congressional Office of Technology Assessment, says that AIDS risk reduc-tion depends on five factors: knowledge, a sense of personal vulnerability, the development of skills needed to change, a sense of personal efficacy (confidence in one's ability to make necessary changes), and community norms supporting the new behaviors.[28]

In the report, Thomas J. Coates and his coworkers suggest that the changes observed in San Francisco demon-strate the importance of these five determinants of behavior. From the beginning of the epidemic, public health officials worked closely with organizations of homosexual men to prevent the dissemination of conflicting messages. Modern market-research techniques were used to identify appropriate messages and the most effective communication channels for reaching different audiences (for example, bisexual men with limited ties to the larger gay community).

The sense of personal vulnerability was relatively easy to convey in San Francisco, because almost everyone had friends or acquaintances who had AIDS. Behavior change may be very difficult to effect without this personal experience. Com-ments from a newly diagnosed AIDS patient in Washington, D.C., illustrate this point. The 35-year-old federal employee told a reporter from the *Washington Post*: "It was inconceivable to me that I might get AIDS. I was the first person I knew who got it. If I had known other people it might have made a real difference."[29] Educational programs in areas with a low incidence of HIV-related disease will have to find other ways to emphasize susceptibility, or efforts might not be sufficient to slow the spread of disease.

The San Francisco campaign also benefited from an early realization by the organizations involved that educational campaigns for high-risk groups have to be specific. Simply stating that sexual intercourse increases the risk of AIDS was not enough, because it was unlikely that those worried about AIDS would stop having sex altogether. The messages had to be explicit about which activities to avoid and how to have sexual contact without transmitting the virus.

A good example of this concept is an early brochure produced by the American Association of Physicians for Human Rights (AAPHR), the national association of gay and lesbian physicians. One section of the brochure focuses on the use of condoms, avoidance of substance abuse, and decreasing the number of sexual partners. Another section, titled "Positive Steps You Should Take," urges readers to ask about the health of sex partners; to increase touching and caressing; and to get adequate rest, nutrition, and exercise. The recommendation, for those who know or suspect that they have AIDS or related conditions, is "don't risk the health of others by having sex. Be sensible. Consult a health care provider who is up to date on gay health care." Materials similar to the AAPHR brochure are available from AIDS hotlines or counseling centers in most major cities in the United States.

Michael Quadland of Mount Sinai School of Medicine in New York compared 4 types of education programs for homosexual men. He found that showing explicit erotic films depicting safer sex practices was more effective in eliciting behavior change than was distributing erotic written materials about safer sex or holding a discussion session at which an AIDS patient described his disease.[30]

Peer discussion and support groups may be the most effective way to achieve the final two goals in AIDS education, developing a sense of personal efficacy and fostering community norms supporting new behaviors. Research from other health promotion efforts suggests that many people cannot sustain changes in behavior unless these goals are met.

Ronald Valdiserri and his coworkers at the University of Pittsburgh are conducting a study of the effects of peer-led, small-group educational sessions promoting risk reduction. Their initial report points out that although preintervention knowledge about AIDS and HIV transmission has been uniformly high, at least 60 percent of the men have reported engaging in unprotected receptive anal intercourse with more than one partner in the preceding 6 months. Questionnaires completed before each group session showed that a substantial number of the men originally had mixed feelings or negative attitudes about risk reduction. The group sessions produced a significant improvement in attitudes; future studies will determine whether the changes in attitude predict long-term changes in sexual behavior.[31]

Most research on AIDS-related behavioral change has focused on self-identified homosexual and bisexual men in large urban settings. A majority of study participants have been white, middle income, and relatively well educated. Coates and his coworkers say that there is an urgent need for more information about the level of high-risk behavior among men who are both homosexual and members of ethnic minorities, among homosexual adolescents, and among homosexuals and bisexuals from smaller urban or rural settings.

The development of broad-spectrum risk-reduction measures also will depend on a better understanding of the relationship between sexual behavior and the use of alcohol and other drugs. Repeated surveys by Communication Technologies, a San Francisco consulting firm, have shown that those who continue to practice unsafe sex are more likely to combine sexual activity with drugs and alcohol than are those who successfully adopt safer sex practices.

Intravenous Drug Abusers

HIV infection poses a major threat to the health of intravenous drug abusers, their sexual partners, and their children. Almost 70 percent of AIDS cases resulting from heterosexual intercourse with a member of a recognized high-risk group involve sexual contact with an intravenous drug abuser. More than 70 percent of children infected with HIV at or before birth have at least one parent who is a drug abuser.

Transmission of HIV among drug abusers results from sharing hypodermic needles and syringes. Options proposed to reduce this practice include (1) decreasing the amount of illegal drug abuse generally (through treatment programs and reduction of drug trafficking), (2) educating drug users about sterilization procedures and the need to seek out clean equipment, and (3) providing sterile needles and syringes.

The Presidential Commission on the Human Immunodeficiency Virus Epidemic wrote in its March 1988 interim report: "The Commission believes that curbing drug abuse, especially IV drug abuse, through treatment is imperative to deter the progression of the HIV epidemic. What is needed is a clear Federal, state, and local government policy, in other words a national comprehensive policy, unequivocally committed to providing 'treatment on demand' for intravenous drug abusers, with a coherent funding structure that provides for an ongoing, stable ten-year commitment to providing drug treatment services and treatment research."[32] The commission estimated that a 10-year funding commitment for such a program would be in the range of 15 billion dollars (approximately 1.5 billion dollars per year). Funding would be accomplished through a 50 percent federal and 50 percent state and local matching program.

The commission's call for "treatment on demand" refers to this country's severe shortage of drug treatment programs. In early 1988 the National Institute on Drug Abuse estimated that there were 1.1 million to 1.3 million IV drug abusers in the United States; publicly financed programs (both methadone maintenance and drug-free residential programs) could accommodate only 148,000 of them. In poor neighborhoods of Los Angeles, San Francisco, and Chicago, addicts have had to wait up to 6 weeks for placement in a treatment program;

in other cities the wait has been up to 6 months.[33] While they wait for treatment, IV drug abusers continue to inject drugs several times each day, increasing their risk of contracting and spreading HIV infection.

Increasing treatment services is an important goal, but it takes time. The president's commission estimated that funding alone could increase treatment capacity by about 20 percent; to go further will require building programs and a major effort to recruit and train new staff. In many communities, attempts to establish new drug treatment facilities have met with local resistance. Public health officials have spent countless hours explaining the need for new programs to local officials and residents.

Meanwhile, the spread of HIV continues. The prevalence of HIV infection among intravenous drug abusers remains relatively low in many U.S. cities, but researchers believe that this could change very rapidly. In Manhattan, blood samples collected over the years from IV drug abusers show that the prevalence of HIV infection rose to more than 40 percent within 3 years after the first antibody-positive sample was collected— today about 60 percent of addicts in New York City test positive. In Edinburgh, Scotland, HIV-seroprevalence levels among IV drug abusers rose to 50 percent within 2 years after the first seropositive sample. Seroprevalence levels among addicts in several Italian cities increased to 50 percent within 4 years after the first positive sample.[34]

To prevent similar patterns in other cities, public health specialists are combining expansion of drug abuse treatment with innovative prevention programs, such as ex-addict outreach activities and self-help groups. The ex-addicts teach current IV drug users how to sterilize their injection equipment and how to use condoms to prevent the spread of HIV to sexual partners. In some areas they dispense vouchers for immediate admission to detoxification programs. The purpose of the self-help groups is to build social support for risk-reduction measures; studies have shown that having acquaintances who try to protect themselves encourages self-protection.

The outreach workers also convey relevant information about current research. For example, Don C. Des Jarlais of the New York State Division of Substance Abuse Services and his coworkers recently conducted a study of the relationship between injection practices and T4 cell loss in IV drug abusers infected with HIV. Over a 9-month period they found that high frequencies of drug injection were associated with an increased loss of T4 cells. Des Jarlais concludes:

The observed relation between frequency of drug injection and T4 cell loss over a defined time period does not necessarily imply differences in ultimate outcomes of HIV infection. Nevertheless, it is clearly appropriate to warn IV drug users that continued drug injection may increase the immunosuppression that precedes development of AIDS. Reduced drug injection may thus protect the health of the HIV infected drug user as well as possibly reducing transmission to other IV drug users through shared drug injection equipment.[35]

In addition, current IV drug abusers are warned about the association between HIV infection and "non-AIDS" deaths. Several studies have shown that the appearance of HIV among IV drug users in New York City was accompanied by an "epidemic level" increase in deaths from a variety of infections not covered by the original CDC surveillance definition of AIDS— infections such as endocarditis (inflammation of cells lining the heart), nonpneumocystis pneumonia, and tuberculosis.

At the beginning of the epidemic many public health officials believed that risk-reduction education for intravenous drug abusers was unrealistic because the target population simply would not listen. But Des Jarlais and his coworkers found that as early as 1984 almost all IV drug abusers in New York City knew about AIDS and its transmission through shared injection equipment and that more than half reported behavior changes to reduce their risk of infection.[36] Concern over the disease produced an increased demand for "new" needles (not previously used for injecting illicit drugs). This demand, in turn, led to the selling of "resealed" needles—

sellers on the street put used, unsterilized needles back into their original wrappings, resealed them, and sold them again.[37]

The final option, the provision of sterile injection equipment, has been adopted quietly by some European countries, but in the United States the concept has aroused considerable controversy. After 3 years of debate, a small pilot program was approved by the state health commissioner of New York in March 1988.[38] The program will take addicts from the waiting lists of existing drug treatment programs and enroll them in a needle-exchange program. Each participant will receive a free sterile needle at a drug counseling session; used needles will be exchanged for new ones at subsequent meetings with a drug counselor. Returned needles will be analyzed to determine whether they have been used by more than one person.[39]

Opponents of the needle-exchange program express concern about the moral dilemma raised when government organizations provide the materials necessary to carry out an illegal act. They worry that programs that provide for continuing drug use may increase the number of addicts or discourage current IV drug users from entering treatment programs.

Des Jarlais says, however, that preliminary data from the Amsterdam needle exchange program and from bleach distribution programs in San Francisco and New York City "all indicate that providing for 'AIDS-safer injection' and treatment to reduce drug injection are complementary rather than contradictory."[40] Drug counselors have found that teaching IV drug users about the need to avoid HIV transmission has led many to decide to seek treatment for their drug problems. Future studies will determine whether the provision of sterile needles and syringes actually reduces the incidence of HIV infection.

Prevention of Heterosexual Spread of HIV Infection

Des Jarlais estimates that three-quarters of IV drug users in the United States are heterosexual males and that the great majority have their primary sexual relationship with a woman who does not inject drugs. Epidemiologic studies indicate that for women with AIDS sexual contact with such men is a risk factor second only to personal IV drug abuse. Among women who have acquired AIDS sexually, almost 5 times as many have been sexual partners of intravenous drug users as of bisexual men.[41]

The women at greatest risk of acquiring HIV infection through heterosexual intercourse are members of large inner-city minority groups. The CDC reports that AIDS occurs 11 to 13 times more often among black and Hispanic women than among white women.

Dramatic increases in the incidence of syphilis among heterosexuals in New York City, Los Angeles, and parts of Florida indicate that the people at risk of heterosexually acquired HIV infection have not adopted safer-sex practices. From 1986 to 1987 the incidence of syphilis in New York City more than doubled; in Los Angeles County it rose by almost 97 percent.[42]

The economic and cultural factors that place poor, inner-city women at risk of HIV infection also interfere with risk-reduction education and behavior change. Many of the women are poorly educated and have little power to alter the circumstances of their lives. The reluctance of such women to assert their own needs in sexual relationships (for example, to insist on the use of condoms) is discussed further in Chapter 8.

In 1987 the National Institute on Drug Abuse (NIDA) began funding a $3.4 million AIDS education project directed at low-income women at risk of HIV infection.[43] Model programs have begun in Los Angeles, Phoenix, and Boston. The goal of these programs is to train natural leaders in the community to provide risk-reduction education and support. Katie Portis, the coordinator of a NIDA-funded program in the Boston area, explains that the outreach workers will seek out women in laundromats, beauty parlors, and other natural gathering places; in addition, they will sponsor house parties with a safer-sex theme. The outreach workers also will help women who want HIV testing but are uncomfortable approaching the health care system on their own. The workers will accompany women to local test sites and help them understand and cope with test results.

A basic premise of the NIDA project is that intervention activities must be culturally specific. A risk-reduction message that is effective among American-born blacks in an inner-city neighborhood may not be meaningful to Haitian-born women in the same community. The Hispanic population in the United States is even more diverse. In Chicago, for example, the Hispanic population includes Mexican Americans, Puerto Ricans, immigrants from several different Central American countries, and immigrants from the Dominican Republic. Each ethnic group has unique social mores that can affect the willingness to accept a particular form of AIDS-related intervention.

Men at Risk Because of HIV-Infected Sexual Partners

The number of men in the United States with heterosexually acquired AIDS remains small (see Chapter 2). Most researchers believe, however, that it will increase as the number of HIV-infected women increases.

Scientists do not have enough data to estimate the number of heterosexual men who do not inject drugs themselves but have regular sexual partners who are IV drug abusers. For now, the only way to provide risk-reduction education for such men is through general public education in areas with a high incidence of HIV infection. The most important messages to convey are that vaginal transmission can occur from woman to man and that proper use of condoms can significantly reduce the risk of infection.

Heterosexual Prostitution as a Risk Factor

Prostitution increases the risk of HIV infection for both prostitutes and their clients; the risk per encounter depends in part on the cumulative incidence of AIDS among heterosexuals in the city or region where the encounter takes place. (Both the prostitute and the client are more likely to be infected in New York City, for example, than in a low-prevalence city such as Colorado Springs.)

A 1987 study conducted by the CDC and collaborators in 7 U.S. cities showed that the greatest risk factor for HIV infection among seropositive prostitutes was IV drug abuse. Half of the prostitutes reported a history of IV drug abuse, including 76 percent of those who were antibody positive. Failure to use condoms also appeared to increase risk. None of 22 prostitutes who reported using a condom with each vaginal exposure (with boyfriends or husbands as well as with clients) was seropositive, compared with 11 percent of those who had unprotected intercourse.[44]

State and local governments have taken a variety of approaches to reducing prostitution-related HIV infection. For example, Florida now requires convicted prostitutes to be tested for sexually transmitted diseases, including HIV infection. (It is a crime in Florida for people who know they have any venereal disease to engage in sexual intercourse.) In Newark, New Jersey, an ordinance requires antibody testing for anyone convicted of a prostitution-related offense—either a prostitute or a client. Some legal experts believe that such measures may be vulnerable to judicial challenge on equal protection grounds or on the grounds that they violate Fourth Amendment limitations on searches.[45]

The goal of programs to minimize prostitution-related HIV transmission should be to encourage counseling and testing of as many potentially infected women and men as possible. In California, the Prostitutes Education Program offers risk-reduction educational sessions on how to prevent HIV infection. Combining such programs with voluntary testing, therapy for drug addiction, medical care referrals, and vocational rehabilitation may produce the best long-term results.

The CDC recommends that prostitutes who are HIV-antibody positive be instructed to discontinue prostitution, and that "local or state jurisdictions . . . adopt procedures to assure that these instructions are followed" (see Appendix E).

Quarantine orders and other restrictive measures are discussed further below.

Sexual Partners of Hemophiliacs

The National Hemophilia Foundation produces a variety of educational materials about HIV infection for hemophiliacs, their families, and health care providers (these materials are available through local chapters or from the national office in New York City). Hemophiliacs and their sexual partners are urged to adopt practices that minimize the exchange of body fluids during sexual intercourse (use condoms) and to delay having children until more is known about the syndrome.

In September 1987 the National Hemophilia Foundation, the Hemophilia Treatment Centers, and the CDC reported the results of a nationwide study to determine whether the sexual partners of known HIV-positive hemophiliac patients were being tested for HIV antibody and the extent of seropositivity among those who had been tested. (The CDC recommends routine counseling and testing for such women.) The researchers found that only about one-third of the 2,276 sexual partners included in the study had been tested. Of those tested, 10 percent were infected with HIV. Twelve percent of the women had been pregnant during the 2 years before the study, including 22 women who were seropositive. The level of infection among the infants was not determined. According to CDC epidemiologist Janine Jason, these results suggest the need for improved counseling of the sexual partners of all hemophiliacs.[46]

Prevention of HIV Infection in Children

The only effective way to prevent HIV infection in children is to prevent HIV infection in women of childbearing age. Every encounter between a health care provider and a woman at risk of HIV infection should be viewed as an opportunity to provide risk-reduction education.

Since 1985 the definition of "woman at risk" has changed

considerably. The first CDC statement on preventing perinatal infection, issued in December of that year, recommended counseling and HIV testing for women in the following groups: (1) those who had evidence of HIV infection, (2) those who had used IV drugs for nonmedical purposes, (3) those who were born in a country where heterosexual transmission plays a major role in infection, (4) those who had engaged in prostitution, and (5) those who had been the sexual partner of a man at high risk of infection. Identifying such women depended on physician interviews and self-reporting.

Several studies of pregnant women in New York City have shown, however, that brief physician interviews in a busy outpatient setting may not be very successful at eliciting information about risk factors.[47] A significant number of women either do not want to admit to risk factors or are unaware of the risk status of their sexual partners. Rather than depend solely on interviews with a health care provider, the CDC now recommends counseling and voluntary testing for all women of childbearing age "living in communities . . . where there is a known or suspected high prevalence of infection among women."[48]

Counseling before Conception

The ideal time to counsel women about the risk of bearing an HIV-infected child is before conception occurs. Potential sites for counseling and testing include family planning clinics, gynecologic services, sexually transmitted disease clinics, methadone maintenance clinics, detoxification programs, and clinics that serve female prostitutes. (If confidentiality cannot be assured in such settings, women should be referred to established counseling and testing centers.)

Women who test positive or who believe that their sexual partners may be infected with HIV should be advised to delay pregnancy until more is known about transmission of HIV in the womb. But health care providers must understand the sensitive nature of such advice. Chapter 8 explores some of the social and personal factors that might interfere with a woman's ability to accept the constraints on childbearing imposed by HIV infection. Religious opposition to contraception also might prevent a woman from complying with current guidelines.

Efforts to promote family planning among inner-city minority populations have sometimes encountered resistance from community leaders because they were regarded as attempts to impose control on the size of minority populations. Widespread awareness of the suffering imposed by pediatric AIDS makes it unlikely that HIV-related childbearing recommendations would be opposed on similar grounds.

Counseling Early in Pregnancy

Early prenatal counseling and testing for HIV allows an infected woman to make an informed choice regarding continuation of her pregnancy. Between 25 and 50 percent of infants born to HIV-infected women also will be infected.

Health care workers report, however, that fewer than half of infected women who know their HIV status early enough to abort choose to do so. Some may be opposed to abortion on religious grounds. Others may believe that the odds of having a healthy child are worth the risk. In many cases, the decision to continue a high-risk pregnancy may be a form of denial—the woman copes with the diagnosis of HIV infection by ignoring it (see Chapter 8).

Physicians caring for HIV-infected women who elect to continue their pregnancies should be alert to the signs and symptoms of disease progression (although pregnancy itself does not appear to accelerate the progression of symptoms; see Chapter 2). Complaints such as "fatigue" and "loss of appetite," which may be dismissed in a normal pregnancy, should be investigated carefully. They may be the first signs of an HIV-related opportunistic infection. If such an infection develops, physicians must weigh the benefits of existing therapies against the potential risks to the fetus.[49]

Pregnant women infected with HIV often require a tremendous amount of psychosocial support, regardless of their disease status. Obstetricians should become familiar with support services available in their communities.

Counseling of infected women also must address the possibility of HIV infection in older children (who might have been infected in earlier pregnancies), the risks to sexual partners, and the likelihood of infection in future pregnancies. Antibody testing should be offered as soon as possible to the pregnant woman's sexual partner and other offspring.[50]

Delivery and Postpartum Care

Maternal HIV infection should not affect labor and delivery if the mother is otherwise well. There is no evidence at this time that the mode of delivery (vaginal or caesarean section) alters the rate of virus transmission from mother to child. Scientists recommend, however, that an effort be made to avoid direct contact between the mother's vaginal secretions and fetal blood. Thus, the use of scalp electrodes to monitor fetal heart rate and fetal blood sampling during labor (which involves inserting a needle into the fetal scalp) should be avoided.[51]

Specific infection control measures should be followed during all deliveries, whether or not the mother is infected with HIV. This includes the use of protective eyewear and water-repellent gowns and gloves. Caregivers handling the baby should continue to wear gloves until all maternal secretions have been removed from the skin.

Breastfeeding is not recommended for HIV-infected mothers in the United States, although breast milk probably is not a major mode of transmission from mother to child. A few cases of HIV transmission through breast milk have been reported in Australia, France, and Zaire. Infants who were nursed by their mothers developed AIDS in the absence of other risk factors—the mothers were infected by blood transfusions administered following delivery.[52] HIV has been isolated both from the fluid portion of breast milk and from blood monocytes transmitted in the milk.

After birth, both mother and child should be followed

carefully by physicians experienced in the treatment of HIV-related diseases.

Prevention of HIV Transmission in Health Care Settings

Chapter 2 describes the very small but definite risk of HIV transmission in health care settings. As of April 1988, 15 health care workers worldwide, including 11 in the United States, had been infected with HIV through documented occupational exposures.

Clinical Care

The CDC now recommends that health care workers (including emergency response personnel) treat blood and other body fluids from *all* patients as potentially infectious (see Appendix D), in contrast to early recommendations, which emphasized precautions for persons perceived to be at risk of AIDS.

Several factors contributed to this change. In May 1987 James Baker and his coworkers at the Johns Hopkins Hospital in Baltimore examined anonymous blood samples from 203 emergency room patients with no history of HIV infection. They found that 6 of the patients were seropositive. All had been trauma victims who were actively bleeding at the time of admission. Two of the seropositive patients had been intravenous drug abusers, but the authors report that a history of intravenous drug abuse was not discriminating in identifying patients who might be infected with HIV.[53]

One week after the Baker study appeared, CDC officials reported that 3 health care workers in different parts of the country had apparently been infected through non-needlestick injuries. In all cases the skin of the health care worker had come into direct contact with blood from an infected patient, and all had skin lesions that may have been contaminated by blood. One also had infected blood splattered into her mouth. At the time of exposure, only one of the 3 suspected that the patient involved might be infected with HIV.[54] In contrast,

more than 2,000 reported skin and mucous-membrane exposures to body fluids of AIDS patients at the National Institutes
of Health have not resulted in any cases of HIV transmission.[55]

The best way to prevent HIV transmission in health care
settings is to make sure that everyone—including students and
trainees—who comes into contact with blood and other body
fluids understands and practices "universal precautions." On
July 23, 1987, the Occupational Safety and Health Administration, a branch of the Department of Labor, announced that
it would begin fining hospitals that do not protect their
employees from occupational exposure to HIV, hepatitis B
virus, and other bloodborne infections.[56] Protection includes
providing an initial orientation and continuing education
about the prevention of bloodborne infections, providing
equipment and supplies necessary to minimize the risk of
infection, and monitoring adherence to recommended protective measures (see Appendix D).

Routine HIV screening of hospital patients. Some physicians and
other health care personnel have called for routine screening of
all hospital patients; others have proposed HIV screening for
specific groups of patients (for example, those undergoing
elective surgery) to minimize risk to health care providers.[57]

Opponents of such testing worry that it would give
health care workers a false sense of security. People who have
been recently exposed to HIV may test negative on standard
antibody tests for a period of weeks to months (see Chapter 2).
If health care workers failed to follow strict precautions based
on a patient's negative antibody test, they might be increasing
their risk of exposure to the virus.

Also, existing tests have a relatively high false-positive
rate in populations with a low risk of infection. Michael Hagen
and his coworkers in the Division of Clinical Decision Making
at Tufts University School of Medicine suggest that the social
costs of labeling uninfected people "seropositive" may be
much higher than the benefits of routine testing in a hospital
setting.[58]

Good medical practice requires that all patients be evaluated for risk factors for HIV infection through careful history taking (including sexual history). If a patient's history indicates that he or she has one or more recognized risk factors for HIV infection, the patient should be counseled about the advisability of an HIV test—how knowledge of the test result improves patient management—and provided with appropriate risk-reduction information. Patient consent to the test should be documented in the medical record. Seropositive patients should receive further counseling from properly trained staff. (Hospital personnel perform a valuable public health service if they also reinforce risk-reduction messages when they convey negative test results.) All staff members should continue to follow universal precautions regardless of the HIV status of patients.

The Centers for Disease Control says that hospitals that decide to institute routine testing of any patient group also should ensure (1) that confidentiality safeguards are in place to limit knowledge of test results to those directly involved in the care of the infected patients or as required by law, and (2) that identification of infected patients will not result in denial of needed care or provision of suboptimal care.

Infected health care workers. No reports exist of HIV transmission to patients from infected health care workers, but transmission during invasive procedures (such as surgery) remains a possibility. According to the Council on Ethical and Judicial Affairs of the American Medical Association, "a physician who knows that he or she is seropositive should not engage in any activity that creates a risk of transmission of the disease to others."[59] It also recommends that a physician who is seropositive or who has AIDS should consult colleagues about which activities he or she can pursue without creating a risk to patients.

Clinical Laboratory

The recommendation to assume that blood and body fluids from all patients are potentially infectious also extends to the clinical laboratory. In the past, health care workers were advised to place "biohazard" labels on specimens they believed might contain HIV or hepatitis B virus. A recent study suggests, however, that the use of such labels may actually increase the risk of infection of health care workers.

H. Hunter Handsfield and his coworkers at Harborview Medical Center in Seattle examined more than 500 blood samples that were about to be discarded in the hospital's clinical laboratories. They found that 1.1 percent of specimens without a "biohazard" label contained HIV antibodies. Handsfield and his colleagues expressed concern that a two-tiered system (distinguishing between "safe" and "unsafe" specimens) could cause laboratory workers to become complacent about the handling of unlabeled specimens—they might be less likely to wear gloves, for example. To avoid such complacency, the Seattle researchers concluded that biohazard labeling should not be employed and that all specimens should be handled with equal precautions. [60]

Research Laboratories

In 1987 public health officials reported that 2 laboratory workers had become infected with HIV after handling culture materials containing very high concentrations of the virus. Both workers were employed in so-called high-containment laboratories (Biosafety Level 3) under contract with the National Institutes of Health.

Molecular analysis of HIV-1 isolates derived from the blood of the first worker demonstrated that he was infected with the same strain of virus he had been handling in the laboratory. [61] The worker did not recall any episode of direct skin exposure to the virus—he always wore gloves and standard cloth laboratory gowns—but he did report frequent spills of contaminated material that could have resulted in unrecognized exposures (potentially contaminated gloves may not always have been changed in accordance with biosafety guidelines). The second worker probably was infected when he cut his gloved finger with a blunt needle while cleaning contaminated equipment.[62]

Biosafety officials who investigated the incidents believe that existing biosafety measures are adequate but that "workers need to adhere to them more strictly."[63] In January 1988, Stanley H. Weiss of New Jersey Medical School and his colleagues proposed that routine, periodic testing for HIV-1 be incorporated into laboratory safety programs for researchers working with concentrated virus. They emphasized that such testing "must be done in an environment that protects the privacy of the worker and, through legal means, protects the worker from discrimination in the workplace."[64]

Risk-Reduction Education for the General Population

The incidence of HIV infection in the general population has remained extremely low. This fact is encouraging, but it also means that it may be harder to make people pay attention to risk-reduction information. A young heterosexual adult who has never met a person with AIDS or known of a case in his circle of friends may question the need to adopt safer-sex practices, even if he understands the ways in which HIV is transmitted.

Another factor that complicates information and education efforts for the general population is that different audiences require very different types of materials. A parent who is worried about the presence of a child with AIDS in the local elementary school, for example, has concerns different from those of the sexually active high school or college student.

The U.S. Public Health Service (PHS) has produced guidelines advising communities how to deal with HIV infection in the classroom (Appendix G) and in the workplace (Appendix H). Both sets of guidelines stress that HIV is not spread by the types of nonsexual, person-to-person contacts likely to occur in schools, offices, and factories. In general, elementary school children and adolescents with AIDS whose physicians believe they are well enough to attend school should be permitted to do so without restrictions. The PHS guidelines recommend that decisions about school attendance be made by using the team approach—including the child's physician and parent or guardian, public health personnel, and personnel associated with the proposed care or educational setting.

Infected preschool-age children and older children with HIV infection who for some reason are unable to control their body secretions, are prone to biting, or have open sores may pose a risk to others. These children should be placed in more restricted school or day care settings. The PHS recommendations provide special guidelines for persons caring for these children (Appendix G). All schools and day-care facilities should adopt routine procedures for handling blood and other body fluids whether or not children with HIV are enrolled.

There is no evidence of transmission of HIV infection in personal service settings such as barbershops and beauty salons. Workers in these fields are advised, however, that transmission theoretically could occur in the highly unlikely event that copious amounts of blood from a person infected with HIV came into contact with an open wound in another person.

Services such as ear piercing and tattooing that involve intentional breakage of the skin may involve a small risk of infection if needles and other tools are not sterilized properly. Clients should assess the cleanliness of the establishments in which these services are provided and should ask about sterilization practices before undergoing the procedures.

Fear of HIV infection has led some people to postpone health care procedures such as dental surgery and eye examinations. Although there is no evidence to date that the virus has been transmitted through medical instruments, the CDC has issued guidelines to ensure that all personnel in these areas understand and follow proper sterilization techniques. These techniques completely eliminate the risk of transmission of HIV from one patient to another.

Donating Blood

Concern about HIV infection also has led some surgical patients to insist upon choosing their own blood donors from among family and friends. Such designated donation is provided by the American Red Cross and by the other major voluntary blood-donor organizations. Several studies have shown, however, that the incidence of HIV infection among designated donors is no different from that among volunteer blood donors; in fact there has been concern that family pressure to donate blood for a sick relative may lead some people to ignore their high-risk status and donate blood when they would not do so otherwise. Donor screening and routine testing of all donated blood and blood products for HIV antibodies have reduced the risk of transfusion-associated AIDS to very low levels.

A common misconception, which arose after the discovery of transfusion-associated AIDS, was that people could contract AIDS by donating blood. It is impossible to get AIDS by giving blood because in this country a new, sterilized needle and collection set are used for each donor and discarded afterward.

AIDS Education in Schools

Over the long term, the best way to stop the spread of HIV infection will be to reduce the development of behavior that leads to transmission of the virus. AIDS education should begin before young people start engaging in risky sexual practices or taking drugs.

By February 1988, 18 states and the District of Columbia had laws mandating education about AIDS in the public schools.[65] The laws vary widely, ranging from simple statements that local school boards must implement some form of AIDS education to highly specific instructions about the content of that education.

According to the CDC's 1988 "Guidelines for Effective School Health Education to Prevent the Spread of AIDS," the "specific scope and content of AIDS education in schools should be locally determined and should be consistent with parental and community values."[66] Most educators agree that the success of an AIDS education program depends on support from parents and community leaders, but in some cases state involvement may be necessary to get an education project moving. Katherine Fraser, codirector of the AIDS education project at the National Association of State Boards of Education, recently told a reporter: "In a lot of instances, state requirements are resented and are counterproductive. But [in] this . . . case . . . many local boards are facing opposition in their communities and they're looking to the state for a requirement. They want to go back to the community and say, 'Look, this is something we're required to do. Let's figure out how.' "[67]

Reaching Adolescents

The CDC guidelines also recommend that deliberations about the need for and content of AIDS education consider the prevalence of behavior that increases the risk of HIV infection among young people.

Conservative educators and policymakers say that AIDS education in the schools should focus on the moral grounds for refraining from sex before marriage. They believe that specific guidelines on how to practice safer sex or avoid drug-related infections simply encourages socially unacceptable behavior.

Past experience suggests, however, that admonitions to "just say no" to sex or drugs probably will not be very effective at reducing the transmission of HIV. Despite extensive programs urging adolescent girls to refrain from sex, U.S. teenagers have one of the highest pregnancy rates in the developed world. In addition, approximately 2.5 million U.S. teenagers contract a sexually transmitted disease each year.

Recent surveys of AIDS-related knowledge and behavior among adolescents indicate that many teens are still misinformed or confused about HIV infection. For example, a random-sample survey of 860 adolescents (16 to 19 years of age) in Massachusetts found that 8 percent did not know that AIDS is transmitted by heterosexual intercourse. Seventy percent of the teens interviewed reported being sexually active, but only 15 percent reported changing their sexual behavior because of concern about contracting AIDS. Of those who had made changes, only 20 percent reported using condoms or abstaining from sex. Lee Strunin and Ralph Hingson of Boston University School of Public Health, who conducted the Massachusetts study, say that 54 percent of those questioned indicated they did not worry about contracting AIDS.[68] This finding is disturbing because previous studies have shown that people who lack a sense of vulnerability are unlikely to change health-related behaviors. Relatively few cases of AIDS have been diagnosed among teenagers, but researchers believe that a substantial portion of AIDS cases occurring in people between 20 and 29 years of age actually resulted from infections acquired during the teen years (because of the long incubation period between HIV infection and the development of symptoms).

A San Francisco study suggests that misperceptions about a partner's willingness to use condoms also limit safer-sex practices among adolescents. Susan Kegeles and her coworkers at the University of California School of Medicine at San Francisco found that adolescent girls were uncertain about their partners' desires regarding condom use when, in reality, adolescent boys were quite positive about using them.[69]

Parents and educators should teach young people that the only completely effective way to avoid HIV infection is to abstain from sex and intravenous drugs, but they also should make sure that adolescents who choose to experiment are not risking their lives because of lack of information. Adolescents must have accurate knowledge about HIV transmission and about effective risk-reduction measures. Behavioral research indicates that intervention programs also may have to alter perceptions about personal vulnerability and provide teens with the social skills necessary to communicate AIDS-related concerns to their peers.

Homosexual adolescents.   The adolescents at greatest risk of sexually transmitted HIV infection are young men who engage in unprotected homosexual intercourse. Some communities that are willing to provide explicit risk-reduction information for heterosexual adolescents in the classroom may be unwilling to do the same for homosexual adolescents.

Most cities now have special community agencies that provide confidential AIDS-related counseling and testing. If all adolescents are made aware of such agencies, those who have questions beyond those raised in the school setting can get the answers they need.

Programs on college campuses.   The level of AIDS education and prevention services on college campuses varies widely. In 1987 Barbara Ann Caruso and John Haig conducted a survey of directors of student health services at 47 colleges in the Philadelphia area to determine (1) their judgment of how campus AIDS programs should be run and (2) their institution's current activities related to AIDS. More than half of the 37 responding colleges already had established coordinated AIDS-related activities, but only one third had adjusted their counseling services to meet the needs of those who perceived themselves to be at high risk of infection. Moreover, only 4 had conducted special AIDS training sessions for staff, and only 1 had budgeted funds for new personnel.

Caruso and Haig concluded that "academic institutions must be encouraged to address AIDS with the attention and resources necessitated by any public health crisis."[70] Options available for AIDS-related education on college campuses include discussion sessions led by peer counselors (trained by the college health center), symposia involving outside speakers, and frequent AIDS-related articles in campus periodicals.

Colleges also can provide specific services to promote risk reduction. Many schools have approved the sale of condoms in bookstores, health centers, and dormitory vending machines. Some colleges offer confidential HIV testing, but most prefer to refer students to off-campus testing sites in the community.

David W. Fraser, president of Swarthmore College in Pennsylvania, says that continuing assessment of AIDS education programs is essential if such programs are to achieve their goal of helping students make informed decisions. College staff should monitor students' reactions to specific programs and expand or modify them as needs change and new topics arise.[71]

Government Initiatives: Beyond Voluntary Measures

The March 1986 PHS recommendations for reducing the risk of HIV transmission focus primarily on education and voluntary testing, but they also express support for state and local actions to regulate or close establishments "where there is evidence that they facilitate high-risk behaviors, such as anonymous sexual contacts and/or intercourse with multiple partners or IV drug abuse (e.g., bathhouses, houses of prostitution, 'shooting galleries')."[72]

This statement of support reflects the fact that potential public health measures cover a wide spectrum of activities —from general education and voluntary testing and counseling to mandatory testing and various forms of quarantine. As measures become more restrictive, public health officials face increasingly difficult decisions regarding the balance between a state's right to protect the health of its citizens and the fundamental civil rights of an infected individual.

Mandatory Screening

In his first speech devoted exclusively to the topic of AIDS, on May 31, 1987, President Ronald Reagan urged states to "offer routine testing for those who seek marriage licenses," called for mandatory HIV testing of federal prisoners, and announced plans to add AIDS to the list of contagious diseases for which immigrants and aliens can be denied access to the United States.[73]

Controversy over mandatory testing has been widespread since the beginning of the epidemic. Some people have called for mandatory screening of the entire U.S. population while others, like President Reagan, have favored screening of selected subgroups. Opponents of mandatory testing believe that the social costs far outweigh the benefits, except in the case of blood, organ, and tissue donors. In its 1986 report *Confronting AIDS*, the Institute of Medicine said:

Mandatory screening of the entire U.S. population for HIV infection would be impossible to justify now on either ethical or practical grounds. Mandatory screening of selected subgroups of the population—for example, homosexual males, IV drug users, prostitutes, prisoners, or pregnant women—raises serious problems of ethics and feasibility. People whose private behavior is illegal are not likely to comply with a mandatory screening program, even one backed by assurances of confidentiality. Mandatory screening based on sexual orientation would appear to discriminate against or to coerce entire groups without justification.[74]

Premarital screening. The problems inherent in widespread screening of populations at low risk of HIV infection are best illustrated by the experience in Illinois with premarital testing. On January 1, 1988, the state of Illinois began requiring applicants for a marriage license to provide proof that they had undergone an HIV antibody test. Immediately, the number of marriage licenses issued in the state began to drop. Surveys of county clerks in adjacent states indicated that many Illinois couples were opting for out-of-state weddings.

Opponents of premarital HIV testing believe that it is based on an unrealistic view of marriage in today's society. The rationale for the concept is that it prevents the infection of unsuspecting spouses and potential offspring. But marriage is no longer a precursor to sexual activity or even to childbearing. Most couples who marry already have been sexual partners for some time. In New York City, which has the highest incidence of pediatric HIV infection in the country, 83 percent of children with AIDS have been born to unwed mothers.

In October 1987 Paul Cleary and his associates at the Harvard School of Public Health estimated that universal premarital screening in the United States would detect fewer than 0.1 percent of HIV-infected individuals at a cost of substantially more than $100 million.[75] Critics of premarital testing laws also have expressed concern about the potential for false-positive results in screening populations with a very low prevalence of infection (see Appendix C).

State Representative Barbara Flynn Currie, who has sponsored one of many bills to repeal the Illinois law, says that the cost of uncovering one case of HIV infection through mandatory premarital testing in Illinois is about $50,000.[76] She and others believe that this money could be better spent in other AIDS prevention and treatment programs.

An alternative to mandatory premarital testing that might have similar benefits but much lower costs is to provide all people considering marriage with information about AIDS, HIV infection, and the availability of counseling and testing.

The military. Some people who oppose mandatory screening in the civilian population accept its application in the military services. Blood tests have been used to screen out new recruits with HIV antibodies since the fall of 1985; testing of all active-duty personnel and those serving in the National Guard and reserves was begun in 1986.

Military sources state that these actions are necessary to ensure the continued strength of the armed forces; to ensure that personnel in combat areas are available to provide transfusions for an injured comrade without the risk of transmitting HIV infection; to protect the health of those whose natural defense mechanisms have been compromised by infection with HIV; and to protect the sexual partners of military personnel in other countries. They note that recruits with weakened immune systems might have severe adverse reactions to the numerous immunizations required for military service. In addition, those who carry the virus might be more susceptible to tropical diseases encountered during overseas assignments.

The decision to initiate widespread screening led to general confusion within the services about what should be done with those who test positive. The activities most often associated with transmission of the virus, homosexuality and drug abuse, are considered grounds for dismissal without benefits by all branches of the military. Department of Defense guidelines make it clear, however, that the services cannot use a positive HIV-antibody test result as a basis for deciding that an individual has engaged in these activities (although they do not prohibit investigation of the possible cause of the presence of the antibodies).

In general, the services have decided that people who test positive and have signs of disease will be processed for medical disability. Those who have evidence of exposure but appear clinically normal will be retained in the military, though with assignment limitations (including no overseas duty and ineligibility for sensitive, stressful jobs).[77] Individual rulings could be affected, however, by evidence of misconduct (that is, homosexuality or drug abuse) independent of the medical evaluation.

Spokesmen for homosexuals have criticized the military screening program on several grounds. They believe that the underlying purpose of testing for exposure to HIV is to identify homosexuals in the armed forces, and that the decision barring recruits who test positive but are otherwise healthy is designed primarily to avoid the costs of caring for these individuals if they should become sick. The provision for limited duty has been viewed as a threat to career advancement for individuals who had planned to spend their entire adult lives in the military.

A more general concern, however, has been that the military's decision would encourage other large organizations to implement similar screening programs. Since January 1, 1987, the Department of State has been testing its own employees and dependents over the age of 15 prior to overseas assignments. In March 1987 the Department of Labor began testing all incoming Job Corps members assigned to residential positions, and in June the Federal Bureau of Prisons began screening all incoming and outgoing federal prisoners. In addition, all immigrants and refugees seeking permanent residence in the United States must be tested for HIV infection.[78]

Legal restraints and an appreciation of the benefits of voluntary as opposed to mandatory testing have kept most institutions in the private sector from following the government's lead. If educational programs fail to effect widespread behavioral change, however, proponents of mandatory screening may become more vocal. Society as a whole must decide whether the health needs of the community justify the infringement on civil liberties associated with such measures.

Quarantine

Concern over civil liberties looms larger as communities across the country seek to reactivate local quarantine laws. Before the development of antibiotics and other wonders of modern medicine, these laws were important tools in the battle against infectious disease. Many older people still remember the starkly lettered signs on the door that warned of diphtheria or whooping cough in a household.

Unlike these other diseases, however, AIDS is not transmitted through casual contact; the types of behavior that spread the syndrome are well understood. AIDS patients and others who know they are infected with HIV and who comply with public health guidelines about transmission of the virus present no danger to the community. Quarantining individuals simply because they are infected with HIV would be totally unnecessary and unjustified, as well as impractical. It would mean quarantining more than a million people for life.

Legal restraints may be necessary, however, for those few people who continue high-risk behaviors without regard for the health of others. This issue has arisen primarily with respect to prostitutes who refuse to leave the streets. Female prostitutes have been quarantined in California, Nevada, and Florida. In one case, a Florida judge confined a female prostitute with AIDS to her home and enforced the order by requiring her to wear an electronic bracelet that would alert police if she strayed too far from the monitoring device placed in her telephone.[79]

The use of quarantine laws to slow the spread of HIV infection raises many ethical, moral, and legal questions. For example, at what point should educational efforts give way to restrictive measures such as house arrest? Does society have a responsibility to provide for those who are confined as a result of quarantine laws? What is society's responsibility to those who knowingly engage in sexual intercourse with prostitutes? What is the likelihood that even the very limited use of quarantine laws would dissuade other potentially infected individuals from seeking counseling and testing?

States must have the authority to act against those who would willfully endanger others, but they should use the authority only when efforts to obtain voluntary compliance have failed. In addition, the measure proposed should be the least restrictive alternative available and should be applied only through legal steps assuring due process.

Conclusion

Public health measures to fight HIV infection consist of a wide range of options, including general education, specific education for those at high risk of infection, voluntary testing and counseling, partner notification, mandatory reporting of test results, mandatory screening, regulations to close establishments associated with high-risk behavior, and various forms of quarantine.

Public health officials continue to place greatest emphasis on voluntary measures to reduce high-risk behavior. Efforts to increase general awareness of risk-reduction measures have been relatively successful, but it appears that many people are not using the information they have. Researchers need to learn more about the factors that motivate behavior change, especially with regard to sexual activity and drug abuse. Studies in other fields indicate that effective education programs must be highly specific and must create a supportive social environment for those willing to change.

An important element of current prevention programs is to encourage as many potentially infected people as possible to seek counseling and voluntary testing. Such programs will be most successful if state and local authorities strengthen measures to assure confidentiality and to protect records from unauthorized disclosure. Several states have reexamined protections afforded to all types of health records. Federal and state lawmakers also are evaluating legislation to prevent discrimination against those who are infected or perceived to be at risk of HIV infection.

The development of reasonable and equitable approaches to the AIDS crisis will require the involvement of government officials at all levels, business leaders, educators, health care professionals, and all others concerned with balancing the needs of the community against those of individuals.

developed symptoms). The ultimate impact of antiviral drugs on the HIV epidemic in the United States may depend on whether society can devise new ways to help patients pay for them.

The need for low-cost, oral drugs is even more urgent in developing countries. In some parts of the world, however, lifelong therapy with antiviral drugs may never be feasible. (The cost of a single day of AZT therapy exceeds the annual per capita health care expenditure in many countries.) Public health education will slow the spread of HIV, as would an effective cure, but the major hope for complete eradication of the disease is widespread immunization.

Recent attempts at vaccine development have been discouraging. Scientists have tried all the "obvious" solutions —solutions based on experience with other types of viral infections—and none of them has worked. Potential vaccines have failed to protect laboratory animals from viral challenges. Despite these results, several vaccine candidates have been approved for human safety trials (phase 1) in the United States and elsewhere.

Drug Development

Since the discovery of HIV, patient advocacy groups have grown increasingly vocal about what they perceive as "foot-dragging" on the part of government officials and others involved in the design, testing, and licensure of potential therapeutic agents. During the early years of the epidemic, the federal government devoted most of its AIDS budget to basic research on the natural history of HIV infection. (In fact, much of what is now known about the structure and life cycle of HIV has resulted from those federally sponsored activities.) The federal agencies responsible for drug development sometimes lacked the resources necessary to respond immediately to new leads. Projects were delayed by staffing problems, difficulties in obtaining experimental drugs, and confusion over who should take responsibility for particular projects.

Enormous efforts by administrators and scientists at the

National Institutes of Health and the Food and Drug Administration (FDA) have resolved some of these issues. The agencies have established new programs to screen existing agents for potency against HIV, organized a nationwide network of medical institutions to conduct clinical trials, streamlined the evaluation process leading to licensure, and formalized procedures to allow very ill patients to obtain drugs before clinical trials have been completed.

Scientists in the Preclinical AIDS Drug Development Program at the National Cancer Institute (NCI), who participated in the development of AZT, now have the capability to screen up to 20,000 compounds per year for specific anti-HIV activity. They are testing compounds from NCI's own repository of 500,000 synthetic chemicals and natural products, as well as substances developed by industry and by the National Cooperative Drug Discovery Groups.

The National Institute of Allergy and Infectious Diseases (NIAID) started the National Cooperative Drug Discovery Group Program in 1986 to stimulate new ideas in AIDS therapy. The first 16 groups, each headed by a university-based principal investigator, include participants from more than 60 independent academic, industrial, and government laboratories. Castanospermine and dideoxycytidine (ddC) are among the compounds developed through this program.

The government also has taken an active role in establishing facilities for clinical trials of AIDS drugs. NIAID supports 35 AIDS Clinical Trial Units (ACTUs) in medical centers in 15 states and the District of Columbia.[2] The ACTUs have enrolled several thousand patients in carefully designed clinical studies. Administrators of the program work closely with industry representatives to minimize duplication. They also try to ensure that all promising agents receive adequate attention.

The FDA, one of the most frequent targets of criticism among those dissatisfied with the pace of drug development in AIDS, has given all potential AIDS drugs a 1-AA classification—the highest possible priority in the drug review system. The role of the FDA is misunderstood by many people in this country. It is responsible for making sure that drugs marketed in the United States meet established standards of safety and efficacy, but it does not initiate or conduct clinical trials on its own. The FDA reviews the design and outcome of studies performed by drug sponsors. The sponsor for a particular drug may be a pharmaceutical manufacturer, a government agency (such as NIAID), or another type of research organization.

If laboratory and animal studies indicate that a drug has the potential to suppress or inactivate an infective agent without damaging healthy tissues, the drug sponsor requests permission from the FDA to begin the first of 3 phases of clinical trials. (This procedure involves filing an investigational new drug application, or IND.) Phase 1 studies usually involve between 20 and 100 volunteers. The goals are to establish the drug's safety in human beings and to begin determination of appropriate dose levels and routes of administration.

In phase 2 trials researchers gather additional information about possible adverse effects and begin to assess a drug's clinical potential. A recent FDA publication explains that most phase 2 studies are randomized, controlled trials. A group of patients receiving the drug, a "treatment" group, is matched with a group that is similar in important respects, such as age, sex, and disease state (factors that could affect the course of the disease or the effect of the investigational drug). The second, or "control," group receives a standard treatment or a placebo (an inert substance). Many phase 2 studies are double blind —that is, neither the patients nor the researchers know who is getting the experimental drug. Double-blind studies help reduce errors in interpretation caused by unwarranted enthusiasm or other forms of bias.

Phase 3 clinical trials involve many more patients— several hundred to several thousand. The larger trials allow researchers to acquire more information about efficacy and to identify some of the less common side effects associated with an experimental drug.

If the results of all three phases of clinical trials are favorable and the sponsor decides it wants to market a drug, it files a new drug application (NDA) with the FDA. The FDA reviews all relevant data to determine whether the benefits of the proposed therapy outweigh the risks for the drug's intended target population. If the benefit–risk ratio is acceptable, the drug is approved for marketing.

The time allotted for FDA review of an IND is 30 days, but agency administrators have pledged to review AIDS-related INDs in only 5 days. The average NDA review takes about 2 years; AZT was approved in less than 4 months. FDA Administrator Frank Young explains that one reason for the rapid approval of AZT was that FDA scientists had an opportunity to work closely with the drug's sponsor from the very beginning of the development process. (Early and consistent communication between FDA officials and drug sponsors is expected to play a central role in new administrative and legislative proposals to improve the drug approval process.)

Clinical Trials

Even with the 1-AA priority and the operational changes made by the FDA, the minimum time required for the development of future AIDS drugs probably will be 2 to 3 years. Many HIV-infected patients believe that this is too long. They question the need for formal clinical trials when thousands of patients are dying for lack of effective medications.

Physicians answer that prospective clinical trials are the only way to obtain definitive information about the relative risks and benefits of new therapies. Well-designed studies prevent people from wasting precious time and money on remedies that are ineffective and perhaps also dangerous.

Gerald Friedland, a professor at Albert Einstein College of Medicine in New York City and a clinician who has treated hundreds of AIDS patients, uses two examples to describe the importance of clinical trials in AIDS therapy. The first involves suramin, a drug employed widely in Africa to treat various parasitic diseases (trypanosomiasis and onchocerciasis). In 1979 Belgian researcher Erik De Clercq reported that suramin inhibited animal retroviruses in the test tube. Subsequent in vitro studies against HIV looked promising. But early clinical trials revealed that suramin was too toxic for use in AIDS patients. In some it caused adrenal insufficiency, and in others it appeared to increase the progression of HIV-related diseases.

Friedland's second example involves alpha interferon, a natural substance that inhibits the replication of many RNA and DNA viruses. The New York physician participated in an AIDS clinical trial comparing 2 different doses of alpha interferon and a placebo. He says that the vast majority of patients who received interferon appeared to experience adverse reactions from the drug. However, when clinical abnormalities in the study group were compared with clinical abnormalities in the control group the differences were not statistically significant. In other words, many of the problems that clinicians had attributed to the drug were actually caused by the disease. Without the placebo control, the effects of interferon might have been seriously misjudged.

These cases demonstrate several important points. First, there is no guarantee that a drug that looks safe and effective in the test tube will work in patients. The FDA recently determined that only 21 percent of all drugs submitted for IND evaluation make it through all 3 phases of clinical trials and the premarket evaluation. Fifty-seven percent are screened out along the way for reasons of safety or efficacy. (The remaining 22 percent are discontinued by their sponsors for "commercial" reasons.)

The second point is that every disease creates a unique set of circumstances. An antimicrobial drug that has an acceptable benefit-risk ratio for patients with one disease may be totally unacceptable for patients with another disease. This is especially true if short-term use of the drug suffices in one case but is not sufficient to eradicate disease in the other.

Groups of patients with the same disease also may respond differently to therapeutic drugs. Age, sex, disease severity, and even socioeconomic factors such as nutrition may affect the way a drug behaves in the body. Most of the clinical trials of AIDS drugs have been conducted in homosexual men. Recently, many scientists have expressed concern that the results of such trials might not be applicable to the growing population of HIV-infected intravenous drug abusers. The latter tend to have more concurrent infections and other characteristics that could alter their ability to tolerate new therapies.

Similarly, drugs found to be effective in adults cannot automatically be approved for use in children, because differences in organ size and metabolism may have an enormous impact on toxicity. In some cases children can tolerate drugs better than adults, but these cases can be identified only through very careful clinical trials.

The interferon story illustrates a third critical point. AIDS is an extremely complex disease involving multiple organ systems. Anecdotal reports of drug efficacy and toxicity are very difficult to interpret. Symptoms wax and wane, often for no apparent reason. Without controlled clinical trials it is impossible to distinguish between disease symptoms and drug-related effects or to determine accurately the relative merits of drug candidates.

Thomas Fleming, professor of biostatistics at the University of Washington, explains that a clinical trial should be designed to meet 3 basic requirements: it should be acceptable on ethical grounds, it should allow unbiased or fair evaluation, and it should be as efficient as possible.

To meet these requirements researchers must answer many complex questions: Should the study be placebo-controlled? How many patients should be included? What should the entry criteria be? What dosage levels are appropriate? What must the patients know before they can give informed consent? How long should the study last? How should physicians define a positive response or an adverse effect? How will adverse effects be distinguished from disease progression? What criteria should a safety monitoring board use to stop the study early?

Defining a positive response is critical in AIDS research. Most AIDS-related research protocols require that physicians monitor the effects of an experimental therapy on the quantity and activity of a patient's immune cells. Patients sometimes misinterpret this attention to laboratory measurements and place unreasonable emphasis on indications of biologic activity, such as a change in the number of circulating T4 lymphocytes.

The goal of clinical studies is to measure clinical efficacy —appropriate outcome measures include delayed progression of disease, increased survival time, pain relief, or improved quality of life. Several early drug candidates produced changes in immune function but did not produce clinical improvement. In contrast, AZT prolongs survival in some patients but does not produce a consistent increase in T4 cells.

Patient participation.   After fulfilling all the requirements necessary to begin a clinical trial, some researchers have had trouble finding suitable volunteers. The issue of patient participation has grown increasingly complex. Patient advocacy groups say that thousands of patients who wish to participate in trials cannot do so, because there are not enough trials available. On the other hand, some trials are stalled by a lack of participants. Part of the problem is geographic—the studies are conducted primarily at medical centers in major urban areas—but there are other issues as well.

In December 1987 reporter Philip Boffey interviewed dozens of people to determine why a study considered by many to be the most important AIDS-related clinical trial in the United States—a placebo-controlled trial of AZT in people with asymptomatic HIV infection—was behind schedule. After identifying a variety of bureacratic and other problems, Boffey added: "There is also, ironically, a reluctance on the part of many AIDS virus carriers to enter the trial, either because they fear they will not get the drug in a random trial or else they fear the toxicity of AZT."[3]

This ambivalence is understandable given the uncertainty surrounding HIV infection. Patients are frustrated and confused. One of the most serious consequences of this frustration is that many people infected with HIV are adopting unproved remedies obtained through an "AIDS underground." Some of these compounds are imported and others are manufactured in makeshift laboratories in kitchens and basements.

Self-medication may fill an emotional need for patients who do not have access to clinical trials or licensed medications—many say that it decreases the feeling of helplessness that can be so overwhelming in the early stages of disease. But physicians worry that patients will become victims of unscrupulous vendors or will expose themselves to dangerous side effects associated with some of the more powerful compounds.

People who believe in the merits of a particular underground drug also may hesitate to give up the drug to participate in clinical trials. The FDA is particularly concerned about patients who enroll in trials but continue to take underground medications; such behavior could invalidate the results of an entire study.

In a report titled *An Agenda for AIDS Drug Development*, based on a meeting at the Institute of Medicine (IOM) in September 1987, participants stressed the importance of informing potential recipients of experimental drugs about the logic and design of clinical trials. Underground remedies are less likely to have appeal if HIV-infected persons and the general public have a better understanding of established therapies and ongoing scientific research.

The IOM panel also recommended consideration of community-based centers for clinical investigation. Community-based organizations in both California and New York have obtained state approval to set up facilities for managing clinical trials. Questions remain about whether the community-based trials will be able to maintain the level of scientific rigor necessary to obtain unequivocal answers.

Treatment IND. The desire to help desperately ill AIDS patients without access to clinical trials was one of the factors behind the FDA's decision to formalize procedures for the early release of certain experimental drugs. Under regulations issued on May 22, 1987, physicians can request permission for access to experimental drugs if a patient has an immediately life-threatening condition and no other satisfactory treatment exists. The new rules are based on the assumption that such patients are willing to accept greater risks (of drug failure or adverse reactions) than those who are less seriously ill.

FDA administrators say that approval of a treatment IND (the official term for permission to use an investigational drug for treatment) is most likely to be granted for a life-threatening condition if the drug involved is nearing the end of the second phase of clinical testing—at that time, the drug's safety and dosage have been established and there is some evidence of therapeutic benefit. Separate criteria exist for diseases that are serious but not immediately life-threatening.

Resource Issues

The IOM report on promoting drug development against HIV stressed the need for greater participation in AIDS research and for expanded laboratory and clinical facilities.

Some major academic institutions have hesitated to become involved in AIDS research because of the cost of developing containment facilities suitable for studies of live HIV. Building funds generally have not kept pace with government-sponsored research grants. Some experienced researchers also have expressed frustration about difficulties in obtaining cell lines and other materials necessary to start AIDS-related programs. To solve this problem, NIAID has put forth 2 major contracts. The first will fund a national respository for HIV-related reagents. The second will support a genetic engineering program to produce large quantities of all known proteins encoded by the HIV genome. The proteins will be available to all investigators in the general biomedical research community, as well as to those in industry.

Increasing facilities for clinical trials is a more difficult problem. The hospitals and clinics that serve large numbers of AIDS patients are often overcrowded and understaffed. Participation in clinical trials increases the workload because staff members must follow very specific guidelines to ensure compliance with research protocols. The identification of subtle treatment-related changes in clinical status often requires extra patient interviews, physical examinations, and laboratory tests.

These problems are aggravated by a shortage of researchers trained to design and manage large clinical trials. In the past, young medical scientists often have been steered away from clinical research by advisers who viewed it as less intellectually challenging than basic science research. This trend has resulted in an imbalance that could adversely affect drug development in the future. To overcome this deficit, the IOM committee recommended new fellowship programs and greater recognition within the academic community for the creativity involved in clinical research.

Animal Models

Another area of great concern to everyone involved in promoting drug and vaccine development is the shortage of good animal models of HIV infection.

The ideal animal model for AIDS would be one in which HIV-1 induced an AIDS-like disease in a species that reproduced rapidly and was inexpensive to maintain in the laboratory. Such a model would allow researchers to obtain rapid answers to questions about disease pathogenesis (how the virus causes disease) and about the potential value of new preventive and therapeutic strategies. Unfortunately, the ideal model does not exist.

Apes. As of September 1988, the only nonhuman species that could be infected with HIV-1 were chimpanzees and gibbons. Following infection, HIV-1 persists in the blood cells of these animals much as it does in human blood cells, but so far none has developed AIDS or a serious AIDS-related disease (several have varying degrees of lymphadenopathy).

Patricia Fultz, a researcher at the Yerkes Regional Primate

Research Center in Atlanta, says that if chimpanzees prove to be inherently resistant to HIV-1 diseases, "then comparisons of immune responses of humans and chimpanzees early after infection may aid in defining the elements of a protective immune response against HIV."[4] Studies of chimpanzees already have provided important, albeit discouraging, insights into the difficulties surrounding the development of an HIV vaccine.

The chimpanzee model is extremely valuable, but it has many practical drawbacks. The endangered status of the animals, as well as their lack of availability and high cost, has prompted growing calls for restraint in the use of chimpanzees. The Public Health Service AIDS Animal Models Committee oversees the utilization of chimpanzees supported by government funds. The committee assesses the scientific merit of experimental protocols involving the animals and attempts to avoid unnecessary duplication.

Other primates.   Fortunately, many AIDS-related questions can be answered in other types of animal models. Fultz notes that one of the most important advances in AIDS research was the discovery of the simian immunodeficiency virus (SIV). SIV was isolated originally from macaques with an AIDS-like disease at the New England Regional Primate Research Center in 1984. Since then, other researchers have isolated closely related viruses from many African species of nonhuman primates, including the sooty mangabey and the African green monkey.

The basic structure of the SIV genome is very similar to that of HIV, and both types of virus bind to the CD4 receptor on the T4 lymphocyte. In addition, SIV causes the same spectrum of disease symptoms in macaques that HIV-1 causes in humans—from swollen glands to full-blown AIDS with involvement of the central nervous system. Macaques breed well in captivity and are available in large numbers. These characteristics make SIV ideal for preclinical studies of certain antiviral drugs and vaccines.

Scientists also are very interested in the way different

isolates of SIV interact with their monkey hosts. For example, researchers have found no evidence of disease in SIV-infected African green monkeys. In experimentally infected macaques, SIV-related disorders usually appear within months to years, but one SIV isolate causes death within a few days. Comparisons of these different models could help scientists (1) identify host factors responsible for protection against disease and (2) localize the segments of the viral genome associated with particular disease manifestations.

Recently several groups have successfully infected macaques with HIV-2, an HIV found primarily among people in certain parts of West Africa (see Chapter 3). An HIV-2-macaque model would have several advantages over an SIV-macaque model, especially for vaccine development. If a vaccine against HIV-2 were found to be successful in monkeys, it could be adapted more quickly for human trials than a comparable SIV vaccine.

Lentiviruses in ungulates and cats. Both HIV and SIV belong to the subfamily of retroviruses called lentiviruses. Before the discovery of the human and nonhuman primate viruses, the only known lentiviruses caused encephalitis, anemia, pneumonia, or arthritis in sheep, goats, and horses.

Researchers have been studying the ungulate lentiviruses for more than two decades. The lessons may seem discouraging. Frequent mutations of the lentivirus that infects horses—equine infectious anemia virus—allow the virus to evade elimination by the immune system. The disease caused by the visna viruses of sheep has a long and erratic clinical course, which may include progressive paralysis or relapses and remissions. Some infected animals remain healthy but can transmit the virus to other sheep. The caprine arthritis-encephalitis virus of goats does not evoke neutralizing or protective antibodies—antibodies and virus persist in apparent harmony. Efforts to develop a vaccine against the animal lentiviruses have been unsuccessful.

The positive side of the association between HIV and the ungulate lentiviruses is that past experience with the animal viruses may help AIDS researchers avoid some of the less productive avenues of investigation. Lentivirus studies generally have not received high funding priority, in part because they appeared to have little relevance to human disease.

Recently researchers have identified 2 new members of the lentivirus family, the bovine immunodeficiency virus (BIV) in cows and the feline immunodeficiency virus (FIV) in cats. The cat model may be particularly useful, because FIV appears to have the same target cell as HIV, the T lymphocyte, and because cats are easy to manage in the laboratory.

Mouse models. The feline, ungulate, and primate diseases described above all have relatively long incubation periods (with the exception of the one SIV isolate) and produce a wide range of symptoms. For some purposes, such as in vivo screening of new drug candidates, researchers need models that give unequivocal answers in a very short time. The ideal model would be a natural lentivirus disease in a mouse, rat, or other small mammal. Researchers have yet to find such a model in the wild, but they have developed 3 interim solutions to the problem.

The first strategy employs diseases in mice that are caused by retroviruses other than lentiviruses. Ruth Ruprecht of the Dana-Farber Cancer Institute in Boston explains that all retroviruses have some viral functions in common; for example, all retroviruses code for reverse transcriptase.

Ruprecht says that a mouse retroviral system can be used as a surrogate model to test both the efficacy and toxicity of potential AIDS drugs if the following conditions are met: (1) the candidate antiviral agent affects a similar viral function in both HIV and the mouse retrovirus; (2) in tissue culture, the test compound inhibits HIV propagation at about the same level that it inhibits the mouse retrovirus; and (3) the metabolism of the drug in human and mouse cells is comparable.

Ruprecht and her colleagues have employed a mouse leukemia model to explore the potential of AZT as a prophylactic agent and to assess the efficacy of certain drug combinations. They also have developed a model to study the impact of antiviral therapy on retroviral diseases transmitted in utero. (The model employs a virus called Cas-Br-E, which causes a rapidly fatal disease of the central nervous system in infected mouse pups.) Such studies can provide important information about the timing of therapy, as well as about efficacy and toxicity. For example, in one study Ruprecht and her coworkers compared the effects of beginning high-dose AZT therapy 4 hours or 4 days after inoculation with the Rauscher murine leukemia virus. (Untreated mice die within 4 to 6 weeks.) They found that all the mice who started getting AZT 4 hours after the virus survived at least one year. In contrast, when AZT therapy was started 4 days after inoculation with the virus, only about half of the animals were long-term survivors.[5]

The second strategy to increase the availability of laboratory models employs the newest techniques in genetic engineering. Researchers at the National Institutes of Health have produced mice that carry the entire HIV-1 genome in every cell. To produce the transgenic mice, scientists use a very fine glass needle to inject the virus's genetic material directly into fertilized mouse eggs. The treated eggs are implanted into surrogate mothers. Genetic studies shortly after birth identify the mice carrying the viral genes. (Normal mice are not susceptible to infection with HIV.)

At the Fourth International Conference on AIDS in Stockholm, John M. Leonard of the National Institute of Allergy and Infectious Diseases, NIH, and his coworkers reported that some of the transgenic mice display immune-cell abnormalities, swollen lymph nodes, psoriasislike skin lesions, and fatal lung disorders similar to those found in children with congenital HIV infection.[6] Researchers are particularly excited about a third potential strategy for using mice in AIDS research. In September 1988, two California research teams announced that they had transplanted the major elements of the human immune system into a strain of mice lacking normal defense mechanisms. These mice could play an important role in future studies to understand how HIV causes disease and how it might be stopped.

Increasing access to animal models. The IOM report on drug development and other documents have emphasized the importance of broadening the research base to fight HIV infection—that is, of involving more scientists from a wider variety of disciplines. An essential component of this effort will be to increase access to animal models. Some progress has already been made. National meetings sponsored by government and professional organizations have led to better communication between AIDS researchers and scientists familiar with the ungulate lentivirus models. Researchers have intensified the search for small rodents with natural lentivirus diseases and for new species susceptible to HIV infection; work with some of the New World primates looks promising.

The shortage of chimpanzees presents a particularly difficult problem. NIH has funded a National Chimpanzee Breeding Program, but the number of animals available will always be limited. Increased emphasis on the macaque model will help reduce pressure on the chimpanzee population; however, the country's leading primate research facilities are already working at or beyond capacity. They need more trained personnel and additional funds to build appropriate containment facilities for macaques infected with SIV and HIV-2.

Rational Drug Design

When it became clear that many severely ill AIDS patients could not tolerate AZT, some people expected to find an equally effective alternative on the market within months. The failure of government and industry researchers to produce such an alternative generated considerable criticism. In fact, these expectations were not realistic.

Historically, medical science has not fared well in the battle against viral infections. At a conference on AIDS drug development in late 1987, George Galasso, associate director of extramural affairs at NIH, noted that AZT was only the seventh antiviral drug licensed by the FDA, despite a 20-year effort by scientists to find effective therapies for herpes simplex virus, hepatitis B virus, cytomegalovirus infection, and other viral diseases. Very few compounds disrupt viral replication without also disrupting essential metabolic processes in the host.

The first 7 antiviral drugs were all discovered serendipitously through screening programs of existing compounds. Most researchers believe that systematic screening of compounds in the libraries of the world's pharmaceutical companies still offers the best short-term prospect for finding new anti-HIV drugs. In time, however, screening will be replaced by a more rational approach to drug design based on new techniques in virology, cell culture, and molecular biology.

Rational drug design requires an intimate knowledge of the structure and function of viral proteins. The ideal target for rational drug design is a protein that (1) plays a crucial role in the life cycle of the virus and (2) has no counterpart among the vast array of protein molecules in the host cell. When researchers identify such a protein, they attempt to find out as much as possible about its chemical and physical structure. The information is used to design compounds that disable or inhibit the protein in some way, preventing it from performing its normal function.

In some cases a single molecule can present multiple targets for rational drug design. For example, the larger envelope protein of HIV has at least 2 active sites: one binds the envelope protein to the virus membrane, and the other attaches to the CD4 receptor on prospective target cells. Blocking either of these active sites could stop replication and spread of the virus.

The structure and life cycle of HIV are described in Chapter 5. The virus's complexity still baffles scientists, but in the long run it may prove beneficial for drug developers. Because the virus produces more proteins than most other retroviruses, it offers more targets for drugs (see Figure 7.1). Potential targets include the 2 envelope proteins, the core proteins, reverse transcriptase, integrase (which allows the virus to insert itself into host-cell DNA), protease (which cuts

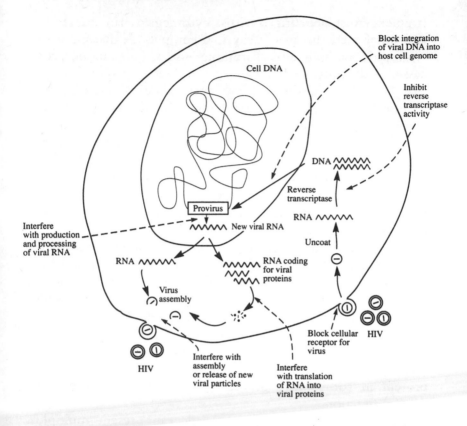

FIGURE 7.1. Preventing replication of HIV. Several of the antiviral drugs now being evaluated for use against HIV act by inhibiting reverse transcriptase activity. Other possible strategies for preventing replication of the virus include blocking specific cellular receptors for the virus, blocking the integration of viral DNA into the host cell genome, interfering with the production and processing of viral RNA, interfering with the translation of viral RNA into new viral proteins, and interfering with the assembly or release of new viral particles.

the precursor of the core proteins into appropriate pieces), the *tat* protein, the *rev* protein, and other regulatory proteins.

Drug Candidates

The FDA reports that it has approved studies to test more than 40 potential AIDS drugs. The descriptions below highlight compounds that have received a large amount of attention from researchers or from groups representing AIDS patients. An up-to-date account of all HIV-related clinical trials is available in the *Directory of Experimental Treatments for AIDS and ARC*, produced by the American Foundation for AIDS Research (AMFAR) and compiled with technical assistance from the Professional Outreach Program of NIAID.

Antiviral Drugs in Clinical Trials

The experimental compounds now undergoing clinical trials act at several different stages in the virus's life cycle. Some prevent viral replication within infected cells; others interfere with the transmission of viral particles from one cell to another.

AL-721. AL-721 is a lipid mixture designed to reduce the cholesterol content of cell membranes. Researchers believe that it may disrupt the organization of the HIV membrane, thereby preventing the virus from binding to and penetrating target cells.

Early clinical trials of AL-721 are under way in both the United States and Israel, where the drug was developed. Preliminary results indicate that it has minimal side effects and that it reduces HIV activity in the body, but it is too early to say whether the drug will have any impact on the clinical course of HIV-infected patients. Despite the lack of definitive information about the drug's efficacy, AL-721 is very popular on the underground market for AIDS drugs.

Ampligen. Ampligen consists of a specific formulation of double-stranded RNA. In a short-term study described in *Lancet,* ampligen appeared to restore immune function and to control HIV replication in 10 patients with AIDS or a pre-AIDS condition.[7] On the basis of these preliminary results, the manufacturer began a placebo-controlled trial involving 330 patients with HIV-related immune dysfunction but not AIDS. The study was halted in October 1988, when an examination

of the data showed that patients receiving ampligen progressed
to AIDS "at least as often" as patients receiving the placebo. A
physician managing the project said that ampligen did not
appear to have an effect on numbers of immune cells, patient
weight loss, or any other clinical signs.[8]

Azidothymidine (AZT). The only licensed antiretroviral drug,
AZT closely resembles one of the natural building blocks of
DNA. Scientists believe that it inhibits replication of HIV by
taking the place of this essential building block during the
conversion of viral RNA into DNA. When the viral enzyme
reverse transcriptase mistakenly places AZT in the DNA chain
instead of the correct molecule, viral DNA formation stops.
Reverse transcriptase appears much more likely to make this
mistake than enzymes that regulate the formation of cellular
DNA.

Following a promising phase 1 trial at the National
Cancer Institute and Duke University, researchers started a
phase 2 study at 12 medical centers across the United States in
February 1986. The study involved AIDS patients who were
within 4 months of their first attack of *Pneumocystis carinii*
pneumonia and ARC patients who had severe clinical signs,
such as significant weight loss or oral thrush.

The phase 2 trial was stopped abruptly in September
1986, when an independent data safety monitoring board
discovered a dramatic difference in outcomes between the 145
patients receiving AZT and the 137 patients receiving place-
bos. Nineteen patients in the placebo arm of the trial had died,
compared with only 1 in the AZT group. The AZT patients
also had significantly fewer opportunistic infections and
showed an increase in several measures of immune function.
Patients in the AZT group generally gained weight, while
those in the placebo group lost weight.

Burroughs Wellcome, the manufacturer, applied for a
new drug application for AZT in December 1986. The NDA
was approved on March 20, 1987. The FDA took the unusual
step of licensing the drug without a phase 3 trial because the
data on safety and effectiveness coming out of the phase 2

study were so strong and because there was no existing therapy for AIDS patients. To answer questions about the long-term effects of AZT, the FDA helped Burroughs Wellcome develop extensive plans for postmarketing studies.

AZT was licensed only for use in adults with the same disease characteristics as those involved in the phase 2 trial. During the study researchers had identified a variety of adverse effects associated with the drug, including bone marrow suppression, nausea, moderate to severe headaches, muscle pain, and insomnia. (Forty of the original AZT recipients in the phase 2 trial required transfusions, compared to 11 patients in the placebo group.) These reversible side effects were considered tolerable for patients with AIDS and severe ARC, but scientists feared the drug might do more harm than good for other groups of patients.

Initially, access to AZT was limited to physicians who requested case-by-case clearance from the manufacturer. This restriction was removed in September 1987, but Burroughs Wellcome cautioned physicians to read the package insert for detailed information before prescribing the drug. Informal surveys among physicians treating AIDS patients revealed that some were following recommended guidelines, while others were prescribing the drug for the entire spectrum of HIV-infected patients. Martin Hirsch, a virologist at the Massachusetts General Hospital in Boston, expressed concern about this practice:

Although it is tempting to extrapolate from the one completed placebo-controlled trial and several anecdotal case reports to other HIV-associated conditions, such extrapolations are dangerous and unwise. Except in carefully controlled trials, it is recommended that AZT be limited to those patients for whom it has been licensed . . . Controlled trials are currently under way in asymptomatic HIV carriers, as well as in patients with early ARC, localized Kaposi's sarcoma, and AIDS dementia complex (HIV encephalopathy). Pediatric trials of AZT are also in progress. Until results from such trials are available, it is impossible to predict accurately whether the potential benefits of AZT in such situations outweigh the considerable risks.[9]

The AMFAR directory notes that preliminary data from some of the long-term AZT studies suggest that patients with early HIV infection may tolerate AZT better than AIDS patients. According to the directory, Samuel Broder and his coworkers at the National Cancer Institute have observed that the incidence of bone marrow suppression among AZT recipients with early HIV infection is about 10 to 15 percent, compared to 40 to 50 percent among AZT recipients with AIDS or severe ARC. Preliminary studies of AZT in HIV-infected children indicate that the drug can produce dramatic improvements in neurologic function, as well as other benefits.[10]

One way to maximize the benefits of AZT may be to combine it with other antiviral or immunomodulatory drugs. Hirsch and his coworkers have demonstrated that the combined effect of AZT and alpha interferon is greater than the sum of their individual effects. The same is true for AZT and castanospermine. Other researchers have reported synergistic antiviral activity when AZT is combined in vitro with acyclovir or granulocyte-macrophage colony stimulating factor (GM-CSF).

Drug combinations also can have an antagonistic effect. In 1987 American and French scientists reported separately that ribavirin inhibits the antiviral activity of AZT in the test tube. Hirsch says that "although in vitro interactions may not necessarily reflect conditions in vivo, combinations showing antagonism in the laboratory should be used clinically only under carefully controlled situations."[11]

The only troublesome drug interaction detected in clinical trials has been an apparent increase in bone marrow suppression associated with the use of acetaminophen (Tylenol) in patients taking AZT. Efforts are under way to learn more about this problem and to assess its impact on the health of HIV-infected patients.

Recombinant soluble CD4 (T4). The first major step toward rational drug design for AIDS therapy was the development of recombinant soluble CD4. Several years ago scientists demonstrated conclusively that cellular susceptibility to HIV infection is determined primarily by the presence of a membrane receptor called CD4, or T4. Infection begins when the viral envelope protein gp120 binds to the CD4 receptor. Cells with numerous CD4 receptors, such as the T4 lymphocyte, are most susceptible to infection with the virus and to HIV-induced cell death.

Recognition of the strong affinity between gp120 and CD4 formed the basis for a novel approach to antiviral therapy. Scientists reasoned that if they could separate the CD4 molecule from the cell membrane and introduce it independently into the body, it might act as a decoy, soaking up viral particles before they could attach to and infect living cells. Such an approach became plausible in 1985 when Richard Axel, professor of biochemistry at the Howard Hughes Medical Institute at Columbia University, cloned the gene for the human CD4 receptor.

Two years later, in late 1987 and early 1988, five independent reseach teams announced that they had produced soluble CD4 and tested its antiviral activity in the laboratory. (The scientists used genetic engineering techniques to insert the CD4 gene into mammalian cells or insect cells in culture. The altered cells secrete recombinant CD4, which is then harvested from the culture medium.) All the scientists found soluble CD4 to be a potent inhibitor of both HIV replication and HIV-induced syncytium formation.

Researchers are enthusiastic about the potential of soluble CD4 in drug therapy, but they caution that several questions must be answered before the compound is ready for large-scale clinical trials. One concern is that soluble CD4 might block the site on monocytes that enables monocytes and lymphocytes to recognize each other during the development of a normal immune response (see Chapter 5). Soluble CD4 does not appear to inhibit T-cell activation in the laboratory, but it could be a problem in vivo.

Another possibility is that recombinant CD4 might stimulate the development of anti-CD4 antibodies. The presence of such antibodies would lead to rapid elimination of the recombinant protein from the body. A more serious concern, however, is that the antibodies might adhere to natural CD4 receptors on cell membranes, triggering the destruction of healthy immune cells. If this occurred, the patient would be more susceptible to infection than before therapy with soluble CD4.

So far, studies of recombinant soluble CD4 in animal models have not shown any of these adverse immunological effects. The first safety trials of the drug in AIDS patients began at the National Cancer Institute, New England Deaconess Hospital in Boston, and San Francisco General Hospital in August 1988.

Dextran sulfate.   Dextran sulfate is a large carbohydrate molecule that has been used since the 1950s as an anticoagulant. Japanese researchers reported in 1987 that the compound could inhibit HIV in the test tube. In April 1988 Hiroaki Mitsuya of the National Cancer Institute and his coworkers reported in *Science* magazine that the principal mode of action of dextran sulfate is to block the the attachment of the virus to target cells. The drug also inhibits the formation of syncytia, the giant cells described in Chapter 5. (In HIV-infected cells in laboratory cultures, syncytium formation is often a major cause of cell death.) Phase 1 trials of the compound are under way in patients with symptomatic HIV infection.

Dideoxycytidine (ddC).   The drug dideoxycytidine is a reverse transcriptase inhibitor with a mechanism of action similar to that of AZT. In the test tube, ddC is about 10 times more potent than AZT.

Results from a phase 1 clinical trial showed that ddC is absorbed well from the gut and that it crosses the blood–brain barrier. In a majority of patients it produced significant immunological improvement and a rapid fall in virus replication (as measured by p24 antigen in the blood).

Initial enthusiasm over ddC paled, however, when patients began developing severe peripheral neuropathy (pains in the legs and feet). Other side effects included a rash, mouth sores, fever, and reduced levels of platelets and neutrophils.

Researchers are exploring several strategies to obtain the benefits of ddC therapy without the problems. One alternative may be to administer smaller doses of the drug. Several groups also have begun preliminary trials in which ddC is alternated on a weekly or a monthly basis with AZT. Robert Yarchoan of the National Cancer Institute and his coworkers report that the weekly regimen was tolerated well by patients participating in a small phase 1 trial.[12]

Foscarnet.   First synthesized in 1924, foscarnet (trisodium phosphonoformate) has been evaluated primarily by European researchers as a treatment for herpes virus infections. Like AZT, it inhibits reverse transcriptase activity. Foscarnet has been shown to block replication of HIV in the laboratory. In the United States, phase 1 studies are under way in AIDS patients with CMV retinitis and in ARC patients. The side effects of foscarnet include metabolic changes that could lead to kidney failure, a reversible decrease in hemoglobin concentration (hemoglobin is the protein that carries oxygen in the blood), tiredness, headache, and some enchephalitislike symptoms. The drug must be given intravenously, a fact that makes it unsuitable for long-term maintenance.

Interferons.   The interferons are natural substances secreted by virus-infected cells to strengthen the defenses of uninfected neighboring cells.[13] Three types of interferon have been identified: alpha interferon, secreted by white blood cells (leukocytes); beta interferon, secreted by fibroblasts; and gamma interferon, secreted by T lymphocytes. All 3 types of interferon have been shown to have anti-HIV activity in the test tube, although the results are more consistent with alpha and beta interferon than with gamma interferon. In mouse retrovirus systems, alpha interferon acts by interrupting the formation and release of new virus particles; it may have a similar mode of action against HIV. All forms of interferon enhance the in vitro function of immune cells, especially the tumor-fighting natural killer (NK) cell.

Alpha interferon has been the most successful of the 3

compounds in AIDS clinical trials. Several research teams have reported that alpha interferon produced by recombinant DNA technology causes regression of Kaposi's sarcoma (KS) lesions. Patients with lesions restricted to the skin or lymph nodes are most likely to have a complete response.

Alpha interferon alone does not appear to be an effective therapy for AIDS patients without KS. However, studies in animal models have shown a dramatic, synergistic antiretroviral effect when alpha interferon is combined with AZT. Clinical trials of the 2-drug combination are under way.

The benefits of beta interferon are less clear. Some KS patients enrolled in a 12-week preliminary trial of the drug showed moderate improvement, but KS lesions in the majority either remained stable or progressed. In a second small study, beta interferon appeared to inhibit HIV replication and prevent the onset of opportunistic infections. Current phase 1 and phase 2 trials are gathering additional information about beta interferon therapy in HIV-positive patients with immunological abnormalities, in KS patients, and in patients with other HIV-related diseases.

Gamma interferon alone has not produced any clinical improvement in patients with AIDS or AIDS-related conditions. The manufacturer reports, however, that gamma interferon combined with a macrophage-derived protein called tumor necrosis factor (TNF) has both antiviral and immune-stimulating effects. Concurrent phase 1 and phase 2 trials of the TNF-gamma interferon combination are under way.

All 3 interferons produce flulike side effects, including fatigue, fever, chills, and muscle pains. Beta and gamma interferon also may cause reversible abnormalities in liver function and a decrease in white blood cells.

Ribavirin. The drug ribavirin inhibits a wide variety of RNA and DNA viruses in the laboratory. Different forms of the drug have been evaluated in the treatment of Lassa fever infection in West Africa and of respiratory syncytial virus (RSV) infection in infants in the United States. Its primary side effect has been a reversible suppression of hemoglobin production. The mechanism of action of ribavirin remains unclear; it may interfere with the processing of viral RNA.

AIDS-related clinical trials of ribavirin have generated tremendous controversy. In January 1987 the manufacturer held a news conference to announce the results of a double-blind, placebo-controlled trial in which ribavirin appeared to delay the progression to AIDS in seropositive patients with very early HIV-related symptoms. However, a subsequent study in patients with more severe pre-AIDS conditions failed to show a significant effect. In fact more deaths occurred among patients receiving ribavirin than among those receiving a placebo.

The commissioner of the FDA, who had recommended against holding the news conference, later charged that the design of the initial study was flawed. When the manufacturer applied for a treatment IND (which would have allowed limited distribution of the drug to severely ill patients not enrolled in clinical trials), the FDA turned down the request.

After reviewing all laboratory and clinical data, the FDA has concluded that further studies of ribavirin are warranted. Federally sponsored trials are in the planning stages.

Immune Modulators

Early in the course of the AIDS epidemic, some scientists speculated that the most effective treatment for the severe immune defects associated with the syndrome might involve techniques to rebuild or stimulate the immune system. Researchers at the National Institute of Allergy and Infectious Diseases, for example, treated several AIDS patients with a combination of bone marrow transplants and lymphocyte transfers from their identical twin brothers. These efforts sometimes resulted in improved immune function, but the patients did not improve clinically, probably because the virus was still present. Additional studies are under way using bone marrow transplantation from an identical twin in combination with antiviral therapy.

Other efforts to stimulate body defense mechanisms have

employed a large variety of natural and synthetic compounds. The natural substances include interleukin-2 (IL-2), an immune-system growth factor produced by T lymphocytes, the white blood cells most often attacked by HIV; granulocyte-macrophage colony stimulating factor (GM-CSF), which induces the proliferation and development of blood-cell precursors in the bone marrow; and Imreg-1. Among the chemically synthesized immune modulators are AS-101 and isoprinosine.

Interleukin-2. IL-2, also called T-cell growth factor, plays a crucial role in the immune response (see Figure 5.4). It causes proliferation of activated T cells and is essential for cell-mediated immunity and other immune functions. Patients with AIDS have markedly reduced levels of IL-2, but efforts to restore immune function with IL-2 alone have been unsuccessful.

Scientists are more optimistic about combining IL-2 therapy with an antiviral agent. When IL-2 is used alone, it may simply create more target cells for replication of HIV (or stimulate replication of latent HIV), resulting in more virus particles. Suppression of viral replication may prevent this from happening. Researchers have begun a phase 1 trial of IL-2 in combination with AZT in patients with very early HIV-related symptoms.

Studies of IL-2 in cancer therapy indicate that side effects of the drug may include fever, chills, exhaustion, loss of appetite, occasional liver abnormalities, and reversible neuropsychiatric disorders. In a study of infectious complications that occur during trials of immunomodulatory agents in AIDS patients, researchers at NIAID also found an unexpectedly large number of nonopportunistic bacterial infections associated with IL-2 therapy.

Granulocyte-macrophage colony stimulating factor. A 1987 study of almost 5,000 HIV-infected men in the United States showed that the loss of T lymphocytes in the blood is often accompanied by reductions in other types of white blood cells, especially neutrophils.[14] Neutrophils are part of the body's first line of defense. They ingest and digest bacteria, damaged host cells, and inorganic toxic substances.

The loss of neutrophils and related immune cells makes HIV-infected patients even more susceptible to infection than they would be from the loss of T cells alone. Researchers do not understand why the cells are depleted, although there is growing evidence that HIV infection causes suppression of blood-forming cells in the bone marrow.

Granulocyte-macrophage colony stimulating factor (GM-CSF) is one of several natural substances that stimulate proliferation and differentiation of blood-cell precursors in the body. In addition, laboratory studies indicate that GM-CSF increases the antibacterial and antitumor activities of some mature blood cells.

Harvard physician Jerome E. Groopman and his coworkers conducted the first clinical trial of GM-CSF in 16 AIDS patients with low white-cell counts. They used human GM-CSF produced by recombinant DNA technology. The researchers found that the drug was well tolerated and biologically active. White-cell counts rose dramatically, although they returned to pretreatment levels within 2 to 10 days after discontinuation of the drug.

The side effects of GM-CSF are closely linked to dosage and frequency of administration. All the patients in the preliminary trial developed mild flulike symptoms. Higher doses may cause severe pain in the muscles and bones.

Groopman and his colleagues believe that GM-CSF may be most effective for AIDS therapy in combination with antiviral drugs such as AZT.[15] GM-CSF and other compounds that stimulate blood-cell production could allow patients to tolerate much higher doses of antiviral drugs whose use has been limited by their effects on the bone marrow.

Imreg-1.   The first new drug application for an immune modulator to treat AIDS patients may be filed by Imreg, Inc., the developer of Imreg-1. Imreg-1 is derived from natural subtances produced by white blood cells. In laboratory studies it enhances the production of IL-2 and gamma interferon by lymphocytes from patients with symptomatic HIV infection.

Company-sponsored clinical trials of Imreg-1 indicate that it may delay the progression of disease in some HIV-infected patients, but these results have not been confirmed.

AS-101.   Laboratory studies indicate that the synthetic drug AS-101 stimulates the production of both IL-2 and GM-CSF by human white blood cells. In a preliminary trial in Mexico, AIDS patients who received the drug showed improvement in several measures of immune function. Side effects included nausea, vomiting, and diarrhea. An FDA-approved phase 1 trial is under way in the United States and Israel, where the drug was developed.

Isoprinosine.   Isoprinosine is an immune system modulator that was developed first as a memory enhancer. Laboratory studies indicate that it enhances many different immune functions, including lymphocyte proliferation, activation of monocytes, and perhaps also IL-2 production.

In short-term clinical studies sponsored by the manufacturer, isoprinosine produced major improvements in T-cell numbers and NK cell activity in patients with early HIV-related symptoms. (In some cases the improvements persisted for months after therapy was withdrawn.) However, the clinical benefits of the drug remain unclear.

Large-scale phase 2 and phase 3 trials are under way in the United States, Norway, Sweden, Denmark, and Australia to determine whether isoprinosine has any effect on the progression of disease in HIV-infected people who are asymptomatic or who have early signs of HIV-related disorders.

Drugs That Failed to Live Up to Expectations

Three years ago, the two drugs most often mentioned in discussions of AIDS therapy were suramin and antimonio-tungstate (HPA-23). Neither of these drugs has lived up to expectations, although HPA-23 is still undergoing clinical trials.

The first clinical trial of suramin produced mixed results. Viral activity decreased markedly in patients who had had evidence of HIV replication before the trial, but physicians did not observe any significant clinical or immunological improvement. Researchers concluded that the results provided a rationale for cautious, experimental trials over longer periods. Ninety-eight patients with HIV-related symptoms were subsequently enrolled in a nationwide phase 1 trial.

The drug-induced adverse effects experienced by patients in that trial ended the prospects for suramin as an anti-AIDS drug in the United States. Almost 25 percent experienced adrenal insufficiency. Scientists believe the drug also may have triggered 3 cases of liver failure in the group. Clinical benefits were limited to 1 patient, who had a complete remission of his non-Hodgkins lymphoma.

HPA-23 is a mineral compound discovered in France about 10 years ago. It has been reported to inhibit reverse transcriptase activity of both mouse and human retroviruses in the test tube. Uncontrolled clinical trials of HPA-23 have been under way in France since 1984. So far, they have failed to produce conclusive evidence that the drug alters the progression of HIV-related diseases. NIAID is working with the manufacturer to develop trials that will provide more definitive information.

Preclinical Studies

The next generation of compounds to enter clinical trials will be more diverse than the current generation. Many will be products of drug screening. Gradually, however, rational drug design will assume a more dominant role. The knowledge acquired by AIDS researchers will shape all future efforts in antiviral drug development.

Chemical relatives of AZT and ddC. Several compounds in the final stages of preclinical testing are reverse transcriptase inhibitors with activities similar to that of AZT. They include CS-87, d4C, and ddA/ddI. All of these compounds are chemically related to DNA building blocks. Researchers hope they will be more effective and less toxic than AZT and ddC.

Castanospermine and other glucosidase inhibitors. In 1987 researchers from the United States, the Netherlands, London, and Australia described the exciting anti-HIV effects of 2 related drugs, castanospermine (a substance extracted from the seeds of an Australian chestnut tree) and dNM (1-deoxynojirimycin). These drugs are glucosidase inhibitors. They inhibit the cellular enzyme required to process or "trim" sugar residues. As described in Chapter 5, the HIV envelope protein gp120 and its precursor are heavily coated with sugar residues. Improper trimming of the sugar residues appears to interfere with the activity of gp120.

In laboratory studies researchers found that the continuous presence of castanospermine or dNM inhibited the infectivity of HIV particles by a factor of almost 100, but it did not stop virus production inside cells already infected with the virus. The drugs appear to prevent newly formed virus particles from completing the binding and fusion reactions necessary to infect new cells.

The most dramatic effect of the two glucosidase inhibitors, however, is their ability to block the formation of "giant cells" or syncytia. Syncytium formation is believed to be important for cell-to-cell spread of HIV; in vitro, it also plays a major role in cell death. In cell culture studies, castanospermine completely blocked syncytium formation for 24 hours and partially inhibited the formation of giant cells for several days. The effect of dNM was similar but somewhat weaker.

Evaluation of the glucosidase inhibitors is continuing with tests in animal models. The Dutch researchers say that "dNM and related compounds are hardly toxic in tissue culture." In addition, derivatives of dNM have been used in humans to control blood glucose levels "with no harmful side effects reported."[16]

Anti-sense DNA sequences. Another new approach to drug design is the development of "anti-sense" oligonucleotides. These are short sequences of DNA that are complementary to pieces of the viral genome. Theoretically, the binding of anti-sense oligonucleotides to viral messenger RNA could inhibit virus replication in 2 ways: it could prevent the messenger RNA from being translated into protein, or it could disrupt the function of HIV regulatory proteins, such as the *tat* and *rev* proteins (see Chapter 5). The limitations and potential side effects of this strategy are not known.

Vaccine Development

The advent of AZT generated tremendous relief among AIDS researchers and clinicians. Despite the drug's limitations, its ability to prolong the lives of some AIDS patients provided much-needed evidence that antiviral strategies could play a role in controlling the epidemic. Scientists had a foundation on which to build—future agents would be safer and more effective.

The story on vaccine development is quite different. In 1986 the Committee on a National Strategy for AIDS, IOM, warned: "The properties of viruses related to HIV suggest that developing a vaccine will be difficult . . . Moreover, even if the scientific obstacles were surmounted, legal, social, and ethical factors could delay or limit the availability of a vaccine. For these reasons, the committee does not believe that a vaccine is likely to be developed for at least five years and probably longer."[17]

Today, the general consensus is that this prediction was overly optimistic. Discouraging results from animal studies and new evidence about the virus's ability to evade the natural immune response suggest that protecting people against HIV-related diseases may require a completely new approach to vaccine development.

Background

Most familiar antiviral vaccines, including those for measles, mumps, and rubella, consist of live viruses that have been weakened (attenuated) in the laboratory so that they elicit a protective response without causing disease. Researchers generally believe that this strategy is not appropriate for HIV because the virus is simply too dangerous. The possibility that an attenuated strain might regain its capacity to cause disease would pose too great a risk.

The traditional alternative to the attenuated vaccine is the killed whole virus vaccine. Examples include the currently licensed influenza vaccines and the Salk poliovirus vaccine. In general, this strategy also has been avoided by AIDS researchers because of uncertainties surrounding the infectivity of genetic material even from a killed retrovirus. (In 1987 Jonas Salk proposed the use of a killed whole virus HIV vaccine to boost the immune responses of people already infected with HIV. This concept is discussed further below.)

Advances in recombinant DNA technology provided AIDS researchers with a third approach—the preparation of a subunit vaccine. Subunit vaccines present no danger of infection because they do not contain any genetic material from the virus; their content is limited to one or more viral proteins or pieces of proteins.

To prepare a subunit vaccine, scientists attempt to identify the viral protein (antigen) most likely to arouse a protective antibody response from the human immune system. (This protein usually is part of the viral envelope, its outer coat.) The researchers pinpoint the portion of the viral genome coding for the protein, isolate it, and insert it into the genetic apparatus of another replicating virus, bacterium, yeast, or animal cell. The outcome is a hybrid organism that replicates and produces the desired protein molecule in large quantities. Purification of the antigen results in a highly specific vaccine. A hepatitis B virus vaccine based on this strategy was licensed in 1987. In addition, a subunit vaccine against feline leukemia virus (an animal retrovirus) is now available for immunization of cats.

In general, subunit vaccines elicit a more limited immune response than whole virus vaccines. To overcome this problem, researchers are experimenting with different types of adjuvants, natural or synthetic substances that can be delivered with an antigen to enhance its potency. Only one adjuvant is licensed for use in the United States; the development of new and safer adjuvants would contribute significantly to vaccine development for many diseases. A variation of the subunit strategy is to take the gene for the desired envelope protein and insert it into the genome of a virus that does not cause disease in human beings. The most obvious choice is the vaccinia virus, which was used to immunize people against smallpox. If the recombinant virus produces the foreign protein, it can elicit a stronger immune response than the foreign protein alone in vaccine recipients.

HIV Vaccines

When scientists first began working on potential vaccines against HIV, their major concern was the diversity of virus isolates. They were worried that antibodies generated against the envelope protein of one isolate of HIV might not recognize the envelope protein of another isolate. As explained in Chapter 5, the most variable segment of the HIV genome is that coding for the envelope protein.

This concern still exists, but it has been overshadowed by a much more serious problem: repeated virus challenge studies in chimpanzees (using HIV) and macaque monkeys (using SIV) have failed to demonstrate that vaccines of any kind can protect against infection with these viruses.[18]

Vaccines evaluated to date have included a killed whole virus vaccine, a variety of subunit vaccines (some containing the HIV envelope protein gp120 and others containing its precursor gp160), and a vaccinia-gp160 recombinant vaccine. In each case the animals were inoculated with a vaccine and then challenged with the same virus isolate used to produce the vaccine. All the animals developed persistent viral infections. As expected, the chimpanzees did not become ill (they do not get AIDS from a natural HIV infection), but the vaccinated macaques developed AIDS and fared no better than unvaccinated controls.

Studies of the immune functions of the immunized animals before they were challenged showed that the vaccines had elicited antibodies and, in some cases, a cell-mediated immune response to the HIV or SIV antigens. In fact the macaques immunized with killed whole virus had neutralizing antibodies (see Chapter 5). Upon challenge, however, the animals became persistently infected.

Some scientists suggested that the first chimpanzee and macaque studies produced negative results because the dose of challenge virus was too high—much higher than the dose of virus transmitted by sexual intercourse with an infected partner or from a contaminated syringe. Challenge studies with smaller doses, however, also have resulted in infection. The underlying issue is that researchers need to learn more about HIV transmission and the natural immune response to the virus.

In people, the presence of antibodies to the core proteins appears to be more closely linked to disease progression than the presence of antibodies to the envelope proteins. (Antibodies to the core proteins diminish as people progress to AIDS.) Perhaps a vaccine consisting of core proteins would be more effective than the envelope vaccines. Researchers also are studying the possibility of making a vaccine that elicits antibodies against reverse transcriptase.

Scientists suspect that HIV infection may be acquired through transmission of already infected lymphocytes and monocytes, as well as from free virus in body fluids. If this is the case, vaccine-induced neutralizing antibodies might be of little value in stopping an initial infection, because the antibodies could not reach the virus. This problem is compounded by the fact that the virus can travel directly from one cell to another through cell-to-cell binding. The destruction of virus-infected cells usually is accomplished by cell-mediated immune mechanisms, but these are less well understood than antibody-mediated phenomena. No one really knows how to elicit a protective cell-mediated immune response.

Safety Trials in Human Beings

The immune responses of chimpanzees and human beings to natural HIV infection differ in several respects. Some researchers believe that these differences may affect the way the two species respond to vaccines. It is possible that a vaccine that failed in chimpanzees could be effective in human beings. The need to compare human and animal responses to different vaccine preparations was one factor in the decision to begin human clinical trials of HIV vaccines. More importantly, however, researchers had to know if potential vaccines would be safe.

The first human trial of an AIDS vaccine was conducted by Daniel Zagury of the Pierre and Marie Curie University in Paris and his coworkers. They demonstrated that a vaccinia-gp160 recombinant virus could induce both antibody-mediated and cell-mediated immunity against HIV. The vaccine did not produce any side effects other than the localized sore normally associated with a satisfactory immune response to vaccinia.

Phase 1 clinical trials of a gp160 subunit vaccine began at NIAID in the summer of 1987. In January 1988 the trial was expanded to include 6 vaccine evaluation units at medical centers around the country. (The vaccine evaluation units were established 5 to 10 years ago to test other, non-HIV, vaccines.) A second U.S. vaccine, a vaccinia-gp160 recombinant similar to the Zagury vaccine, is being tested by researchers associated with the University of Washington.

These trials will not provide any evidence about vaccine efficacy in human beings. Clearly, it would be unethical to challenge the recipients with live virus. The trials are designed only to answer questions about safety and to acquire some preliminary information about the effects of the vaccines on the immune system.

Scientists and reporters who cover science have a responsibility to make it very clear that these trials are preliminary safety trials. They do not signal the advent of an effective solution to the AIDS problem. Raising false hopes could diminish educational efforts that are essential to control the epidemic.

Recruiting subjects. The pace of the U.S. vaccine trials has been slowed somewhat by difficulties associated with recruiting subjects. One problem is that the people who are most motivated to volunteer—people engaging in high-risk behavior—are not suitable for the trials. Researchers need volunteers who are healthy and highly unlikely to become infected with HIV during the course of the study. Symptoms created by HIV or other infections could be wrongly interpreted as adverse reactions to a potential vaccine.

Most of the early volunteers have been homosexual men who do not practice high-risk behavior. Researchers have spent hundreds of hours interviewing and counseling these men and their steady sexual partners to make sure they understand the goals and requirements of the studies.

One of the biggest concerns for prospective subjects has been fear of discrimination. Vaccine recipients test positive on standard tests for exposure to HIV because they develop antibodies against the virus. Volunteers have expressed concern that they will face the same types of discrimination as people infected with HIV—discrimination in housing, employment, insurance, and other vital areas of their lives. To overcome this problem, researchers have developed notarized documents that subjects can use to prove they have participated in the trials, and that their antibodies are a result of immunization rather than infection.[19]

Risk. One of the most difficult factors to assess in early vaccine trials is the amount of risk involved in a study. None of the immunized chimpanzees or macaque monkeys has exhibited adverse reactions from the vaccine candidates, but their numbers have been limited.

Researchers studying subunit vaccines are primarily concerned about 2 types of adverse effects. The first involves interactions between viral proteins and the immune system. Laboratory evidence suggests that some of the immune suppression associated with HIV infection may be caused by free molecules of the HIV envelope protein released from infected cells. The binding of these free molecules of gp120 to uninfected immune cells could impair their function or lead to their destruction by the immune system. The concern is that subunit vaccines consisting of viral envelope proteins might have a similar effect. However, there has been no evidence of vaccine-related immune suppression in any of the immunized chimpanzees, monkeys, or people studied so far.

The second type of adverse effect would not become evident until a vaccine recipient was exposed to a natural HIV infection. Several different models are available of a phenomenon called immunoenhancement, in which antibodies elicited by a vaccine increase the severity of a subsequent infection rather than suppress it. (One form of immunoenhancement occurs when the dominant antibodies elicited by a vaccine are not neutralizing antibodies. The nonneutralizing antibodies block access to critical neutralization sites on the virus particle and enhance its survival.) French researchers Axel Ellrodt and Philippe Le Bras have noted that goats injected with inactivated caprine arthritis-encephalitis virus, a lentivirus described above, develop more severe lesions than unvaccinated goats when later challenged with live virus.[20]

In the HIV and SIV vaccine challenge studies described above, the vaccinated animals fared no worse than their unvaccinated counterparts, but the potential for immunoenhancement cannot be ignored.

The recombinant vaccinia vaccine raises 2 additional issues. Vaccinia does not cause symptoms in people with a normal immune system, but it may cause a severe smallpox-like disease in immunosuppressed individuals. In 1986 physicians at the Walter Reed Army Medical Center reported the case of an army recruit with an unsuspected HIV infection who developed disseminated vaccinia following routine immunization for smallpox. Some researchers are concerned that the use of a vaccinia-based vaccine against HIV might be dangerous in populations with large numbers of people at high risk of infection (because some undoubtedly would have unrecognized HIV-related immune deficiencies). To reduce this risk, researchers at NIAID are attempting to develop a more attenuated vaccinia virus (laboratory studies indicate that recombinant vaccinia viruses containing the HIV envelope gene already are less virulent than the original vaccinia virus). The weakened virus would have the same ability to stimulate the immune system as the natural virus, but would be less likely to cause disease.

Researchers also need to determine whether the live recombinant vaccinia virus can be transmitted from one person to another. This is important for 2 reasons. First, potential recipients of the vaccine may be in contact with HIV-infected immunosuppressed persons, who might be in danger from the vaccinia virus.[21] Second, transmission of the vaccinia recombinant might cause contacts of the recipient who were previously HIV-seronegative to develop HIV antibodies. These contacts would have no way of knowing that they had been infected with the recombinant virus rather than with HIV itself. The developers of the recombinant vaccinia vaccine believe that transmission of the virus is highly unlikely, but they have not ruled it out completely.

Liability issues. For more than a decade the United States has been struggling to develop a just approach to the issues of liability for vaccine-related injury and of compensation for those who are injured. In general, however, the emphasis has been on postmarketing liability. Very little attention has been paid to liability issues surrounding vaccine trials.

Participants in vaccine trials usually sign a statement of informed consent that includes a phrase limiting compensation for injuries related to the trial. Often compensation is provided only for medical care costs associated with an acute or immediate reaction to an experimental vaccine. This practice has not been challenged in the courts.

Some researchers have become uneasy, however, about the ethical and legal problems that would arise if an AIDS vaccine candidate were found to have long-term adverse effects. David Karzon, a professor of pediatrics and infectious diseases at Vanderbilt University, told participants at a meeting on vaccine development: "The institutional review board from my own institution, in reviewing a proposal for an AIDS vaccine clinical trial, felt strongly that the AIDS vaccine volunteers would be subject to a higher level of risk than subjects in other vaccine trials the board had reviewed over the years. Our board approved the proposal with the caveat that the investigators must actively pursue methods of compensation for 'serious, long-term, and expensive complications of the vaccine.' " Karzon suggested that the board's conclusions about risk were based on the general lack of experience with HIV—still less than 10 years—and the potential duration of vaccine-related problems.

Scientists, government policymakers, industry representatives, and the general public must decide whether HIV infection represents a special case in vaccine development and, if so, who should take responsibility for risks incurred in the testing of vaccine candidates.

Efficacy Trials

The issues of volunteer recruitment and vaccine liability will grow more complex as potential vaccines move into larger trials. Phase 2 trials, designed to produce detailed information about safety in specific high-risk populations, will require hundreds of volunteers.

Researchers disagree about when it will be appropriate to begin phase 3 trials to determine whether a vaccine candidate actually protects people from HIV infection.[22] Some believe that efficacy studies should not be conducted until animal studies have provided some evidence of protection. Others question the validity of the chimpanzee model and believe that phase 3 trials should begin as soon as a vaccine candidate successfully completes phase 2 tests. Data from current studies may help resolve this controversy. In the meantime, researchers are beginning to plan for the enormous logistical problems that will be created by the large-scale trials.

Efficacy trials will require thousands of willing, thoroughly informed research subjects who are at high risk but are still uninfected. After immunization it will be necessary to follow them for years to detect signs of HIV-related disease or adverse reactions to a vaccine.

At a recent meeting of the Presidential Commission on the Human Immunodeficiency Virus Epidemic, Anthony Fauci, director of NIAID, said that efficacy studies might have to take place in central Africa, where HIV infection continues to spread rapidly in some urban areas. Researchers originally had planned to conduct phase 3 trials among male homosexuals in the United States, but the level of new infections has dropped so low that such studies may not be feasible (see Chapter 2). Many years and tens of thousands of subjects would be required to show a statistically significant difference between vaccinated and unvaccinated subjects in this population. (HIV infection continues to spread rapidly among intravenous drug abusers in the United States, but scientists worry that they would have difficulty keeping track of such people for the length of a study.)

Even after all the trials have been completed, scientists and policymakers will still face many very difficult questions: What is the ultimate target population for an AIDS vaccine? Is the American public prepared for another attempt at mass immunization after the swine flu experience? Is mass immunization warranted, given the very low risk of infection for heterosexuals in the United States? Who will take responsibility for postmarketing vaccine liability?

The problems of vaccine development discussed above are not insurmountable. Cooperative efforts between government and industry have made for extraordinary progress in other areas of AIDS research and may bring solutions to some of these problems. For the present, however, immunization should not be viewed as an imminent solution to the worldwide epidemic of HIV-related diseases.

Immunizing Seropositive People

Most people think of vaccines only in terms of pre-exposure immunization. The vaccine is administered to induce specific antibodies against an agent in the environment. It prepares the body to defeat the offending agent should exposure occur in the future.

Two vaccines, the rabies and hepatitis B virus vaccines, also are administered to people immediately after exposure to the respective viruses. Rabies and hepatitis B virus have longer incubation periods than those associated with most viral diseases. (The incubation period for influenza is measured in days, whereas the incubation period for rabies is measured in weeks and the incubation period for hepatitis B virus in weeks to months.) The postexposure vaccines are effective because they elicit neutralizing antibodies before the viruses have had time to multiply in the body.

Some researchers believe that postexposure immunization also might prevent the development of symptoms in HIV-infected persons, although the rationale is somewhat different from the rationale for postexposure immunization in rabies and hepatitis. Jonas Salk, who developed the killed polio vaccine, explained the concept in an article in *Nature* in June 1987:

The long incubation period between infection and the development of clinical AIDS may be due to an immune response to the initial infection which persists with health and wanes with disease. If this response can be boosted, it may be possible to reduce the viral burden, prevent the development of disease, and reduce contagiousness . . .

From an epidemiological perspective the prospects for the control of AIDS by immunization of seropositive individuals—if this proved to be successful in preventing the development of disease in those who are asymptomatic—would have a greater and more rapid impact in reducing HIV morbidity and mortality than would an immunization strategy directed at the seronegative population. If immunization of seropositive virus carriers would also reduce their contagiousness then the virus reservoir in the population would be rapidly reduced, as would the frequency of newly acquired infections. The prospect of producing such effects would increase the frequency of blood-testing, for reasons of self-interest, without the need for coercion. This would have the further advantage of accelerating case-finding and early treatment of those so identified.[23]

Salk and his coworkers have begun limited tests of a killed whole virus vaccine in people who are seropositive but have not yet developed symptoms. The goal of the study is to determine whether the vaccine is safe. Some scientists have expressed concern that the vaccine might stimulate the patients' infected immune cells to produce new viral particles, increasing the progression of disease instead of slowing it.

Zagury and his collaborators have conducted preliminary trials of a different form of immunization in 10 seropositive subjects in Zaire. They report that none of the subjects experienced adverse effects.

The ultimate value of postexposure immunization will not be known for some time. If the results of early trials are favorable, efficacy studies will follow the same course as large-scale tests for other HIV therapies.

Conclusion

Scientists have demonstrated that antiviral strategies can prolong the lives of AIDS patients, but the search for effective agents has only begun. Candidate drugs must be suitable for oral administration, must be able to cross the blood-brain barrier, and must be inexpensive and safe enough for lifelong use. Physicians probably will have to use combinations of drugs to minimize long-term toxicity.

The prospects for a vaccine against HIV appear less promising. In addition to the technical problems associated with initial development, the logistics and expense of clinical trials and associated liability issues present great obstacles. Mass immunization against HIV should not be regarded as a reasonable option for the near future.

Antiviral drugs may reduce the contagiousness of HIV, but the most realistic approach to slowing the epidemic remains a combination of health education and other public health measures.

8

Individual and Societal Stress

The psychological and social effects of HIV infection are as varied as the physical symptoms produced by the virus. During the early years of the epidemic, feelings of isolation and anguish experienced by patients and their families and friends were compounded by fear and hostility in their communities:

• A successful attorney loses his job and his closest friend less than a week after the doctor tells him he has Kaposi's sarcoma; his physician recommends a local AIDS support group, but when he enters the group's meeting room he is overwhelmed by the signs of advanced disease and turns to leave.
• A suburban couple and their grown children sit on the edge of the living-room sofa, straining to hear the voice of the youngest son; they know that he is ill, but the revelation that he has AIDS leaves some of them in tears and the rest in stony silence.
• Infants in the nursery of a metropolitan hospital, victims of AIDS acquired in the womb, cry for mothers who do not come, either because they themselves are ill or because they cannot face the burden of caring for a child with such tremendous needs.
• Fire destroys the home of 3 young brothers exposed to HIV through blood products used to treat their hemophilia. The fire follows a week of bomb and death threats and a boycott of the school where the boys had returned after a

federal court ruled that they could not be barred from attending classes with other children.

Increasingly such scenes are giving way to others, characterized by compassion and understanding:

• Two practical support volunteers from the Shanti Project in San Francisco help a man with AIDS pack his belongings and prepare to move into one of the 12 independent living residences maintained by the Shanti Project for men and women with AIDS who need permanent low-cost housing.

• A volunteer "buddy," trained by the AIDS Action Committee in Boston to provide emotional support for AIDS patients and their families, reads a favorite story to the young son of a woman with AIDS.

• A woman from the Houston organization Pet Patrol hurries past a waiting ambulance and runs up the steps of a nearby apartment complex. An AIDS patient has refused to leave for the hospital until he knows that his small dog is in good hands. Pet Patrol volunteers have helped him care for the dog for several months and will now provide a foster home for the animal.

• A hospice worker in New York City sits for hours by the bedside of a man whose only remaining fear is that he will be alone when he dies.

These are just a few examples of the types of support provided to AIDS patients by volunteers across the country. Their actions do not compensate for the discrimination and prejudice that still prevail in some areas, but they do provide a foundation for a just and humane response to the AIDS epidemic. HIV infection has changed our society; its full impact on patients, their families, healthy members of high-risk groups, and the general population is only now beginning to be understood.

AIDS Patients

The psychological impact of a diagnosis of AIDS is similar in some respects to that elicited by diagnoses of other fatal illnesses. The first response is often denial—in some cases so strong that patients refuse medical care. For most, however, the denial is tempered by realism. The result may be behaviors that seem contradictory, such as arranging to meet with a lawyer but refusing to sign a will. Whatever their initial reactions, AIDS patients need immediate and continuous access to counseling and a compassionate and understanding health care team.

The patient's response to AIDS depends in part on his or her psychological condition before the appearance of the syndrome. Patients with a history of psychiatric disorders are less likely than others to adjust to their illness and imminent death. Their inability to cope may become particularly evident when the physician recommends risk-reduction measures such as avoidance of sexual behaviors that could transmit the virus, reduced alcohol consumption, or elimination of drug abuse. In some cases these proscribed behaviors may be the patient's principal ways of handling stress.

After the initial period of denial, most patients pass through a period characterized by alternating episodes of anger and depression, combined with fear about the future course of the disease and the effects of therapy. The anger may be especially severe in AIDS patients because of their relative youth. (Almost 90 percent of AIDS patients are between the ages of 20 and 49.) Death is difficult to face at any age, but a premature death seems especially unfair. The fear may be exacerbated by recent experiences involving friends or acquaintances who succumbed to AIDS. Indeed, many patients have lost an entire social network to AIDS and are left without support for some of the most difficult months or years of their lives.

In some cases the combination of psychosocial stresses associated with AIDS may lead to suicide. Researchers at Cornell University Medical College and the Office of the Chief Medical Examiner of New York found that the suicide rate in 1985 among men with AIDS in New York City was 36 times higher than that among men of the same age without AIDS. Most documented AIDS-related suicides occurred within 6 months of receiving the diagnosis.[1]

Health care professionals can help AIDS patients through these turbulent times by encouraging them to express their fears, providing accurate information, directing anger into constructive pathways (such as volunteer activities), prescribing appropriate medications (ranging from mild antianxiety drugs to stronger antidepressants, depending on the needs of the patient), and encouraging the development of new social contacts.

Eventually, most AIDS patients who are not overwhelmed by neurological problems begin to accept the limitations imposed by the disease and assume an active role in decisions about their future health care. Those who remain mobile often use the time to work at AIDS crisis centers or to participate in other community projects. As the disease progresses, the focus gradually shifts to preparations for death.

Several factors—some social, others physiological—may make AIDS patients psychologically more vulnerable than people with other fatal illnesses.

Coping with Discrimination

The distribution of AIDS cases in the United States —more than 70 percent among homosexual men and 19 percent among intravenous drug abusers—has fostered the belief in some segments of society that AIDS is a form of punishment for socially unacceptable behavior. One AIDS patient recalls that his sister's first response upon hearing he had AIDS was "You should be ashamed of yourself."

The concept of a "gay disease" has been extremely hard to change, despite knowledge that the syndrome is a viral illness transmitted by heterosexual as well as homosexual intercourse. The social stigma attached to the syndrome may be especially overwhelming for homosexual or bisexual men who have hidden their sexual orientation for years from family and friends.

Homosexual men who have internalized society's disapproval of their sexual orientation may accept discrimination from others without complaint. Some patients with AIDS have lost both their jobs and their homes within weeks of the diagnosis, although these actions increasingly are being challenged successfully in court. An employer or landlord who goes to great lengths to help a person with cancer or heart disease may be unwilling to exhibit the same compassion for a person with AIDS.

For AIDS patients, the trauma of being fired or evicted quickly becomes subordinate to practical concerns about how and where they will live the last months of their lives. Many need immediate legal and financial counseling, as well as more conventional social services. Boston, Los Angeles, New York, Philadelphia, San Francisco, and Washington, D.C., are among the cities that have comprehensive networks of AIDS-related agencies to deal with the psychosocial effects of the AIDS crisis. Working together, these agencies offer emergency housing and food services, free legal advice, practical support for daily living, substance abuse counseling, and individual counseling for patients and their families.

Minorities. The premier AIDS service organizations, the Gay Men's Health Crisis in New York City, the San Francisco AIDS Foundation, and the Shanti Project in San Francisco, have helped thousands of homosexual men overcome the isolation and fear associated with a diagnosis of AIDS. They have attempted to respond with equal compassion to the needs of other groups with a high incidence of HIV infection. Some experts believe, however, that services developed primarily for white homosexual men may not be capable of solving the more diverse problems of the predominantly black and Hispanic populations infected through intravenous drug abuse.

Blacks represent about 12 percent of the U.S. population, but they account for more than 25 percent of AIDS cases in this country. Hispanics, who represent about 7 percent of the population, account for almost 15 percent of AIDS cases. More than 40 percent of black and Hispanic adults with AIDS report a history of intravenous drug abuse, compared with only 14 percent of white adults with AIDS. Minority AIDS patients also are more likely to be among the poor or nearly poor. California psychologists Vickie Mays and Susan Cochran have noted the lack of information about the specific psychosocial needs of black AIDS patients: "The vast majority of articles on the psychosocial impact of AIDS address the emotional and behavioral responses of white gay men with AIDS . . . Black Americans differ in respect to the resources available and the cultural norms at work in coping with their illness. These differences may be manifested in such areas as help-seeking behavior, perceptions of the severity of medical or psychological problems, perceived barriers to the use of health care facilities, or the use of informal help systems."[2]

Mays and Cochran believe that the consequences of AIDS-related discrimination may be more severe for low-income black patients than for white patients. They note that people in lower socioeconomic groups tend to depend more heavily on family and friendship networks for support during health crises than do people in higher socioeconomic groups (who are more likely to seek professional care). If family members and friends reject a black AIDS patient—because of fear of HIV infection or negative attitudes toward the stigmatized behaviors associated with the disease—the patient may have difficulty finding alternative sources of emotional and physical support. Lack of financial resources, cultural barriers to communication, and an unwillingness to appear vulnerable to "outsiders" may delay efforts to seek professional help.

Beginning in 1985, church-based organizations in several cities began providing services specifically for minority AIDS patients, but much more needs to be done.

Women.   Women with AIDS face the same psychological problems as men with the disease, but their isolation may be more profound. Constance Wofsy, a physician at San Francisco General Hospital, notes that because the disease has occurred predominantly among men, women with AIDS may have trouble finding primary care physicians, gynecologists, counselors, and other health professionals who are aware of their needs.[3] Physicians may fail to diagnose AIDS and other

HIV-related problems in women who are not IV drug abusers or prostitutes.

Many women first learn they are infected with HIV after the birth of an affected child. The combination of intense grief and guilt may impair their ability to care for the sick child and any healthy children already in their homes. For women who subsequently develop an HIV-related disease, the emotional toll becomes even greater. Most are single parents with extremely limited financial resources. They have to plan for the welfare of surviving children as they prepare themselves for death.

Children. Growing up with HIV infection may be the most difficult battle created by the epidemic. Newspapers and magazines have devoted much attention to the plight of infants with AIDS, especially those abandoned in hospitals by impoverished parents. Fear of contagion has denied some of these extremely ill babies the cuddling and close contact essential for even a very short life.

But the focus on infants with AIDS has left many people with the mistaken impression that all children with congenital HIV infection die in infancy. In fact new studies indicate that the incubation period for maternally transmitted pediatric AIDS is much more variable than previously reported.[4] Some HIV-infected children have reached their fifth and sixth birthdays with few signs of illness. The tremendous psychosocial needs of these children, and of the smaller group of children who have been infected through contaminated blood or blood products, is just beginning to be understood.

In New York City at least 80 percent of children with AIDS have parents who are IV drug abusers. Few of the children remain with their own families. Some are placed in loving foster homes, but even the more fortunate suffer from developmental problems characteristic of children who have been denied a consistent, one-on-one caregiver. These developmental problems may be difficult to distinguish from those caused directly by HIV infection. As the children grow, some begin to exhibit emotional problems common to youngsters with other serious chronic diseases. They may be angry and frustrated because they cannot play the games other children play. Some become obsessed with thoughts of death.

All children with HIV–related diseases and their caregivers suffer from the stigma associated with AIDS. Parents and foster parents of older children with AIDS worry constantly that their children will mention their illness to "the wrong person," such as a landlord who could force the family to leave their home. No one really knows how the children interpret these pleas for secrecy, but it would be surprising if the enforced silence did not exacerbate feelings of fear and isolation.

Special day-care centers for children with AIDS and parent support groups help alleviate some of the fear. One New York widow, who has 3 foster children with AIDS, described the importance of these support services to a reporter for the *New York Times*: "These are the only places we can use that word [AIDS] or talk about what's really going on. Before I met these people, it was like I was on a mountaintop, high as can be. It was lonely and it was terrifying."[5]

Physical Limitations

Two characteristics of infection with HIV also interfere with patients' efforts to cope with AIDS. The first is the many different clinical signs and symptoms associated with disruption of the immune system. A man with Kaposi's sarcoma may learn to accept the disfigurement of this cancer and adapt to cancer therapy, but when he suddenly develops *Pneumocystis carinii* pneumonia, his resiliency may disappear. Each new manifestation of disease may elicit the same anger and fear associated with the original diagnosis and require a new period of adjustment.

The second problem, which is potentially much more serious, is the effect of HIV on the nervous system. Neurologic disease caused by the virus may lead to gradual deterioration of mental faculties over a period of months. Health care providers must learn to watch for this process, which can affect the patient's ability to cope with the illness in a variety of ways.

In some cases, mild memory loss or an inability to accomplish simple tasks may cause depression, in other cases the depression itself may be a symptom of the infection. Subtle personality changes may alter the way the patient relates to medical and nursing staff or result in an inability to comply with therapeutic regimens.

Samuel Perry and Paul Jacobsen from Cornell University Medical College in New York City group the psychiatric symptoms associated with HIV infection into 2 clusters. The first cluster includes the mild chronic depression. It may be accompanied by apathy, social withdrawal, fatigue, weight loss, anxiety, impaired concentration, and complaints of forgetfulness. The second cluster encompasses a variety of rapid-onset psychotic disorders. Symptoms, which often appear in conjunction with a medical crisis, may include grandiosity, suspiciousness, hallucinations, rambling and repetitive speech, and confusion.[6]

The New York scientists stress that mental health professionals can intervene in many different ways to help patients with both types of psychiatric syndromes. They can work with family members and friends to marshal resources for long-term maintenance care; they can help the patient establish a comfortable daily routine that is realistic in terms of the remaining cognitive and physical capabilities; and they can provide a surrogate relationship to reduce the severe alienation that often accompanies AIDS. The AIDS Health Project of the University of California at San Francisco has published a resource guide for mental health professionals called *Working with AIDS*, which contains suggestions for specific interventions and numerous examples of counseling plans.[7]

Perry and Jacobsen note that drug therapy for patients with HIV-related psychiatric symptoms is similar to that for patients with other diseases that cause diminution of brain function. They caution, however, that dosage requirements are generally lower and that side effects, including sedation and confusion, may be more severe.

Diagnosis of HIV-related mental disorders.   Accurate diagnosis is essential for proper treatment of HIV-related mental syndromes. Researchers are developing a battery of neuropsychological and behavioral tests to assist physicians in differentiating between central nervous system disorders caused by HIV and stress-related psychological problems.

Initial assessments of both psychological distress and mental status may be complicated by a variety of sociocultural factors. For example, Mays and Cochran refer to non-AIDS-related studies showing that mental health professionals tend to underdiagnose affective disorders (involving mood or emotional feeling) and overdiagnose schizophrenia in blacks, especially black men. They explain: "The tendency for black males to be somewhat remote, withdrawn, and formal in the presence of white professionals may be misinterpreted as the patient's attempt to cope with an underlying thought disorder or schizophrenic psychotic process rather than a culturally relevant stance when dealing with a nearly foreign white world. The patient may, in fact, be quite depressed but deem it culturally inappropriate to reveal this emotional distress."[8]

Cultural differences also may hamper efforts to assess cognitive deficiencies. Questions about politics and current events, often used to measure cognitive abilities, might be meaningless to a patient preoccupied by the problems of poverty. Health care workers must make sure that the questions used to evaluate mental functions are within the patient's realm of experience.

Decision making.   When dementia resulting from HIV infection becomes severe, the patient may be unable to participate in decisions about future care. One aspect of this problem is determining when an individual is capable of giving informed consent for an experimental drug regimen.

More complex questions arise over the very difficult choice between aggressive life-prolonging measures and simple supportive care in the final stages of AIDS. When does a peaceful death become more desirable than further efforts to prolong life?

In most other diseases, if a severely ill patient is mentally incompetent the physician turns to the family for guidance on how the patient would have handled this choice. Physicians and family members share the decision-making process. But many AIDS patients are estranged from their families of origin. If asked, some indicate that they would prefer to have friends or lovers take the part of other family members in health care decisions.

Unresolved questions about the use of cardiopulmonary resuscitation and similar measures can cause extreme anguish for friends and family during the final days of an AIDS patient's life. Physicians and nurses can prevent such turmoil by taking time to learn a patient's views about the desirability of heroic medical treatments before the onset of dementia. The initial approach may be difficult, because the patient may not be emotionally ready to enter into such discussions when the disease appears to be under control. However, with appropriate reassurances and compassion health care providers can help the patient explore his own feelings about these very difficult issues.

Formal directives may take the form of a living will or a durable power of attorney for health care. The latter allows a competent patient to designate a proxy to make decisions about medical care if he should become incompetent to make decisions.[9]

Patients with Milder Symptoms of HIV Infection

People with less severe symptoms of HIV infection face many of the same stress factors as people with AIDS: physical limitations, social prejudice, potential loss of economic self-sufficiency, and the need to change high-risk behavior. In fact a 1985 study by Susan Tross and Jimmie Holland of Memorial Sloan-Kettering Cancer Center in New York City found that patients with ARC (AIDS-related complex) exhibited a higher level of social and psychological distress than AIDS patients.[10] The authors speculated that this more intense distress reaction probably resulted from the uncertainty associated with ARC.

Some patients diagnosed with ARC appeared to remain stable for years, while others progressed rapidly to AIDS.

Knowledge acquired from long-term studies of people at high risk of AIDS has begun to answer some of the questions about the natural history of HIV infection. For example, several groups of researchers have demonstrated that, in the absence of other symptoms, persistently swollen glands are not indicative of a declining immune system in people infected with HIV. This information and similar findings could help some patients cope with the uncertainty of their symptoms.

Healthy People in High-Risk Groups

The manner in which people respond to the knowledge that they are at high risk for AIDS depends on many factors: their feelings about the activities or circumstances that place them at high risk, their general level of psychological functioning, and their ability to seek out and obtain emotional support. Chapter 6 explores these issues as they relate to AIDS education and testing. This section takes a more specific look at some of the social forces shaping the response to the AIDS crisis.

Homosexual Men

Imagine the psychological impact of watching a dozen friends under the age of 45 succumb to a fatal illness. For tens of thousands of homosexual men in the United States, the death of loved ones and friends has become a common occurrence. For most of these men, the stress of constant grief has been amplified by fear—fear that the next cough or skin blemish will signal the beginning of their own battle with HIV infection.

Homosexual communities have responded to the crisis by creating social and political organizations to aid the sick and to lobby for financial support of research and treatment facilities. Many of the men involved in these organizations had not publicly identified themselves as homosexuals before the crisis began—thus, the communities may be stronger and more unified than ever before. But anxiety levels are high. Conversations about AIDS have become a part of every social gathering. Some men develop physical symptoms that mimic those of HIV infection. Others make frequent trips to the doctor seeking unrealistic guarantees.

The desire to know one's antibody status may conflict with another type of fear—fear of personal exposure should the results become known. Brett Cassens, former president of the American Association of Physicians for Human Rights, says that confidentiality "is considered by most gay persons to be the most important if not the only true defense against social discrimination." (Confidentiality with respect to HIV testing is discussed in Chapter 6.)

Researchers studying the psychosocial consequences of being at high risk for AIDS report growing concern among homosexual men that the United States is moving toward the adoption of extreme measures in the fight against HIV infection. David Ostrow and his colleagues at the University of Michigan School of Medicine note that their subjects—homosexual and bisexual men enrolled in the Chicago cohort of the national Multicenter AIDS Cohort Study—have responded with increasing anger and fear to the question "Is there anything else about AIDS and how it has affected you which you would like to tell us?" Ostrow says that expressions of alarm about society's reactions to the AIDS crisis have increased in parallel with media coverage of proposals for mass HIV-antibody screening and quarantine. He concludes that fear of quarantine is "a very real part of the psychiatric picture of AIDS today in the United States."[11]

Growing reports of AIDS-related violence also contribute to the alarm. The number of incidents of antigay violence or harassment recorded by the National Gay and Lesbian Task Force increased from 2,042 in 1985 to 7,008 in 1987. Fifteen percent of the 1987 incidents involved verbal references to AIDS, some of them directed against people with AIDS.[12]

Women

The vast majority of women who are at high risk for AIDS are either intravenous drug abusers or the sexual partners of intravenous drug abusers. For many, the day-to-day demands of poverty and drug abuse were overwhelming before the appearance of AIDS. The threat of disease simply increases the burden; often the women feel they have no control over their own lives.

In a report on a day-long AIDS prevention forum for women in October 1986 in New York City, Caroline Sparks of the Feminist Institute in Bethesda, Maryland, noted that participants repeatedly expressed reluctance to assert their own needs and wishes in relationships.[13] The women feared rejection if they urged their sexual partners to practice safer sex. They consistently viewed themselves as less powerful than the men in their lives.

This sense of dependence causes psychological conflicts on many different levels. Female partners of intravenous drug abusers may be angry at their partners for exposing them to the risk of HIV infection, but they may be unable to express the anger for fear of losing the relationship. If the partner becomes ill, the desire to leave may conflict with feelings about the woman's role as caregiver.

Accepting the constraints on childbearing imposed by HIV infection also tends to be more difficult for women than for men. Many segments of society continue to view childbearing as the ultimate goal of womanhood. As noted in Chapter 6, more than half of pregnant women who know they are infected with HIV early enough to abort choose not to do so; in addition, some women become pregnant repeatedly even after having given birth to an infected child.

Constance Wofsy recently outlined some of the reasons for this behavior.[14] She notes that many HIV-seropositive women who are healthy are in a strong state of denial. Subconsciously or consciously they choose to ignore their antibody status and continue their lives accordingly. Alternatively, a woman may feel incapable of taking the measures necessary to prevent conception. Her partner's aversion to condoms may preclude their use; or her partner may insist on having children for reasons of his own.

Counselors who work with women at high risk for HIV infection must provide them with the skills necessary to make and implement informed decisions about protecting their own lives and about childbearing. In some cases, role-playing may help women overcome apprehensions about discussing sex and contraception with male partners. Support groups consisting of women with similar problems may reduce fears of rejection and social isolation. The most important goal of counseling is to help women at high risk for AIDS develop a sense of independent control over their own lives.

Older Children and Adolescents

A 1987 study exploring the impact of the fear of AIDS on hemophiliacs and their families produced one very alarming finding: parents reported more distress from the AIDS fear than did hemophiliacs or their mates. (The study population included 116 hemophiliacs, age 16 or older, and 40 mates and 94 parents of hemophiliacs.) The study's authors, including David Agle of Case Western Reserve University, noted that parents were twice as likely as their sons to report the highest level of preoccupation with health concerns and the need for a safer life-style, and twice as likely to experience the fear that any illness might be the start of AIDS. In addition, 7 percent of parents reported the highest level of fear that they themselves could acquire AIDS and 7 percent reported the highest degree of reluctance to be close to their children.[15]

These findings provide important insights into the potential effects of HIV infection on childrearing. Agle and his colleagues suggest that the intense anxiety experienced by parents of children who are HIV seropositive but otherwise healthy can "enhance the tendency toward overprotective parenting as well as the avoidance of healthful intimacy with the child."[16]

Older children and adolescents who are seropositive for

HIV cannot be shielded from news reports and other reminders of the AIDS epidemic. Fears about being viewed as contagious can lead to social isolation and increase doubts about self-worth common to all young teenagers. Strong parental support can minimize the effects of these outside influences, but if the parent-child relationship is distorted by anxiety, the child may be at risk for severe psychological problems. Agle and his coworkers encourage mental health workers to pay particular attention to the evaluation of parental distress in caring for the families of hemophiliacs and other adolescents at high risk for HIV-related diseases.

The General Population

Media polls in 1987 indicated that most adults in the United States were concerned but not panic-stricken about AIDS. School boycotts (protesting the attendance of children with AIDS in elementary schools) and job discrimination against those believed to belong to high-risk groups have been the exception rather than the rule. Frequent reassurances from the CDC have contributed to this relative calm, but perhaps the most important explanation for the public's behavior to date has been the relatively low prevalence of disease nationwide.

No one is quite sure how the general public will respond to the large increase in AIDS cases expected over the next 4 years, when a quarter of a million Americans are predicted to have the disease. Will the population take up the cry of elderly Florida homeowners who protested the placement of a group home for teenagers with AIDS by putting up a sign "Danger AIDS—Keep Away," or will it show the compassion demonstrated by a Massachusetts town that rallied around the family of a young hemophiliac dying from AIDS?

A telephone poll of 1,000 adults released in January 1988 by the SRI Gallup company indicated that 81 percent supported federally financed research to find a cure for AIDS, up from 70 percent one year earlier. The poll also showed an increase in the number of respondents who knew that AIDS is transmitted through sexual contact (76 percent versus 61 percent) and an increase in the number opposed to quarantining AIDS patients (39 percent versus 34 percent).[17]

In an interview with the Associated Press, pollster Steven Steiber interpreted these results as an indication that "Americans have become more enlightened and less fearful in terms of a reactionary response [to AIDS]."[18] He suggested that the increased public support for AIDS research might be a result of increased personal exposure to people with AIDS. Six percent of respondents indicated that they personally knew an AIDS patient—an increase of 50 percent from the previous year.

On the surface, the SRI Gallup poll seems reassuring. It suggests that public education programs about HIV are having a beneficial effect. But the fact that almost 30 percent of those polled still favor quarantine, and that another 27 percent say they are neutral on the issue, indicates that the "epidemic of fear" continues to play a major role in public opinion.

Charles Turner, a study director with the National Research Council's Commission on Behavioral and Social Sciences and Education, has shown that support for quarantine and other restrictive measures is strongly linked to beliefs about how HIV is transmitted. In an analysis of several national polls taken in 1985, Turner found that people who believed that HIV infection could be transmitted by sharing a drinking glass were almost twice as likely to oppose having HIV-infected students in school as those who did not believe in such transmission. Similarly, people who answered "yes" to the question "Do you think you could get AIDS by being sneezed or coughed on by someone who has AIDS?" were more than twice as likely to support quarantining of AIDS victims as those who answered "no."[19]

At times, lack of unanimity within the medical community has adversely affected public understanding of AIDS risk factors. Some of the most serious problems have occurred when physicians who lacked knowledge about the syndrome aired their own fears in an open forum. For example, in mid-1985 3 physicians in a major southwestern city stood before the city council and warned members of their community to stop shaking hands with strangers because they might catch AIDS from sweaty palms. This advice probably had much more impact locally than published statements by CDC epidemiologists.

The damage can be even more severe when a politician carelessly adopts ideas not supported by scientific evidence. On December 17, 1987, the *Boston Globe* reported that Republican presidential candidate Pat Robertson had told interviewers that AIDS could spread through the air. (The headline read "Robertson says AIDS spreads easily.") A follow-up story by *Globe* reporter John Ellement revealed that Robertson's comments were based on a quick reading of 2 pages from a report by British physician John Seale.[20] Seale's views on AIDS, including the belief that HIV can be transmitted by coughing or sneezing, have been discredited by many prominent AIDS researchers.[21] Robertson's adoption of Seale's position represented a setback to efforts to provide the public with accurate information.

The problems associated with HIV infection will continue to be part of American society for the foreseeable future. The major unanswered question is whether or not the disease will begin to spread more rapidly into the so-called general population.

If the epidemic does begin to spread more widely among heterosexuals, strong leadership will be necessary to counteract the search for scapegoats that has accompanied countless epidemics in the past. The increase in antigay violence described above indicates that such a tendency already exists. Added pressure on hospitals, schools, and other social institutions could tip the balance of power in favor of those who would blame the victims rather than the disease.

Other issues will arise if the epidemic does not spread far beyond the established risk groups. Some policy experts worry that the public will lose interest in supporting AIDS research and educational programs if HIV infection is viewed as a problem affecting only homosexuals and impoverished minorities. The capacity to view those who are at risk of HIV infection as fundamentally different could increase the likelihood of inappropriate restrictions and decrease the chances of developing measured, humanitarian responses to the crisis. Ronald Bayer, an associate for policy studies at the Hastings Center, asks: "In the face of an extended microparasitic siege, will American social institutions respond on the basis of reason guided by a scientific understanding of how HTLV-III transmission occurs, or will anxieties overwhelm the capacity for measured responses? . . . At stake is not only the question of how and whether it will be possible to weaken, if not extirpate, the viral antagonist responsible for AIDS, but the kind of society America will become in the process."[22]

Health Care Personnel

The impetus created by the AIDS epidemic to reexamine basic value systems has been greatest for the health care professions. In a September 1987 speech before the Presidential Commission on the Human Immunodeficiency Virus Epidemic, Surgeon General C. Everett Koop assailed the "unprofessional conduct" of physicians and others who withhold care from persons with AIDS. "Such conduct," he said, "threatens the very fabric of health care in this country."[23]

Six months before Koop's statement, Milwaukee surgeon W. Dudley Johnson, a pioneer of coronary artery bypass surgery, had announced that he would no longer operate on patients who were HIV positive. "It puts all of us around the table at too much risk," Johnson had explained. "There are simply too many unknowns, too many questions."[24] (Chapter 2 describes the very small, but measurable, risk of infection for health care providers.)

Opinions about Johnson's statement varied widely both inside and outside the medical profession. A handful of surgeons followed his example and closed their practices to HIV-infected patients. But many others insisted that physicians have an ethical responsibility to care for all patients, regardless of risk status.

The debate prompted the American Medical Association

to take a very unusual step. For the first time in its 140-year history, the organization issued specific guidelines pertaining to a single disease. The 4-page document, prepared by the AMA Council on Ethical and Judicial Affairs, states: "A physician may not ethically refuse to treat a patient whose condition is within the physician's current realm of competence solely because the patient is seropositive. The tradition of the AMA, since its organization in 1847, is that 'when an epidemic prevails, a physician must continue his labors without regard to the risk to his own health.' "[25]

Recognizing that physicians have a responsibility to care for patients with HIV infection is not enough to ensure that AIDS patients receive high-quality care. Physicians, nurses, mental health workers, and others involved in direct patient services need regular access to new information about HIV and established avenues for handling the stress that invariably accompanies working with AIDS patients.

AIDS education for health care providers involves more than a simple recitation of facts. In early 1986, researchers from the University of California at Los Angeles interviewed 1,000 randomly selected primary care physicians throughout California to assess their AIDS-related experiences and knowledge.[26] They concluded that a majority of those interviewed lacked the knowledge and skills required to carry out their roles in dealing with HIV infection (both caring for patients at high risk and providing adequate advice and reassurance to patients at low risk). One of the most important variables associated with competence on AIDS-related issues was the way a physician felt about treating homosexual patients. Those who reported "moderate" or "a good deal" of discomfort in dealing with homosexuals in their practices were less likely to respond correctly to basic medical questions about AIDS.

A revealing 3-city study conducted by researchers at the University of Mississippi highlights the manner in which physicians tend to stigmatize AIDS patients. Jeffrey Kelly and his colleagues sent 1 of 4 vignettes describing a patient to physicians in Columbus, Ohio; Phoenix, Arizona; and Memphis, Tennessee. The vignettes were identical except that the patient's illness was identified as either AIDS or leukemia and the patient's sexual preference as either heterosexual or homosexual. After reading the vignette, the physicians were asked to complete a set of objective attitude measures concerning their reactions to the patient.

Analysis of the physicians' answers indicated that some had strong negative feelings about interacting socially with AIDS patients, even if the interaction were limited to a single conversation. In general, they considered AIDS patients to be more deserving of their illness and less deserving of sympathy than those with leukemia. Kelly and his coworkers conclude: "In addition to training in medical aspects of AIDS prevention, diagnosis, and management, it will be important for health care providers who will soon be treating AIDS-affected patients to examine their own attitudes toward these persons, become knowledgeable about lifestyle issues that influence the health of gay patients, and be sensitive to the stigmatization that AIDS patients too often face."[27]

The rapid evolution in the care of HIV-infected patients dictates that education about AIDS must be a continuous process. Donna Gallagher, clinical coordinator for the AIDS and Oncology Program at Harvard Community Health Plan in Boston, says that one of her biggest problems is counteracting the hopelessness engendered by the early years of the AIDS epidemic.

She cites a recent case in which patients with their first episode of *Pneumocystis carinii* pneumonia were being told by physicians in a hospital emergency room that admission to the intensive care unit would only prolong their suffering—that most patients with AIDS die rapidly despite the use of aggressive life-sustaining measures.

Although it is true that AIDS is a fatal disease, new treatment regimens have made a dramatic difference in the life expectancy of patients with *P. carinii* pneumonia: 85 to 90 percent now survive their first episode, and some return to independent living after a second or third episode. The information conveyed to patients by the physicians in that particular emergency room did not present an accurate picture of available alternatives.

Support Groups

Helping patients and family members maintain a balanced perspective about the outcome of AIDS is one of the most challenging aspects of providing care for HIV-infected patients, primarily because it requires health care providers to deal effectively with their own feelings about the disease. Watching the gradual deterioration and death of men and women who should be in the prime of life requires tremendous emotional stamina, especially for those accustomed to winning medical battles against an array of lesser pathogens.

Frequent staff meetings at which workers feel comfortable expressing their concerns about patient interactions, personal safety, and related issues are essential for any institution providing regular services for AIDS patients. Such meetings may prevent the AIDS-related "burnout" of one of this country's most vital resources—highly trained, compassionate health care providers.

Career Choices

Leaders in medical, dental, and nursing education worry that fear of HIV infection may discourage young people from entering the health care professions at a time when staff shortages could prove disastrous for the urban centers most affected by the AIDS epidemic.

Michael Specter, a staff writer for the *Washington Post*, noted in a recent article that medical school applications are at their lowest point in years and that some of the best resident training programs in the country have been unable to fill all of their positions. "Over the past few years," Specter says, "a growing percentage of the nation's brightest medical school graduates have been shopping for specialties requiring little real contact with patients."[28] Officials cite a variety of reasons for these trends, but many physicians believe that fear of AIDS plays a dominant role.

Educators in all the health fields are exploring ways to convey to students that the risk of HIV infection for those following recommended procedures is *extremely* small and that the rewards of providing care are substantial.

Conclusion

The psychosocial impact of HIV infection should not be underestimated. AIDS transforms the lives of patients, their families, and friends, but its effects are not limited to those who know AIDS firsthand. Fear of the syndrome, of its devastating complications and high mortality rate, affects all of us.

For now, prevention through risk-reduction education and other public health measures is the only effective weapon against the AIDS epidemic. Data on homosexual groups indicate that behavioral change is possible with appropriate educational interventions, but researchers still know very little about whether such changes will last or how to reach other segments of society. Studies of the factors that influence sexual behavior and drug abuse among both high- and low-risk groups should be given high priority.

Psychosocial factors also may play a role in determining a person's susceptibility to infection or to disease once the virus has entered the body. For example, scientists in other fields have shown a direct link between stress and immune function. Researchers at the National Institute of Mental Health and other organizations have begun long-term studies to determine the relationship between psychological status and immunological and clinical function in people at high risk of HIV infection.

Efforts to plan for the future health care needs of patients infected with HIV also depend on greater knowledge about the range of neuropsychiatric problems caused by the virus. Clinicians need better tests to monitor changes in mental function. Without these tests, it may be very difficult to assess the patient's capabilities with respect to self-care and compliance with therapeutic regimens. Unrealistic expectations in these areas could be a source of extreme frustration for both the patient and the medical staff.

The majority of AIDS cases in the United States have been concentrated in urban centers in New York, California, Florida, New Jersey, the District of Columbia, and Texas, but other parts of the country will become more heavily burdened as those who are now HIV-seropositive begin to develop symptoms. These new patients and the communities in which they live will require knowledgeable physicians, nurses, dentists, psychologists, social workers, and a vast array of support services. Education of these professionals, encompassing both the psychosocial and the health effects of the syndrome, should be given high priority by educational institutions, professional societies, and the government.

9

The Impact of AIDS on the Health Care System

Nowhere has the impact of AIDS on the health care system been more dramatic than in New York City. In May 1986 the city's hospitals were operating at 81.6 percent of capacity. For 1987 the average was 90 percent, and by the end of the year some inner-city hospitals were more than 100 percent full. In January 1988 an article in the *New York Times* described hospital emergency rooms in which critically ill patients waited as many as 5 days for admission to hospital wards.[1]

The reasons for the severe hospital bed shortage in New York City are complex—not all of them are a result of the AIDS epidemic. Unexpected increases in other patient groups contributed to the problem. Some people believe that a 10-year effort to trim health care costs by reducing the number of hospital beds in the city went too far. But the growth in AIDS cases has pushed the system to its limits. New York City has 24 percent of the AIDS caseload in the United States. In 1987 the number of AIDS patients hospitalized in public and private city hospitals increased by more than 40 percent. Public health experts believe that by 1991 almost 9 percent of all patients in New York City will be hospitalized for AIDS, up from 3 percent in 1985.

Efforts to find solutions to the overcrowding in New York hospitals have been stymied by the national shortage of health care workers, especially nurses. In March 1988 state health officials approved plans to increase the capacity of hospitals in New York City by 475 beds for AIDS patients. At the time, the president of the Greater New York Hospital Association said that it could take up to 2 years to hire the estimated 750 nurses required for the expansion.[2]

San Francisco, which ranks second in the number of AIDS cases, has not experienced this overcrowding. Experts say that San Francisco is better off than New York in part because of the comprehensive support system for AIDS patients established by the city's homosexual community. This system includes home nursing and hospice care. The availability of alternative care facilities reduces the number of AIDS patients who need hospitalization at any one time. (New York's state health commissioner estimates that 30 percent of New York City's AIDS patients could leave their hospital beds if they had somewhere else to go.)[3]

Public health experts warn, however, that the San Francisco model does not represent a long-term solution to the problem of AIDS care. Many of the community-based services in San Francisco have been provided by volunteers. Since early 1987 it has been clear that the volunteer pool would not expand sufficiently to keep pace with the epidemic. Some experienced volunteers have shown signs of the same type of emotional burnout seen in health care workers; the task of replacing them grows increasingly difficult.[4]

In 1986 New York City and San Francisco accounted for about 40 percent of all AIDS cases in the United States; experts estimate that by 1991 they will account for only 20 percent. Other major metropolitan areas will soon face their own battles with AIDS.

Meeting the Needs of HIV-Infected Patients

The relatively sudden appearance of large numbers of patients with complex HIV-related diseases has highlighted inadequacies in both the organization and financing of health care in the United States. The Institute of Medicine (IOM) report *Confronting AIDS: Update 1988* outlines a model for AIDS care that includes "appropriate inpatient services for those most acutely ill and comprehensive outpatient care operating at the interface of hospitals and community-based agencies."[5] The model is based on the principle that, to the extent possible, care should be delivered in community settings, rather than in hospitals, to make it more humane and cost-effective.

Public health officials say that one of the biggest impediments to providing adequate care is the lack of established long-term care facilities, especially for patients with AIDS-related dementia, for IV drug abusers with AIDS, and for HIV-infected children.

Patients with AIDS-Related Dementia

Patients with AIDS-related dementia often are too disoriented to live on their own but do not require the intense level of services provided by an acute care hospital. They need an intermediate level of care comparable to that provided for the elderly in nursing homes.

Existing nursing homes generally have been reluctant to admit AIDS patients, in part because of unfounded fears of contagion. In addition, few nursing homes have experience handling patients with severely compromised immune systems, and some may not be staffed adequately to deal with the rapid fluctuations in clinical status characteristic of advanced HIV-related disorders.[6]

Limited reimbursement for costs associated with skilled nursing care contributes to the difficulties in placing patients with dementia. In a 1988 report on AIDS and nursing homes, A. E. Benjamin of the Institute for Health Policy Studies at the University of California, San Francisco, estimated that the true cost of long-term care for AIDS patients is between $200 and $300 per day; yet the typical reimbursement for nursing home care is about $50 per day.[7]

Efforts to place AIDS patients in established hospices also have encountered problems. Hospice care generally has been reserved for patients who have chosen to forgo all treatment except pain relief. But many young AIDS patients are not willing to cut themselves off from new treatment alternatives.

They want to continue radiation therapy or chemotherapy until the last possible moment. Also, reimbursement for hospice care has been based on the premise that patients will receive 80 percent of their care at home. Public and private insurance has not been available to fund hospice care for patients who cannot stay at home.

Skilled nursing facilities must be provided for the growing number of patients with AIDS-related dementia and other neuropsychological deficits. The needs of these patients may be served best at AIDS-dedicated facilities with strong ties to acute care hospitals experienced in the treatment of HIV-related disorders. If such facilities are not available, incentive payments to existing nursing homes may encourage them to provide the necessary services.

Intravenous Drug Abusers

One of the main reasons for the success of the San Francisco system in the short term has been the homogeneous nature of the AIDS population in that city. About 95 percent of AIDS patients in San Francisco are homosexual or bisexual men. In contrast, more than 35 percent of the AIDS patients in New York City are intravenous drug abusers.

Intravenous drug abusers with AIDS are more likely to become totally dependent on the medical care system than are other HIV-infected patients. They are generally sicker when they enter the system, and they are less likely to have a support network of family and friends. The fact that many are homeless contributes to extended hospitalizations. In addition, their often-continuing use of illegal drugs makes the development of community-based group care programs very difficult.[8]

Social workers and physicians in New York City say that "despite a longstanding New York City policy to provide housing other than shelters for homeless AIDS patients, hundreds of people suffering with symptoms of AIDS are living in such shelters."[9] Reporter Gina Kolata describes the overwhelming despair of these homeless men and women who are "among the poorest, least educated and most troubled members of society." She says that most try to hide their illness because they fear they will be ostracized or physically abused by other shelter residents.

There is an urgent need for more long-term residential facilities or group homes for AIDS patients who are IV drug abusers. Those who remain on the streets or in shelters are at extreme risk of acquiring life-threatening secondary infections. They also are more likely to continue high-risk behavior, and therefore are more likely to transmit HIV infection to others.

HIV-Infected Children

Every day at least 10 infants and children with AIDS wait in the hospitals of New York City for someone who will give them an opportunity to experience a normal home life.[10] In the past, some children have waited for several years.

Almost 80 percent of infants who are infected with HIV at birth come from families in which one or both parents are IV drug abusers. In an environment dominated by the combined problems of drug abuse and extreme poverty it is extremely difficult to meet the needs of a chronically ill child. Some mothers abandon their babies in the hospital; others visit often but are too debilitated by their own battles with HIV to take their children home.

In devising long-term care plans for chronically ill children, health care providers usually try to find solutions that preserve the family unit. This may be particularly difficult in AIDS cases, but experts believe the concept should not be abandoned. A mother who is too weak to care for her child on a full-time basis may be able to keep her child at home with the assistance of a special day-care or respite care program. For more serious cases, the IOM Committee for the Oversight of AIDS Activities recommends the establishment of "family" homes that "would allow children and their mothers (who may require medical and drug abuse treatment services) to remain together."[11]

Some HIV-infected infants will never be able to live with their parents. The problems of finding suitable foster care for such children have been described numerous times in the press. Some foster parents are unwilling to take HIV-infected babies because of unfounded fears of disease transmission through household contact. Many others fear the emotional devastation of caring for a child who is unlikely to survive more than a few years. Those who have accepted the challenge say that the rewards more than outweigh the difficulties. They speak proudly of weight gains, improvements in health status, and developmental achievements that occur when a child who has spent most of his life in a hospital crib moves into a loving foster home.

Unfortunately, the demand for foster homes probably will continue to exceed the supply. State officials have predicted that more than 700 HIV-infected babies will be born in New York in 1988. Midway through the year, agencies had recruited fewer than 100 foster parents willing to accept an HIV-infected child.[12]

To overcome the problem of scarce foster care, nonprofit agencies in several communities have developed innovative group homes for HIV-infected children. Some of the best known include Hale's Cradle in New York City, the Farano Center for Children in Albany, and Grandma's House in Washington, D.C. Professional staff members and volunteers work together in these homes to provide a warm and stimulating environment.

The group homes are less expensive than long-term hospitalization but more expensive than foster care. In May 1988 the director of the Farano Center said that the cost of caring for a child at the center was $162 per day, compared with $700 to $900 per day for acute-care hospitalization.[13]

Physicians and other health care providers must be aware of the complete range of services provided for HIV-infected patients by medical and social service agencies in their communities. For adults as well as children, continuity of care must be ensured from the earliest stages of HIV infection.

AIDS-Related Costs

Officials estimate that the annual cost of treating people with AIDS in New York City alone will be at least $1 billion by 1991. Most other regions of the country have just begun to assess the potential economic consequences of the epidemic.

Direct Costs of Care

Studies of the range of costs associated with AIDS have been surprisingly limited. David Bloom of Columbia University and Geoffrey Carliner of the National Bureau of Economic Research have reviewed the 7 most widely cited studies of the personal medical costs of AIDS.[14] Personal medical costs include expenditures for hospital services, physician inpatient and outpatient services, other outpatient care, and nursing home, home nursing, and hospice services. Most studies have focused primarily on the cost of hospital-based care, because specific data on the costs of other types of services are limited or nonexistent.

Bloom and Carliner compared the 7 studies on the basis of the authors' estimates of the cumulative medical costs of AIDS through 1991. The totals ranged from $6.3 billion to $45.4 billion (1986 dollars). Most of the variation reflects differences in estimates of the total number of days AIDS patients spend in the hospital after diagnosis (ranging from 34 days to 168 days). The highest estimate comes from a January 1986 report by Ann Hardy of the Centers for Disease Control and her coworkers.[15] It is based on an early and very small sample of AIDS patients in New York City. Scientists generally agree that this estimate and the figures based on it— including the widely quoted estimate for lifetime hospital costs of $147,000 per AIDS patient—do not accurately reflect current conditions. Bloom and Carliner conclude from their analysis that "the lifetime cost of medical care per patient will not exceed $80,000 . . . If current projections of future AIDS cases are accurate, the cumulative lifetime costs of 270,000 cases diagnosed between 1981 and the end of 1991 will not exceed $22 billion."[16]

The caveat about the accuracy of current projections is extremely important. Anne Scitovsky, chief of the Department of Health Economics at the Palo Alto Medical Foundation/Research Institute, warns that all projections of health care costs associated with AIDS must be interpreted cautiously because of uncertainties about the actual number of AIDS cases. The most obvious source of uncertainty at the moment concerns the number of patients with AIDS-related dementia and AIDS wasting syndrome, 2 conditions added to the CDC definition of AIDS in August 1987.[17] No data exist on the costs of treating these disorders.

A survey by the National Association of Public Hospitals and the Association of Americal Medical Colleges Council of Teaching Hospitals reveals striking regional variations in AIDS costs.[18] The costs per patient per year appear to be highest in the Northeast ($23,421 in 1985), followed by the Midwest ($19,530), the South ($16,902), and the West ($14,858). Dennis P. Andrulis and his coworkers, who conducted the study, explain that at least part of the variation may be explained by the higher proportion of IV drug abusers among AIDS patients in the Northeast (3.5 times higher than in other regions). Intravenous drug abusers with AIDS tend to require more days of hospital care and possibly also more expensive care per day than other AIDS patients.[19]

Some of this difference may be associated with differences in the manifestations of disease. Annual medical care costs are lowest for AIDS patients with an initial diagnosis of Kaposi's sarcoma, which occurs primarily among AIDS patients who acquire HIV through homosexual activity.[20] Intravenous drug abusers are more likely to have *Pneumocystis carinii* pneumonia or some other life-threatening infection when they enter the health care system.

All the studies described so far assume that methods of delivering care and treatment techniques will not change. This assumption represents another important source of uncertainty in cost estimates. Studies in California and Massachusetts show that medical care costs for people with AIDS have declined since the early days of the epidemic, primarily because physicians have learned to treat patients more efficiently and because coordinated care systems are making people less dependent on hospital services.[21]

Treatment methods also are changing rapidly, although the economic impact of these changes remains unclear. Costs associated with the drug azidothymidine (AZT) provide a useful example. Current studies indicate that AZT reduces the need for hospitalization for *P. carinii* pneumonia and perhaps lessens the severity of pneumonia episodes, which should lower costs. On the other hand, the drug is expensive (the annual cost is about $8,000 per patient), it has relatively severe side effects (one-third of patients on AZT require regular blood transfusions for anemia), and it may prolong the period during which patients require skilled nursing care (for example, if the drug protects patients against opportunistic infections but does not prevent AIDS-related dementia).

In the first study to incorporate the cost of AZT in an economic forecast, Fred Hellinger of the National Center for Health Services Research and Health Care Technology Assessment projects that the lifetime costs of treating an AIDS patient will increase from $57,000 in 1988 to $61,800 in 1991 because of the wider use of AZT (costs estimated in 1985 dollars).[22] The economic impact of other new forms of treatment, such as prophylactic antibiotic therapy to reduce the likelihood of future episodes of *P. carinii* pneumonia, has not been examined.

Treatment costs will become an even bigger issue if current studies show that AZT can prevent or slow the onset of disease in people who are infected with HIV but not yet sick. Michael Specter, a reporter for the *Washington Post*, quotes one "senior federal scientist" about the impact of such a finding: "When that happens, we are in for a very bad day. We don't have enough AZT for a million people and the country could not afford it if we did."[23]

Animal studies suggest that a whole range of future anti-HIV therapies may be most effective if begun before the onset of clinical symptoms. Thus, health care planners must look beyond those with full-blown disease to the vast number of people with asymptomatic HIV infections to assess the true medical care costs of the AIDS epidemic.

Nonpersonal Costs

The spread of HIV has created the need for a variety of nonpersonal services that must be included in the direct costs of the epidemic. Scitovsky and Dorothy P. Rice, former director of the National Center for Health Statistics, explain that these nonpersonal costs include expenditures for biomedical research, health education, blood screening services (for blood donors, commercial plasma donors, individuals who believe themselves at high risk of infection, military personnel, and apprehensive members of the general population), counseling and other services providing spiritual and emotional support to patients and their families, housing, and assistance with the chores of daily living (such as shopping).[24]

Scitovsky and Rice estimate that the nonpersonal direct cost of AIDS was $542 million in 1986 and will be $2.3 billion in 1991 (costs expressed in 1986 dollars). The 1991 figure should be considered a low estimate because Scitovsky and Rice's paper appeared before health care experts began calling for large-scale expansion of drug abuse treatment programs in the United States. Increasing the availability of education and treatment programs for IV drug abusers is now recognized as a key to controlling the spread of HIV infection. In 1988 the Presidential Commission on the HIV Epidemic estimated that a national commitment to providing treatment on demand for IV drug abusers would cost about $1.5 billion per year.[25]

Indirect Costs

The personal and nonpersonal direct costs of AIDS pale in comparison with the indirect costs of the epidemic. Indirect costs reflect the loss to society of individual productivity as a result of disability or death. The indirect costs of AIDS are particularly high because the disease strikes young adults in their most productive years.

Two groups of researchers have estimated the indirect costs of the epidemic. Both limited their analyses to AIDS patients. Hardy and her coworkers estimated the indirect costs associated with the first 10,000 cases of AIDS at $4.8 billion (about 3.5 times their estimate of direct hospital costs).[26] Scitovsky and Rice estimated indirect costs for AIDS cases prevalent in 1985, 1986, and 1991 at $3.9 billion, $7.0 billion, and $55.6 billion, respectively. Estimates for 1986 and 1991 are about 7 times the estimated direct medical care costs for the same years.

Scitovsky explains that these estimates are very rough because they assume that people with AIDS have the same age- and sex-specific average earnings as other Americans. Very few data are available to test the validity of this assump tion. In fact researchers believe that homosexual and bisexual men may have above-average earnings, while IV drug abusers probably have lower or no earnings or derive their income from illegal sources. These errors may offset each other in the final calculations.

Despite the uncertainties, both studies clearly demonstrate that loss of future output represents a major share of the economic impact of AIDS. Bloom and Carliner conclude that for the 270,000 AIDS cases projected to arise between 1981 and the end of 1991, forgone earnings could total $146 billion. [27]

Nonpecuniary Costs

No one has attempted to place a value on the tremendous pain and suffering endured by AIDS patients, their families, and their friends. Other nonmonetary factors that might be considered in an assessment of the total costs of the epidemic include the need to behave differently to avoid contracting or transmitting HIV; the rise in discriminatory practices against groups with large numbers of AIDS cases (based on unfounded fears about transmission through casual contact); and the apparent decrease in the number of young people seeking careers in some fields of primary health care.

Placing AIDS Costs in Perspective

The lifetime medical cost per AIDS patient is similar to costs for other serious illnesses, such as heart disease, cancer of the digestive system, and end-stage renal disease.[28] Because the number of cases has been relatively small, AIDS has not yet had a major impact on total national health care expenditures in this country. Bloom and Carliner estimate that the direct cost of AIDS in 1986 was only 0.4 percent of total health expenditures. (According to the National Center for Health Statistics, total national health care expenditures for 1986 were $458.2 billion.) The estimated indirect cost of AIDS was about 2.1 percent of the indirect costs of all illnesses in 1986.

The rate of increase in the prevalence of AIDS is greater, however, than the rate of increase in the prevalence of other diseases that are expensive to treat. Bloom and Carliner estimate that "the direct costs of AIDS will represent 1.5 percent of total national health care expenditures in 1991, over four times higher than the ratio in 1986."[29] The difference in indirect costs will be even greater. Scitovsky and Rice estimate that by 1991 AIDS will represent almost 12 percent of the estimated total indirect costs of all illnesses.[30]

Even with these increases, AIDS will not constitute a major shock to the national economy in the early 1990s. But it will prove a tremendous financial burden for AIDS patients and their families and for municipalities with a high prevalence of HIV infection.

Inequities in the burden of AIDS costs have been a major concern of national committees studying the AIDS crisis.[31] Researchers estimate that the lifetime cost of treating AIDS patients in New York City in 1991 will equal about $100 for each New York City resident; in San Francisco the figure will be about $350 per resident. Private insurance companies, the federal government, and patients themselves will share the burden with local taxpayers, but tax increases required to cover the cost of AIDS could make some communities less desirable places to live. Jo Ivey Boufford, president of New York City's Health and Hospitals Corporation, estimates that local tax revenues paid 27 percent of the total cost of AIDS care in the city in fiscal 1987.[32]

Efforts to determine who pays AIDS medical bills on a national basis have been hampered by insufficient data. In the most comprehensive report to date, Andrulis and his coworkers found that 54 percent of AIDS patients in their study were covered by Medicaid, 2 percent by Medicare (because AIDS patients generally do not live long enough to qualify for Medicare benefits), and 17 percent by private insurance. Twenty-four percent were categorized as "self-pay" or "other," terms often used to indicate "no-pay" or indigent patients.[33] Bloom and Carliner suggest that these figures may overestimate the extent of Medicaid coverage and underestimate private insurance coverage, in part because public hospitals are overrepresented in the sample. Researchers at the Health Care Financing Administration estimate that Medicaid covers 40 percent of AIDS patients.[34]

Andrulis and his associates found that the proportion of self-pay patients was greatest in the South, where states tend to have very restrictive Medicaid eligibility requirements. The public hospitals that treat AIDS patients in these localities must absorb a significant share of the cost and in the future may find it impossible to remain solvent unless some mechanism is developed to provide them with economic relief.

Evidence from several studies indicates that the proportion of AIDS patients who are covered by private health insurance has declined over time.[35] This trend probably will continue as the demographics of the epidemic change. In addition, a recent survey by the congressional Office of Technology Assessment (OTA) found that commercial insurance companies, Blue Cross/Blue Shield plans, and health maintenance organizations plan to reduce their exposure to the financial impact of AIDS.[36] Possible strategies include reducing sales to individual and small group markets through tighter underwriting guidelines, expanding the use of HIV and other testing, adding AIDS-related questions to enrollment applications, and denying applicants with a history of sexually transmitted diseases. In states that prohibit the use of HIV antibody testing to determine health insurance eligibility, insurers may refuse to sell insurance to residents of cities with a high prevalence of AIDS. OTA researchers report that one commercial carrier has withdrawn from the District of Columbia as a result of the AIDS epidemic, that some have placed dollar limits on AIDS coverage in new policies, and that others have introduced waiting periods for AIDS benefits.

The IOM Committee for the Oversight of AIDS Activities examined a variety of short- and long-term proposals to improve health care coverage for all people with HIV infection. It concluded that the extreme adverse effects of AIDS on health care delivery systems in high-prevalence areas necessitate an immediate response from the federal government in the form of a federal grant program. Such a program would (1) offer financial relief to states and medical institutions currently bearing a disproportionate burden of AIDS care, (2) remove financial impediments to adequate medical care for HIV-infected people who are uninsured or unable to obtain insurance through conventional means, (3) enable federal officials to offer technical assistance to states and localities in designing new health service delivery patterns, and (4) create an incentive for the most cost-effective use of existing resources. This program, however, would be only a short-term solution. The committee urged the federal government "to take the lead in developing a comprehensive and coherent national plan for delivering and financing care for HIV-infected and AIDS patients."[37] Elements of such a plan might include encouraging private insurers through government subsidy, modifying Medicaid to make it more uniform among the states, and setting up state insurance risk pools.

The Need for Leadership

Both the IOM committee and some members of the Presidential Commission on the HIV Epidemic concluded that there has been a lack of strong federal leadership on AIDS with regard to health care planning and financing, as well as in other areas. In *Confronting AIDS: Update 1988*, the IOM panel reaffirms an earlier recommendation to establish a permanent national commission on AIDS and HIV infection.

The commission would have an advisory role and would be responsible for monitoring the epidemic as it affects all components of the public and private sector; evaluating research, health care, and public health needs; formulating recommendations for modifying the direction and intensity of health care, public health, and research efforts as the AIDS problem evolves; setting the tone for educational campaigns; assuming an advisory and catalytic role in stimulating appropriate action by federal, state, and local governments, industry, the academic scientific community, and private foundations and organizations; encouraging greater U.S. contributions to international efforts; monitoring and advising on legal and ethical questions raised by the epidemic, reporting to the American public to clarify points of possible confusion, such as the extent of the spread of HIV through heterosexual activity or the effectiveness of condoms; and providing a forum for all involved and interested parties.

As envisioned by the IOM committee, the 9-member commission would have a five-year renewable term. It would have ample staff and funding and possibly also a $10 million discretionary fund that would be spent through existing agencies to permit a rapid response to any new or unforeseen opportunity or problem.

Such a commission would provide the consistent national leadership that has been lacking in this country's initial efforts to prevent and control HIV infection.

National AIDS Hotline:
1-800-342-AIDS

The National AIDS Hotline is a toll-free service available to callers 24 hours a day, 7 days a week. Operated by the American Social Health Association (ASHA), the hotline provides callers with confidential information and referrals. A variety of printed materials are available upon request, free of charge.

Hotline operators are trained to answer basic AIDS-related questions. They also have extensive referral lists for

- state and local AIDS hotlines
- HIV testing and counseling centers
- AIDS educational organizations
- public health clinics/hospitals
- organizations that provide local physician referrals
- legal services
- financial services
- patient and family support groups
- drug abuse counseling
- state AIDS coordinators

Appendix B

August 1987 CDC Surveillance Case Definition for Acquired Immunodeficiency Syndrome

Introduction

The following revised case definition for surveillance of acquired immunodeficiency syndrome (AIDS) was developed by CDC in collaboration with public health and clinical specialists. The Council of State and Territorial Epidemiologists (CSTE) has officially recommended adoption of the revised definition for national reporting of AIDS. The objectives of the revision are a) to track more effectively the severe disabling morbidity associated with infection with human immunodeficiency virus (HIV) (including HIV-1 and HIV-2); b) to simplify reporting of AIDS cases; c) to increase the sensitivity and specificity of the definition through greater diagnostic application of laboratory evidence for HIV infection; and d) to be consistent with current diagnostic practice, which in some cases includes presumptive, i.e., without confirmatory laboratory evidence, diagnosis of AIDS-indicative diseases (e.g., *Pneumocystis carinii* pneumonia, Kaposi's sarcoma).

The definition is organized into three sections that depend on the status of laboratory evidence of HIV infection (e.g., HIV antibody) (Figure 1). The major proposed changes apply to patients with laboratory evidence for HIV infection: a) inclusion of HIV encephalopathy, HIV wasting syndrome, and a broader range of specific AIDS-indicative diseases (Section II.A); b) inclusion of AIDS patients whose indicator diseases are diagnosed presumptively (Section II.B); and c) elimination of exclusions due to other causes of immunodeficiency (Section I.A).

Application of the definition for children differs from that for adults in two ways. First, multiple or recurrent serious bacterial

Source: Reprinted from Council of State and Territorial Epidemiologists and CDC, Center for Infectious Diseases, AIDS Program, "Revision of the CDC Surveillance Case Definition for Acquired Immunodeficiency Syndrome," *Morbidity and Mortality Weekly Report*, 36, supp. 1 (August 14, 1987), 3S–15S.

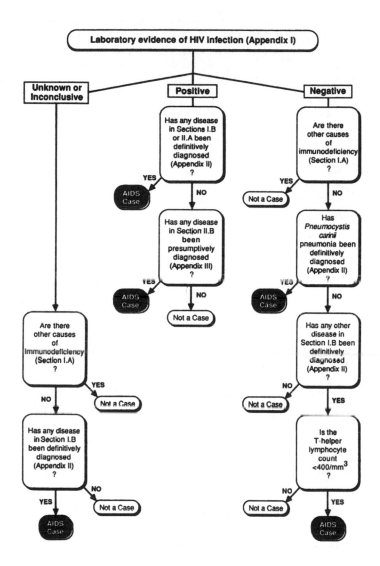

FIGURE 1. Flow diagram for revised CDC case definition of AIDS, September 1, 1987

infections and lymphoid interstitial pneumonia/pulmonary lymphoid hyperplasia are accepted as indicative of AIDS among children but not among adults. Second, for children <15 months of age whose mothers are thought to have had HIV infection during the child's perinatal period, the laboratory criteria for HIV infection are more stringent, since the presence of HIV antibody in the child is, by itself, insufficient evidence for HIV infection because of the persistence of passively acquired maternal antibodies <15 months after birth.

The new definition is effective immediately. State and local health departments are requested to apply the new definition henceforth to patients reported to them. The initiation of the actual reporting of cases that meet the new definition is targeted for September 1, 1987, when modified computer software and report forms should be in place to accommodate the changes. CSTE has recommended retrospective application of the revised definition to patients already reported to health departments. The new definition follows:

1987 Revision of Case Definition for AIDS for Surveillance Purposes

For national reporting, a case of AIDS is defined as an illness characterized by one or more of the following "indicator" diseases, depending on the status of laboratory evidence of HIV infection, as shown below.

I. Without Laboratory Evidence regarding HIV Infection

If laboratory tests for HIV were not performed or gave inconclusive results (See Appendix I) and the patient had no other cause of immunodeficiency listed in Section I.A below, then any disease listed in Section I.B indicates AIDS if it was diagnosed by a definitive method (See Appendix II).

A. *Causes of immunodeficiency that disqualify diseases as indicators of AIDS in the absence of laboratory evidence for HIV infection*
   1. high-dose or long-term systemic corticosteroid therapy or other immunosuppressive/cytotoxic therapy ≤3 months before the onset of the indicator disease
   2. any of the following diseases diagnosed ≤3 months after diagnosis of the indicator disease: Hodgkin's disease, non-Hodgkin's lymphoma (other than primary brain lymphoma), lymphocytic leukemia, multiple myeloma, any other cancer of lymphoreticular or histiocytic tissue, or angioimmunoblastic lymphadenopathy

3. a genetic (congenital) immunodeficiency syndrome or an acquired immunodeficiency syndrome atypical of HIV infection, such as one involving hypogammaglobulinemia
B. *Indicator diseases diagnosed definitively (See Appendix II)*
   1. candidiasis of the esophagus, trachea, bronchi, or lungs
   2. cryptococcosis, extrapulmonary
   3. cryptosporidiosis with diarrhea persisting >1 month
   4. cytomegalovirus disease of an organ other than liver, spleen, or lymph nodes in a patient >1 month of age
   5. herpes simplex virus infection causing a mucocutaneous ulcer that persists longer than 1 month; or bronchitis, pneumonitis, or esophagitis for any duration affecting a patient >1 month of age
   6. Kaposi's sarcoma affecting a patient <60 years of age
   7. lymphoma of the brain (primary) affecting a patient <60 years of age
   8. lymphoid interstitial pneumonia and/or pulmonary lymphoid hyperplasia (LIP/PLH complex) affecting a child <13 years of age
   9 *Mycobacterium avium* complex or *M. kansasii* disease, disseminated (at a site other than or in addition to lungs, skin, or cervical or hilar lymph nodes)
   10. *Pneumocystis carinii* pneumonia
   11. progressive multifocal leukoencephalopathy
   12. toxoplasmosis of the brain affecting a patient >1 month of age

II. With Laboratory Evidence for HIV Infection

Regardless of the presence of other causes of immunodeficiency (I. A), in the presence of laboratory evidence for HIV infection (see Appendix I), any disease listed above (I.B) or below (II.A or II.B) indicates a diagnosis of AIDS.

A. *Indicator diseases diagnosed definitively (see Appendix II)*
   1. bacterial infections, multiple or recurrent (any combination of at least two within a 2-year period), of the following types affecting a child <13 years of age: septicemia, pneumonia, meningitis, bone or joint infection, or abscess of an internal organ or body cavity (excluding otitis media or superficial skin or mucosal abscesses), caused by *Haemophilus, Streptococcus* (including pneumococcus), or other pyogenic bacteria
   2. coccidioidomycosis, disseminated (at a site other than or in addition to lungs or cervical or hilar lymph nodes)

3. HIV encephalopathy (also called "HIV dementia," "AIDS dementia," or "subacute encephalitis due to HIV") (*See* Appendix II for description)
4. histoplasmosis, disseminated (at a site other than or in addition to lungs or cervical or hilar lymph nodes)
5. isosporiasis with diarrhea persisting >1 month
6. Kaposi's sarcoma at any age
7. lymphoma of the brain (primary) at any age
8. other non–Hodgkin's lymphoma of B-cell or unknown immunologic phenotype and the following histologic types:
   a. small noncleaved lymphoma (either Burkitt or non-Burkitt type) (*See* Appendix IV for equivalent terms and numeric codes used in the *International Classification of Diseases,* Ninth Revision, Clinical Modification)
   b. immunoblastic sarcoma (equivalent to any of the following, although not necessarily all in combination: immunoblastic lymphoma, large-cell lymphoma, diffuse histiocytic lymphoma, diffuse undifferentiated lymphoma, or high-grade lymphoma) (*See* Appendix IV for equivalent terms and numeric codes used in the *International Classification of Diseases,* Ninth Revision, Clinical Modification)

   Note: Lymphomas are not included here if they are of T-cell immunologic phenotype or their histologic type is not described or is described as "lymphocytic," "lymphoblastic," "small cleaved," or "plasmacytoid lymphocytic"

9. any mycobacterial disease caused by mycobacteria other than *M. tuberculosis,* disseminated (at a site other than or in addition to lungs, skin, or cervical or hilar lymph nodes)
10. disease caused by *M. tuberculosis,* extrapulmonary (involving at least one site outside the lungs, regardless of whether there is concurrent pulmonary involvement)
11. *Salmonella* (nontyphoid) septicemia, recurrent
12. HIV wasting syndrome (emaciation, "slim disease") (*See* Appendix II for description)

B. *Indicator diseases diagnosed presumptively (by a method other than those in Appendix II)*
   Note: Given the seriousness of diseases indicative of AIDS, it is generally important to diagnose them definitively, especially when therapy that would be used may have serious side effects or when definitive diagnosis is needed for eligibility for antiretroviral therapy. Nonetheless, in some

situations, a patient's condition will not permit the performance of definitive tests. In other situations, accepted clinical practice may be to diagnose presumptively based on the presence of characteristic clinical and laboratory abnormalities. Guidelines for presumptive diagnoses are suggested in Appendix III.

1. candidiasis of the esophagus
2. cytomegalovirus retinitis with loss of vision
3. Kaposi's sarcoma
4. lymphoid interstitial pneumonia and/or pulmonary lymphoid hyperplasia (LIP/PLH complex) affecting a child <13 years of age
5. mycobacterial disease (acid-fast bacilli with species not identified by culture), disseminated (involving at least one site other than, or in addition to lungs, skin, or cervical or hilar lymph nodes)
6. *Pneumocystis carinii* pneumonia
7. toxoplasmosis of the brain affecting a patient >1 month of age

III. **With Laboratory Evidence against HIV Infection**

With laboratory test results negative for HIV infection (see Appendix I), a diagnosis of AIDS for surveillance purposes is ruled out *unless:*

A. *all the other causes of immunodeficiency listed above in Section I.A are excluded; AND*

B. *the patient has had either:*
   1. *Pneumocystis carinii* pneumonia diagnosed by a definitive method (see Appendix II); *OR*
   2. a. any of the other diseases indicative of AIDS listed above in Section I.B diagnosed by a definitive method (see Appendix II); *AND*
      b. a T-helper/inducer (CD4) lympocyte count <400/mm^3.

Commentary

The surveillance of severe disease associated with HIV infection remains an essential, though not the only, indicator of the course of the HIV epidemic. The number of AIDS cases and the relative distribution of cases by demographic, geographic, and behavioral risk variables are the oldest indices of the epidemic, which began in 1981 and for which data are available retrospectively back to 1978. The original surveillance case definition, based on then-available knowledge, provided useful epidemiologic data on severe HIV disease (1). To ensure a reasonable predictive value for underlying immunodeficiency caused by what was then an unknown agent, the indicators of AIDS in the old case definition were restricted to particular opportunistic diseases diagnosed by reliable methods in patients without specific known causes of immunodeficiency. After HIV was discovered to be the cause of AIDS, however, and highly sensitive and specific HIV-antibody tests became available, the spectrum of manifestations of HIV infection became better defined, and classification systems for HIV infection were developed (2–5). It became apparent that some progressive, seriously disabling, and even fatal conditions (e.g., encephalopathy, wasting syndrome) affecting a substantial number of HIV-infected patients were not subject to epidemiologic surveillance, as they were not included in the AIDS case definition. For reporting purposes, the revision adds to the definition most of those severe non-infectious, non-cancerous HIV-associated conditions that are categorized in the CDC clinical classification systems for HIV infection among adults and children (4,5).

Another limitation of the old definition was that AIDS-indicative diseases are diagnosed presumptively (i.e., without confirmation by methods required by the old definition) in 10%–15% of patients diagnosed with such diseases; thus, an appreciable proportion of AIDS cases were missed for reporting purposes (6,7). This proportion may be increasing, which would compromise the old case definition's usefulness as a tool for monitoring trends. The revised case definition permits the reporting of these clinically diagnosed cases as long as there is laboratory evidence of HIV infection.

The effectiveness of the revision will depend on how extensively HIV-antibody tests are used. Approximately one third of AIDS patients in the United States have been from New York City and San Francisco, where, since 1985, <7% have been reported with HIV-antibody test results, compared with >60% in other areas. The impact of the revision on the reported numbers of AIDS cases will also depend on the proportion of AIDS patients in whom indicator diseases are diagnosed presumptively rather than definitively. The use of presumptive diagnostic criteria varies geographically, being more common in certain rural areas and in urban areas with many indigent AIDS patients.

To avoid confusion about what should be reported to health departments, the term "AIDS" should refer only to conditions meeting the surveillance definition. This definition is intended only to provide consistent statistical data for public health purposes. Clinicians will not rely on this definition alone to diagnose serious disease caused by HIV infection in individual patients because there may be additional information that would lead to a more accurate diagnosis. For example, patients who are not reportable under the definition because they have either a negative HIV-antibody test or, in the presence of HIV antibody, an opportunistic disease not listed in the definition as an indicator of AIDS nonetheless may be diagnosed as having serious HIV disease on consideration of other clinical or laboratory characteristics of HIV infection or a history of exposure to HIV.

Conversely, the AIDS surveillance definition may rarely misclassify other patients as having serious HIV disease if they have no HIV-antibody test but have an AIDS-indicative disease with a background incidence unrelated to HIV infection, such as cryptococcal meningitis.

The diagnostic criteria accepted by the AIDS surveillance case definition should not be interpreted as the standard of good medical practice. Presumptive diagnoses are accepted in the definition because not to count them would be to ignore substantial morbidity resulting from HIV infection. Likewise, the definition accepts a reactive screening test for HIV antibody without confirmation by a supplemental test because a repeatedly reactive screening test result, in combination with an indicator disease, is highly indicative of true HIV disease. For national surveillance purposes, the tiny proportion of possibly false-positive screening tests in persons with AIDS-indicative diseases is of little consequence. For the individual patient, however, a correct diagnosis is critically important. The use of supplemental tests is, therefore, strongly endorsed. An increase in the diagnostic use of HIV-antibody tests could improve both the quality of medical care and the function of the new case definition, as well as assist in providing counseling to prevent transmission of HIV.

References

1. World Health Organization. Acquired immunodeficiency syndrome (AIDS): WHO/CDC case definition for AIDS. WHO Wkly Epidemiol Rec 1986;61:69–72.
2. Haverkos HW, Gottlieb MS, Killen JY, Edelman R. Classification of HTLV-III/LAV-related diseases [Letter]. J Infect Dis 1985;152:1095.
3. Redfield RR, Wright DC, Tramont EC. The Walter Reed staging classification of HTLV-III infection. N Engl J Med 1986;314:131–2.
4. CDC. Classification system for human T-lymphotropic virus type III/lymphadenopathy-associated virus infections. MMWR 1986;35:334–9.
5. CDC. Classification system for human immunodeficiency virus (HIV) infection in children under 13 years of age. MMWR 1987;36:225–30,235.
6. Hardy AM, Starcher ET, Morgan WM, et al. Review of death certificates to assess completeness of AIDS case reporting. Pub Hlth Rep 1987;102(4):386–91.
7. Starcher ET, Biel JK, Rivera-Castano R, Day JM, Hopkins SG, Miller JW. The impact of presumptively diagnosed opportunistic infections and cancers on national reporting of AIDS [Abstract]. Washington, DC: III International Conference on AIDS, June 1–5, 1987.

Appendix I. Laboratory Evidence for or against HIV Infection

1. *For Infection*
   When a patient has disease consistent with AIDS:
   a. a serum specimen from a patient ≥15 months of age, or from a child <15 months of age whose mother is not thought to have had HIV infection during the child's prenatal period, that is repeatedly reactive for HIV antibody by a screening test (e.g., enzyme-linked immunosorbent assay [ELISA]), as long as subsequent HIV-antibody tests (e.g., Western blot, immunofluorescence assay), if done, are positive; *or*
   b. a serum specimen from a child <15 months of age, whose mother is thought to have had HIV infection during the child's perinatal period, that is repeatedly reactive for HIV antibody by a screening test (e.g., ELISA), plus increased serum immunoglobulin levels and at least one of the following abnormal immunologic test results: reduced absolute lymphocyte count, depressed CD4 (T-helper) lymphocyte count, or decreased CD4/CD8 (helper/suppressor) ratio, as long as subsequent antibody tests (e.g., Western blot, immunofluorescence assay), if done, are positive; *or*
   c. a positive test for HIV serum antigen; *or*
   d. a positive HIV culture confirmed by both reverse transcriptase detection and a specific HIV-antigen test or in situ hybridization using a nucleic acid probe; *or*
   e. a positive result on any other highly specific test for HIV (e.g., nucleic acid probe of peripheral blood lymphocytes).

2. *Against Infection:*
   A nonreactive screening test for serum antibody to HIV (e.g., ELISA) without a reactive or positive result on any other test for HIV infection (e.g., antibody, antigen, culture), if done.

3. *Inconclusive (Neither for nor against Infection):*
   a. a repeatedly reactive screening test for serum antibody to HIV (e.g., ELISA) followed by a negative or inconclusive supplemental test (e.g., Western blot, immunofluorescence assay) without a positive HIV culture or serum antigen test, if done; *or*
   b. a serum specimen from a child <15 months of age, whose mother is thought to have had HIV infection during the child's perinatal period, that is repeatedly reactive for HIV antibody by a screening test, even if positive by a supplemental test, without additional evidence for immunodeficiency as described above (in 1.b) and without a positive HIV culture or serum antigen test, if done.

Appendix II. Definitive Diagnostic Methods for Diseases Indicative of AIDS

Diseases	Definitive Diagnostic Methods
cryptosporidiosis cytomegalovirus isosporiasis Kaposi's sarcoma lymphoma lymphoid pneumonia or hyperplasia *Pneumocystis carinii* pneumonia progressive multifocal leukoencephalopathy toxoplasmosis	Microscopy (histology or cytology)
candidiasis	Gross inspection by endoscopy or autopsy or by microscopy (histology or cytology) on a specimen obtained directly from the tissues affected (including scrapings from the mucosal surface), not from a culture
coccidioidomycosis cryptococcosis herpes simplex virus histoplasmosis	Microscopy (histology or cytology), culture, or detection of antigen in a specimen obtained directly from the tissues affected or a fluid from those tissues
tuberculosis other mycobacteriosis salmonellosis other bacterial infection	Culture
HIV encephalopathy* (dementia)	Clinical findings of disabling cognitive and/or motor dysfunction interfering with occupation or activities of daily living, or loss of behavioral developmental milestones affecting a child, progressing over weeks to months, in the absence of a concurrent illness or condition other than HIV infection that could explain the findings. Methods to rule out such concurrent illnesses and conditions must include cerebrospinal fluid examination and either brain imaging (computed tomography or magnetic resonance) or autopsy

HIV wasting syndrome*

Findings of profound involuntary weight loss >10% of baseline body weight plus either chronic diarrhea (at least two loose stools per day for ≥30 days) or chronic weakness and documented fever (for ≥30 days, intermittent or constant) in the absence of a concurrent illness or condition other than HIV infection that could explain the findings (e.g., cancer, tuberculosis, cryptosporidiosis, or other specific enteritis)

* For HIV encephalopathy and HIV wasting syndrome, the methods of diagnosis described here are not truly definitive, but are sufficiently rigorous for surveillance purposes.

Appendix III. Suggested Guidelines for Presumptive Diagnosis of Diseases Indicative of AIDS

Diseases	*Presumptive Diagnostic Criteria*
Candidiasis of esophagus	a. recent onset of retrosternal pain on swallowing; *and* b. oral candidiasis diagnosed by the gross appearance of white patches or plaques on an erythematous base or by the microscopic appearance of fungal mycelial filaments in an uncultured specimen scraped from the oral mucosa.
Cytomegalovirus retinitis	a characteristic appearance on serial ophthalmoscopic examinations (e.g., discrete patches of retinal whitening with distinct borders, spreading in a centrifugal manner, following blood vessels, progressing over several months, frequently associated with retinal vasculitis, hemorrhage, and necrosis). Resolution of active disease leaves retinal scarring and atrophy with retinal pigment epithelial mottling.
Mycobacteriosis	microscopy of a specimen from stool or normally sterile body fluids or tissue from a site other than lungs, skin, or cervical or hilar lymph nodes, showing acid-fast bacilli of a species not identified by culture.

Kaposi's
sarcoma

a characteristic gross appearance of an erythematous or violaceous plaque-like lesion on skin or mucous membrane.

(*Note:* Presumptive diagnosis of Kaposi's sarcoma should not be made by clinicians who have seen few cases of it.)

Lymphoid
interstitial
pneumonia

bilateral reticulonodular interstitial pulmonary infiltrates present on chest X ray for ≥2 months with no pathogen identified and no response to antibiotic treatment.

*Pneumocystis
carinii*
pneumonia

a. a history of dyspnea on exertion or nonproductive cough of recent onset (within the past 3 months); *and*

b. chest X-ray evidence of diffuse bilateral interstitial infiltrates or gallium scan evidence of diffuse bilateral pulmonary disease; *and*

c. arterial blood gas analysis showing an arterial pO_2 of <70 mm Hg or a low respiratory diffusing capacity (<80% of predicted values) or an increase in the alveolar-arterial oxygen tension gradient; *and*

d. no evidence of a bacterial pneumonia.

Toxoplasmosis
of the brain

a. recent onset of a focal neurologic abnormality consistent with intracranial disease or a reduced level of consciousness; *and*

b. brain imaging evidence of a lesion having a mass effect (on computed tomography or nuclear magnetic resonance) or the radiographic appearance of which is enhanced by injection of contrast medium; *and*

c. serum antibody to toxoplasmosis or successful response to therapy for toxoplasmosis

Appendix IV. Equivalent Terms and International Classification of Disease (ICD) Codes for AIDS-Indicative Lymphomas

The following terms and codes describe lymphomas indicative of AIDS in patients with antibody evidence for HIV infection (Section II.A.8 of the AIDS case definition). Many of these terms are obsolete or equivalent to one another.

ICD-9-CM (1978)

Codes	Terms
200.0	Reticulosarcoma
	lymphoma (malignant): histiocytic (diffuse) reticulum cell sarcoma: pleomorphic cell type or not otherwise specified
200.2	Burkitt's tumor or lymphoma
	malignant lymphoma, Burkitt's type

ICD-O (Oncologic Histologic Types 1976)

Codes	Terms
9600/3	Malignant lymphoma, undifferentiated cell type
	non-Burkitt's or not otherwise specified
9601/3	Malignant lymphoma, stem cell type
	stem cell lymphoma
9612/3	Malignant lymphoma, immunoblastic type
	immunoblastic sarcoma, immunoblastic lymphoma, or immunoblastic lymphosarcoma
9632/3	Malignant lymphoma, centroblastic type
	diffuse or not otherwise specified, or germinoblastic sarcoma: diffuse or not otherwise specified
9633/3	Malignant lymphoma, follicular center cell, non-cleaved
	diffuse or not otherwise specified
9640/3	Reticulosarcoma, not otherwise specified
	malignant lymphoma, histiocytic: diffuse or not otherwise specified
	reticulum cell sarcoma, not otherwise specified malignant lymphoma, reticulum cell type
9641/3	Reticulosarcoma, pleomorphic cell type
	malignant lymphoma, histiocytic, pleomorphic cell type reticulum cell
	sarcoma, pleomorphic cell type
9750/3	Burkitt's lymphoma or Burkitt's tumor
	malignant lymphoma, undifferentiated, Burkitt's type malignant lymphoma, lymphoblastic, Burkitt's type

Appendix C
Existing Tests for HIV Infection

Tests to detect evidence of HIV infection were first licensed in 1985, primarily to help prevent transmission of AIDS through the blood supply.[1] Since then their use has expanded tremendously. Voluntary testing and counseling are recommended for people seeking treatment for sexually transmitted diseases, for intravenous drug abusers, for all people who consider themselves at risk for HIV infection, for prostitutes, and for women of childbearing age with identifiable risks for HIV infection (see Appendix E). Mandatory testing has been instituted in the United States for applicants for military service, for active-duty military personnel, for Job Corps applicants, and for federal prisoners. HIV tests also are employed by public health officials in blinded surveys to assess the level of HIV infection in specific populations (for example, mothers of newborn infants), and by researchers tracking the effects of experimental antiviral drugs.

The 9 tests currently licensed for clinical diagnosis of HIV infection include 8 enzyme-linked immunosorbent assay (ELISA) tests and one Western blot test-kit. Both the licensed ELISA tests and the Western blot detect the presence of antibodies produced in response to HIV infection. Many other types of tests, including tests that measure specific viral proteins or viral DNA, are used for research purposes.

Licensed Tests

The standard ELISA tests employ either a plastic sheet or plastic beads coated with an extremely thin layer of viral proteins. (The proteins are produced from purified inactivated virus grown in tissue culture.) When human serum is added to this system, any HIV antibodies present in the serum stick to the proteins on the sheet or beads. After an incubation period of about 2 hours the test materials are washed and 2 additional reagents are added to the system. A color reaction occurs if the specimen contains HIV antibodies. Reactions are read with a spectrophotometer and graded to indicate the strength of any positive results. A standard ELISA test takes from 2 to 4 hours and costs from $1 to $4.[2]

The licensed Western blot also employs disrupted purified virus, but the viral proteins are separated by electrophoresis and then transferred to a strip of nitrocellulose paper. The test serum is applied to the paper and incubated overnight. Following the addition of several other reagents, color bands appear on the paper strip wherever HIV antibodies have bound to the separated viral proteins. By comparing the test strip against a laboratory standard (a Western blot from a specimen containing antibodies to all the HIV proteins), it is possible to identify specific HIV antibodies present in the serum. The cost of processing a specimen with the licensed Western blot test is about $45.[3]

The accuracy of currently marketed HIV antibody tests compares very favorably with that of other medical diagnostic tests.[4] The terms used to describe the accuracy of such tests are *sensitivity* and *specificity*. The sensitivity is the percentage of people with a given condition who test positive for that condition (in this case, the percentage of HIV-infected people who have a positive HIV antibody test). The specificity is the percentage of uninfected persons with a negative test result. An ideal test would be 100 percent sensitive and 100 percent specific, but no biological system is perfect. The developers of a test attempt to balance sensitivity and specificity in a manner that is compatible with the rationale for performing the test.

Scientists at the Centers for Disease Control explain that a test for HIV antibody is considered positive when a sequence of tests, starting with a repeatedly reactive ELISA and including an additional, more specific assay, such as a Western blot, are "consistently reactive." Multiple tests are necessary because the ELISA tests are designed to be extremely sensitive. (False-negative results are very unlikely except during the early weeks of infection, when HIV antibodies may not be detectable; see Chapters 2 and 5).

The high sensitivity of the ELISA antibody tests helps ensure that HIV-contaminated blood does not enter the blood supply. The trade-off in attaining this assurance is that a small proportion of those who test positive are not actually infected. Data submitted by the manufacturers to the U.S. Food and Drug Administration indicate that all the licensed ELISA tests have a specificity greater than 99 percent when performed under ideal conditions.[5] But the medical and social consequences of a false-positive HIV test are so serious that such specificity is not considered sufficient. A reactive ELISA must be repeated and then validated with a more specific test before a person is determined to be infected with HIV.

The likelihood that an entire testing sequence (repeated ELISA tests followed by a Western blot) will be false positive depends on the population being tested, the nature of the confirmatory test, and the proficiency of the laboratory performing the test. Estimates of the minimum number of false-positive results that can be expected in a population with a low prevalence of HIV infection range from 1 in 100,000 to 5 in 100,000; one study suggests, however, that in practice the joint false-positive rate may be as high as 1 in 1,250.[6]

The Western blot is highly specific when strict criteria are used to interpret the results, but interpretation varies from one laboratory to the next. Before 1987 some laboratories reported a positive result for specimens demonstrating reactivity against just one HIV protein band. Now most laboratories consider a test positive only if it reveals antibodies against 2 or 3 different HIV proteins. If fewer bands are present, the test is considered indeterminate; it is interpreted as negative only if no bands are present. Retesting after 6 months usually provides a more definitive answer for people with indeterminate test results. Those whose test results are initially indeterminate because they had a relatively new HIV infection are likely to have a positive blot pattern after 6 months. Follow-up testing on an uninfected person should produce a blot pattern identical to the first one.

In its report *Confronting AIDS: Update 1988,* the Institute of Medicine urged the federal government to "give more attention to establishing standards for laboratory proficiency in HIV antibody testing, setting criteria for interpreting assays, and instituting quality assurance procedures."[7]

Other Types of Tests

Although the licensed HIV tests have made a major contribution to protecting the blood supply in the United States, they are not well suited for certain other tasks, such as screening potential blood donors in developing countries (where both laboratory facilities and trained personnel are in short supply) or following the clinical course of HIV-infected patients. More than 25 biotechnology companies are working to develop new strategies to meet these needs.[8]

Second-Generation Antibody Tests

One strategy used by several companies involves substituting HIV proteins produced by recombinant DNA technology for the inactivated natural viral proteins employed in the original antibody tests. Researchers believe that second-generation ELISA tests using the recombinant proteins will prove to be more specific than current tests because they do not contain cellular antigens (which appear to cause some false-positive reactions). The new tests also may be more sensitive because of the high concentration of viral proteins available to react with HIV antibodies in serum specimens.

Second-generation antibody tests now in clinical trials include a 30-minute assay, in which a positive reaction appears as a blue dot on a small plastic card, and a 5-minute test involving microscopic latex beads (visual clumping of the beads indicates a positive response).

Antigen Tests

All antibody tests are limited by their dependence on the immune response to HIV infection. Almost all people infected with HIV go through a brief period in which they have virus in their blood but no antibodies. To improve detection of these early infections, researchers are evaluating tests that measure replicating virus and viral proteins (antigens) shed by infected cells.

In practice, the antigen tests are very similar to the ELISA tests for antibody. A plastic base is coated with purified HIV antibodies. The bound antibodies are incubated with human serum and then treated with a series of reagents. A color change in the system indicates that the specimen contains HIV antigens.

Antigen tests probably will complement rather than replace antibody tests in HIV screening, because many HIV-infected patients do not have detectable levels of free virus or viral antigens in their blood.[9] The antigen tests already have been useful on an experimental basis for following patients during drug therapy.

Detection of Viral DNA or RNA

Recent studies indicate that certain cells can harbor latent HIV in the form of a DNA provirus. Latently infected cells do not produce viral proteins and probably do not elicit antibodies. Thus, it would be useful to be able to detect the DNA provirus directly. One method for doing this involves a new technique called polymerase chain reaction (PCR). PCR tests use recombinant DNA technology to greatly amplify and then identify minute amounts of targeted genetic material.[10]

Early reports indicate that the PCR test may be most useful for early detection of HIV in infected infants. The test also could be invaluable for tracing the course of HIV infection in the body.

In the future many different tests will be available for detection of exposure to HIV. Public health officials, clinicians, and researchers will have to become familiar with the technical characteristics of these tests to ensure that they are used and interpreted properly. Factors other than test performance that must be considered in selecting an appropriate technique include cost, the technical competence of people who will use a particular test, the test's shelf life under varying conditions of heat and humidity, and the availability of appropriate laboratory backup procedures.

Notes

1. John C. Petricciani and Jay S. Epstein, "The Effects of the AIDS Epidemic on the Safety of the Nation's Blood Supply," *Public Health Reports* 103 (1988):236–241.
2. Ron Dagani, "The Problem of Diagnostic Tests," *Chemical and Engineering News* 65, no 47 (1987):35–40.
3. Deborah M. Barnes, "New Questions about AIDS Test Accuracy," *Science* 238 (1987):884–885.
4. Institute of Medicine, *Confronting AIDS: Update 1988* (Washington, D.C.: National Academy Press, 1988).
5. Centers for Disease Control, "Update: Serologic Testing for Antibody to Human Immunodeficiency Virus," *MMWR* 36 (1988):833–840, 852.
6. Michael D. Hagen, Klemens B. Meyer, and Stephen G. Pauker, "Routine Preoperative Screening for HIV: Does the Risk to the Surgeon Outweigh the Risk to the Patient?" *JAMA* 259 (1988):1357–1359.
7. Institute of Medicine, *Confronting AIDS: Update 1988*, p. 71.
8. Sandra Blakeslee, "Pressure for Wider AIDS Testing Fuels Search for Better Methods," *New York Times,* June 19, 1987, p. C14.
9. Thomas F. Zuck and Jay S. Epstein, "The Human Immunodeficiency Virus: Testing for Its Presence and Strategies for Its Inactivation," in *Transfusion-Transmitted Viruses: Epidemiology and Pathology,* ed. S. J. Insalaco and J. E. Menitove (Arlington, Va.: American Association of Blood Banks, 1987).
10. Chin-Yih Ou, Shirley Kwok, Sheila W. Mitchell, David H. Mack, John J. Sninsky, John W. Krebs, Paul Feorino, Donna Warfield, and Gerald Schochetman, "DNA Amplification for Direct Detection of HIV-1 in DNA of Peripheral Blood Mononuclear Cells," *Science* 239 (1988):295–297.

Appendix D
Prevention of HIV Transmission in Health Care Settings

Recent recommendations from the Centers for Disease Control emphasize the need for health care workers to consider *all* patients as potentially infected with human immunodeficiency virus (HIV) and/or other bloodborne pathogens and to adhere rigorously to infection-control precautions for minimizing the risk of exposure to blood and body fluids of all patients. The recommendations with full explanation appear in two documents:

• "Recommendations for Prevention of HIV Transmission in Health-Care Settings," *Morbidity and Mortality Weekly Report* 36, supp. 2 (August 21, 1987).
• "Update: Universal Precautions for Prevention of Transmission of Human Immunodeficiency Virus, Hepatitis B Virus, and Other Bloodborne Pathogens in Health-Care Settings," *Morbidity and Mortality Weekly Report* 37 (June 24, 1988), 377–382, 387–388.

Copies of these documents may be obtained free of charge through the National AIDS Information Clearinghouse, P.O. Box 6003, Rockville, Md. 20850 (or call 1-800-458-5231).

The Occupational Safety and Health Administration (OSHA), Department of Labor, requires that employers protect their workers from occupational exposure to HIV, hepatitis B virus, and other bloodborne infections. For information on OSHA requirements see:

• "Enforcement Procedures for Occupational Exposure to Hepatitis B Virus (HBV) and Human Immunodeficiency Virus (HIV)," OSHA Instruction CPL2-2.44A.

This document may be obtained from the OSHA Publications Distribution Office, Room N3101, U.S. Department of Labor, 200 Constitution Ave. N.W., Washington, D.C. 20210.

Appendix E

Public Health Service Guidelines for Counseling and Antibody Testing to Prevent HIV Infection and AIDS

These guidelines are the outgrowth of the 1986 recommendations published in the *MMWR* (*1*); the report on the February 24–25, 1987, Conference on Counseling and Testing (*2*); and a series of meetings with representatives from the Association of State and Territorial Health Officials, the Association of State and Territorial Public Health Laboratory Directors, the Council of State and Territorial Epidemiologists, the National Association of County Health Officials, the United States Conference of Local Health Officers, and the National Association of State Alcohol and Drug Abuse Directors.

Human immunodeficiency virus (HIV), the causative agent of acquired immunodeficiency syndrome (AIDS) and related clinical manifestations, has been shown to be spread by sexual contact; by parenteral exposure to blood (most often through intravenous [IV] drug abuse) and, rarely, by other exposures to blood; and from an infected woman to her fetus or infant.

Persons exposed to HIV usually develop detectable levels of antibody against the virus within 6–12 weeks of infection. The presence of antibody indicates current infection, though many infected persons may have minimal or no clinical evidence of disease for years. Counseling and testing persons who are infected or at risk for acquiring HIV infection is an important component of prevention strategy (*1*). Most of the estimated 1.0 to 1.5 million infected persons in the United States are unaware that they are infected with HIV. The primary public health purposes of counseling and testing are to help uninfected individuals initiate and sustain behavioral changes that reduce their risk of becoming infected and to assist infected individuals in avoiding infecting others.

Source: Reprinted from *Morbidity and Mortality Weekly Report,* 36 (August 14, 1987), 509–515.

297

Along with the potential personal, medical, and public health benefits of testing for HIV antibody, public health agencies must be concerned about actions that will discourage the use of counseling and testing facilities, most notably the unauthorized disclosure of personal information and the possibility of inappropriate discrimination.

Priorities for public health counseling and testing should be based upon providing ready access to persons who are most likely to be infected or who practice high-risk behaviors, thereby helping to reduce further spread of infection. There are other considerations for determining testing priorities, including the likely effectiveness of preventing the spread of infection among persons who would not otherwise realize that they are at risk. Knowledge of the prevalence of HIV infection in different populations is useful in determining the most efficient and effective locations providing such services. For example, programs that offer counseling and testing to homosexual men, IV-drug abusers, persons with hemophilia, sexual and/or needle-sharing partners of these persons, and patients of sexually transmitted disease clinics may be most effective since persons in these groups are at high risk for infection. After counseling and testing are effectively implemented in settings of high and moderate prevalence, consideration should be given to establishing programs in settings of lower prevalence.

Interpretation of HIV-Antibody Test Results

A test for HIV antibody is considered positive when a sequence of tests, starting with a repeatedly reactive enzyme immunoassay (EIA) and including an additional, more specific assay, such as a Western blot, are consistently reactive.

The *sensitivity* of the currently licensed EIA tests is 99% or greater when performed under optimal laboratory conditions. Given this performance, the probability of a false-negative test result is remote, except during the first weeks after infection, before antibody is detectable.

The *specificity* of the currently licensed EIA tests is approximately 99% when repeatedly reactive tests are considered. Repeat testing of specimens initially reactive by EIA is required to reduce the likelihood of false-positive test results due to laboratory error. To further increase the specificity of the testing process, laboratories must use a supplemental test—most often the Western blot test—to validate repeatedly reactive EIA results. The sensitivity of the licensed Western blot test is comparable to that of the EIA, and it is highly specific when strict criteria are used for interpretation. Under ideal circumstances, the probability that a testing sequence will be falsely positive in a population with a low rate of infection ranges from less than 1 in 100,000 (Minnesota Department of Health, unpublished data) to an estimated 5 in 100,000 *(3,4)*. Laboratories using different Western blot reagents or other tests or using less stringent interpretive criteria may experience higher rates of false-positive results.

Laboratories should carefully guard against human errors, which are likely to be the most common source of false-positive test results. All laboratories should anticipate the need for assuring quality performance of tests for HIV antibody by training personnel, establishing quality controls, and participating in performance evaluation systems. Health department laboratories should facilitate the quality assurance of the performance of laboratories in their jurisdiction.

Guidelines for Counseling and Testing for HIV Antibody

These guidelines are based on public health considerations for HIV testing, including the principles of counseling before and after testing, confidentiality of personal information, and the understanding that a person may decline to be tested without being denied health care or other services, except where testing is required by law *(5)*. Counseling before testing may not be practical when screening for HIV antibody is required. This is true for donors of blood, organs, and tissue; prisoners; and immigrants for whom testing is a Federal requirement as well as for persons admitted to state correctional institutions in states that require testing. When there is no counseling before testing, persons should be informed that testing for HIV antibody will be performed, that individual results will be kept confidential to the extent permitted by law, and that appropriate counseling will be offered. Individual counseling of those who are either HIV-antibody positive or at continuing risk for HIV infection is critical for reducing further transmission and for ensuring timely medical care.

Specific recommendations follow:

1. *Persons who may have sexually transmitted disease.* All persons seeking treatment for a sexually transmitted disease, in all health-care settings including the offices of private physicians, should be routinely* counseled and tested for HIV antibody.

2. *IV-drug abusers.* All persons seeking treatment for IV-drug abuse or having a history of IV-drug abuse should be routinely

---

* "Routine counseling and testing" is defined as a policy to provide these services to all clients after informing them that testing will be done. Except where testing is required by law, individuals have the right to decline to be tested without being denied health care or other services.

counseled and tested for HIV antibody. Medical professionals in all health-care settings, including prison clinics, should seek a history of IV-drug abuse from patients and should be aware of its implications for HIV infection. In addition, state and local health policy makers should address the following issues:

• Treatment programs for IV-drug abusers should be sufficiently available to allow persons seeking assistance to enter promptly and be encouraged to alter the behavior that places them and others at risk for HIV infection.
• Outreach programs for IV-drug abusers should be undertaken to increase their knowledge of AIDS and of ways to prevent HIV infection, to encourage them to obtain counseling and testing for HIV antibody, and to persuade them to be treated for substance abuse.

3. *Persons who consider themselves at risk.* All persons who consider themselves at risk for HIV infection should be counseled and offered testing for HIV antibody.
4. *Women of childbearing age.* All women of childbearing age with identifiable risks for HIV infection should be routinely counseled and tested for HIV antibody, regardless of the health-care setting. Each encounter between a health-care provider and a woman at risk and/or her sexual partners is an opportunity to reach them with information and education about AIDS and prevention of HIV infection. Women are at risk for HIV infection if they:

• Have used IV drugs.
• Have engaged in prostitution.
• Have had sexual partners who are infected or are at risk for infection because they are bisexual or are IV-drug abusers or hemophiliacs.
• Are living in communities or were born in countries where there is a known or suspected high prevalence of infection among women.
• Received a transfusion before blood was being screened for HIV antibody but after HIV infection occurred in the United States (e.g., between 1978 and 1985).

Educating and testing these women before they become pregnant allows them to avoid pregnancy and subsequent intrauterine perinatal infection of their infants (30%–50% of the infants born to HIV-infected women will also be infected).

All pregnant women at risk for HIV infection should be routinely counseled and tested for HIV antibody. Identifying pregnant women with HIV infection as early in pregnancy as possible is important for ensuring appropriate medical care for these women; for planning medical care for their infants; and for providing counseling on family planning, future pregnancies, and the risk of sexual transmission of HIV to others.

All women who seek family planning services and who are at risk for HIV infection should be routinely counseled about AIDS and HIV infection and tested for HIV antibody. Decisions about the need for counseling and testing programs in a community should be based on the best available estimates of the prevalence of HIV infection and the demographic variables of infection.

5. *Persons planning marriage.* All persons considering marriage should be given information about AIDS, HIV infection, and the availability of counseling and testing for HIV antibody. Decisions about instituting routine or mandatory premarital testing for HIV antibody should take into account the prevalence of HIV infection in the area and/or population group as well as other factors and should be based upon the likely cost-effectiveness of such testing in preventing further spread of infection. Premarital testing in an area with a prevalence of HIV infection as low as 0.1% may be justified if reaching an infected person through testing can prevent subsequent transmission to the spouse or prevent pregnancy in a woman who is infected.

6. *Persons undergoing medical evaluation or treatment.* Testing for HIV antibody is a useful diagnostic tool for evaluating patients with selected clinical signs and symptoms such as generalized lymphadenopathy; unexplained dementia; chronic, unexplained fever or diarrhea; unexplained weight loss; or diseases such as tuberculosis as well as sexually transmitted diseases, generalized herpes, and chronic candidiasis.

Since persons infected with both HIV and the tubercle bacillus are at high risk for severe clinical tuberculosis, all patients with tuberculosis should be routinely counseled and tested for HIV antibody (6). Guidelines for managing patients with both HIV and tuberculous infection have been published (7).

The risk of HIV infection from transfusions of blood or blood components from 1978–1985 was greatest for persons receiving large numbers of units of blood collected from areas with high incidences of AIDS. Persons who have this increased risk should be counseled about the potential risk of HIV infection and should be offered antibody testing (8).

7. *Persons admitted to hospitals.* Hospitals, in conjunction with state and local health departments, should periodically determine the

prevalence of HIV infections in the age groups at highest risk for infection. Consideration should be given to routine testing in those age groups deemed to have a high prevalence of HIV infection.

8. *Persons in correctional systems.* Correctional systems should study the best means of implementing programs for counseling inmates about HIV infection and for testing them for such infection at admission and discharge from the system. In particular, they should examine the usefulness of these programs in preventing further transmission of HIV infection and the impact of the testing programs on both the inmates and the correctional system (9). Federal prisons have been instructed to test all prisoners when they enter and leave the prison system.

9. *Prostitutes.* Male and female prostitutes should be counseled and tested and made aware of the risks of HIV infection to themselves and others. Particularly prostitutes who are HIV-antibody positive should be instructed to discontinue the practice of prostitution. Local or state jurisdictions should adopt procedures to assure that these instructions are followed.

Partner Notification/Contact Tracing

Sexual partners and those who share needles with HIV-infected persons are at risk for HIV infection and should be routinely counseled and tested for HIV antibody. Persons who are HIV-antibody positive should be instructed in how to notify their partners and to refer them for counseling and testing. If they are unwilling to notify their partners or if it cannot be assured that their partners will seek counseling, physicians or health department personnel should use confidential procedures to assure that the partners are notified.

Confidentiality and Antidiscrimination Considerations

The ability of health departments, hospitals, and other health-care providers and institutions to assure confidentiality of patient information and the public's confidence in that ability are crucial to efforts to increase the number of persons being counseled and tested for HIV infection. Moreover, to assure broad participation in the counseling and testing programs, it is of equal or greater importance that the public perceive that persons found to be positive will not be subject to inappropriate discrimination.

Every reasonable effort should be made to improve confidentiality of test results. The confidentiality of related records can be improved by a careful review of actual record-keeping practices and by assessing the degree to which these records can be protected under applicable state laws. State laws should be examined and strengthened when found necessary. Because of the wide scope of "need-to-know" situations, because of the possibility of inappropriate disclosures, and because of established authorization procedures for releasing records, it is recognized that there is no perfect solution to confidentiality problems in all situations. Whether disclosures of HIV-testing information are deliberate, inadvertent, or simply unavoidable, public health policy needs to carefully consider ways to reduce the harmful impact of such disclosures.

Public health prevention policy to reduce the transmission of HIV infection can be furthered by an expanded program of counseling and testing for HIV antibody, but the extent to which these programs are successful depends on the level of participation. Persons are more likely to participate in counseling and testing programs if they believe that they will not experience negative consequences in areas such as employment, school admission, housing, and medical services should they test positive. There is no known medical reason to avoid an infected person in these and ordinary social situations since the cumulative evidence is strong that HIV infection is not spread through casual contact. It is essential to the success of counseling and testing programs that persons who are tested for HIV are not subjected to inappropriate discrimination.

References

1. CDC. "Additional recommendations to reduce sexual and drug abuse-related transmission of human T-lymphotropic virus type III/lymphadenopathy-associated virus." MMWR 1986;35:152–5.
2. CDC. Recommended additional guidelines for HIV antibody counseling and testing in the prevention of HIV infection and AIDS. Atlanta, Georgia: US Department of Health and Human Services, Public Health Service, 1987.
3. Burke DS, Brandt BL, Redfield RR, et al. Diagnosis of human immunodeficiency virus infection by immunoassay using a molecularly cloned and expressed virus envelope polypeptide. Ann Intern Med 1987;106:671–6.
4. Meyer KB, Pauker SG. Screening for HIV: can we afford the false positive rate? N Engl J Med 1987;317:238–41.
5. Bayer R, Levine C, Wolf SM. HIV antibody screening: an ethical framework for evaluating proposed programs. JAMA 1986;256:1768–74.
6. CDC. Tuberculosis provisional data—United States, 1986. MMWR 1987;36:254–5.
7. CDC. Diagnosis and management of mycobacterial infection and disease in persons with human T-lymphotropic virus type III/lymphadenopathy-associated virus infection. MMWR 1986;35:448–52.
8. CDC. Human immunodeficiency virus infection in transfusion recipients and their family members. MMWR 1987;36:137–40.
9. Hammett TM. AIDS in correctional facilities: issues and options. 2nd ed. Washington, DC: U.S. Department of Justice, National Institute of Justice, 1987.

Appendix F

The Chronology of AIDS Research

This statement from Robert Gallo and Luc Montagnier constitutes part of the agreement between the U.S. and French AIDS research groups. This history is by no means exhaustive. It outlines the main contributions of the two central parties and of some other groups to the determination of the causative agent of AIDS (acquired immune deficiency syndrome). This is not to diminish the important contribution made in this field (either independently or in collaboration with us) by other laboratories and clinicians distributed worldwide.

Both sides wish it to be known that from the beginning there has been a spirit of scientific cooperation and a free exchange of ideas, biological materials and personnel between Dr. Gallo's and Dr. Montagnier's laboratories. The spirit has never ceased despite the legal problems and will be the basis of a renewed mutual cooperation in the future.

The parties also believe that some clarification is needed regarding their position on nomenclature. Various generic names have been given to the AIDS virus. Dr. Gallo and his collaborators named it HTLV-III in their May 1984 publications according to a recommendation made in September 1983 at the Cold Spring Harbor meeting on HTLVs by a group of ten European, Japanese and American retrovirologists. They suggested that names of human retroviruses discovered in the future related to but distinct from human T-leukaemia virus be named sequentially, numbered HTLV-III, IV, and so on.

Dr. Montagnier and his collaborators first reported in May 1983 the identification of a novel human retrovirus not closely related to HTLV-I and II and in public meetings from September 1983 and subsequently in publications from 1984, they named this virus LAV for lymphadenopathy-associated virus because the first patient from which it was isolated had lymphadenopathy syndrome.

The US Department of Health and Human Services officially assumed a double generic name, HTLV-III/LAV, in recognition of the contributions of both sides.

Source: Reprinted from *Nature,* 326 (April 2, 1987), 435–436, by permission of Macmillan Magazines Ltd.

When the genome structure of the AIDS virus was determined in 1985, the results showed some major differences in the organization of the genetic information from HTLV-I and II. This prompted another and more formal nomenclature committee to suggest a simpler and new generic name as the virus belonged to an entirely new class of human retroviruses. Their suggestion was to use the generic term HIV—human immunodeficiency virus. They also suggested maintaining specific strain names (LAV-1$_{BRU}$, LAV-1$_{LOI}$, HTLV-III$_B$, HTLV-III$_{RF}$, ARVI . . .) in the interest of continuity and appreciation of the biological differences of the strains. Both groups agree with this recommendation.

We set out a brief chronological history of some critical published facts, in the period up to May 1985, on the discovery and demonstration of AIDS as a retroviral disease.

Retroviruses

1970–73. Following Temin's hypothesis that RNA tumour viruses replicate via a provirus DNA intermediate, Temin and Mitzutani (1970),[1] and independently Baltimore (1970)[2], discover reverse transcriptase. Later, the existence and integration of infectious proviral DNA is demonstrated by Hill and Hillova (1971)[3] and confirmed by Montagnier and Vigier (1972)[4], Svoboda and co-workers (1973)[5], and others. Spiegelman (1970)[6], Gallo (1971, 1972)[7,8], Gerwin et al. (1972)[9] and others independently develop useful sensitive specific assays for reverse transcriptase of retroviruses.

1976. Morgan, Ruscetti and Gallo (1976)[10] discover T-cell growth factor, or interleukin-2 (IL-2), necessary for long-term in vitro cultivation of human T cells.

1979. Barre-Sinoussi, Montagnier, Lidereau, Sisman, Wood and Chermann (1979)[11] show that antibody against alpha interferon allows significant increase in mouse retrovirus production by infected cells.

Human Retroviruses

1980–82. Gallo, Poiesz and co-workers (1980) isolate[12] and (1981) characterize[13] the first human retrovirus, called human T-cell leukaemia virus type I (HTLV-I). Hinuma et al. (1981)[14] identify C-type virus in a cell line isolated by Miyoshi from a patient with adult T-cell leukaemia (ATL) and detect antibodies against antigen-bearing cells in patients with ATL. Yoshida and co-workers (1982)[15] isolate and characterize adult T-cell leukaemia virus (ATLV) and demonstrate clonal integration of ATLV proviral DNA in leukaemic cells of patients. In a cooperative study, Gallo and co-workers together with Miyoshi and co-workers (1982)[16] show ATLV to be identical with HTLV-I. In collaborative studies, Catovsky, Blattner, Gallo and co-workers (1982)[17,18] show HTLV-I to be a contributing aetiological factor in T-cell leukaemia in the Caribbean region. Gallo and co-workers (1982)[19] isolate a second type of retrovirus, HTLV-II, from a cell line obtained from a patient with hairy-cell leukaemia.

AIDS

1981. Gottlieb and co-workers (1982)[20], Friedman-Kien and co-workers (1981)[21], Siegel and co-workers (1981)[22], Masur and co-workers (1981)[23] and Mildvan and co-workers (1982)[24] independently diagnose a new disease, AIDS, in groups of young homosexual men.

1982. Epidemiological evidence suggesting that AIDS is a new infectious disease is developed by the Centers for Disease Control (1982)[25].

February 1983. At the Cold Spring Harbor Workshop on AIDS, Gallo proposes that AIDS is probably caused by a retrovirus, presumably a variant of HTLV-I or II.

May 1983. Barre-Sinoussi, Chermann, Montagnier and co-workers (1983)[26] publish: (1) the isolation and identification of a non-transforming retrovirus (later called lymphadenopathy-associated virus (LAV)), different from HTLV-I and HTLV-II, in cultures of T lymphocytes derived from a patient with lymphadenopathy syndrome; (2) the continuous passage of the virus by its transient growth in cultures of T lymphocytes of normal blood donors; (3) the identification of a major protein associated with this virus, p25, not immunologically cross-reactive with the p24 of HTLV-I; and (4) the detection by immunoprecipitation of antibodies against this protein in two patients.

Essex and co-workers (1983)[27] detect antibodies cross-reactive with HTLV-I membrane protein in 25–30% of AIDS patients.

Gelman and co-workers (Gallo's group) (1983)[28] find evidence for presence of the viral genome of HTLV-I or an HTLV-I variant in 2 of 33 AIDS patients.

September 1983. At the Cold Spring Harbor meeting on human T-cell leukaemia-lymphoma viruses:

Montagnier and co-workers (1984)[29] report: (1) the identification of LAV-like viruses from 5 patients with lymphadenopathy and 3 patients with AIDS (homosexual, haemophiliac, Haitian); (2) the selective affinity of LAV for CD4(T4) helper lymphocytes: (3) the presence of antibodies (enzyme-linked immunosorbent assay, ELISA) against the main LAV antigens in patients with lymphadenopathy-associated syndrome (LAS) (63%) and AIDS (20%); (4) that LAV is morphologically similar to equine infectious anaemia virus (EIAV) and different from HTLVs; and (5) the antigenic cross-reactivity between core proteins of EIAV and LAV (virus isolates from LAS patients are called LAV, and from AIDS patients are called IDAV).

Gallo and co-workers (1984)[30] report the presence of HTLV-I antibodies in 10% of AIDS patients and isolates of HTLV-I or HTLV-II or variants of it in fewer than 10% of such cases.

March–April 1984. Montagnier *et al.* (1984)[31] by using more sera of horses infected with EIAV confirm cross-reactivity of the core proteins of LAV with that of EIAV and identify a second viral protein, p18. Vilmer, Chermann, Montagnier and co-workers (1984)[32] confirm previous isolation of an LAV-like virus from one haemophiliac and isolate another one from his asymptomatic brother.

May 1984. Gallo's group (1984) reports: (1) mass and continuous production in a clone of a permanent cell line (H9) of HTLV-III from two AIDS patients and four additional isolates (SN, BK, CS, WT) also infectious for another clone (H4) derived from the same parental cell line (Popovic, Sarngadharan, Gallo and co-workers[33]).

(2) 48 virus isolations, that is, 18 of 21 patients with pre-AIDS, 3 of 4 clinically normal mothers of juveniles with AIDS, 26 of 72 juveniles and adults with AIDS, 1 of 22 healthy male homosexuals, and 0 of 115 heterosexual subjects (Gallo, Salahuddin, Popovic and colleagues[34]). The use of anti-p24 hyperimmune sera proves that the 48 isolates belong to the same kind of virus;

(3) The introduction of the Western blot technique for clinical detection of antibodies in 88% of 48 patients with AIDS, 79% of 14 homosexuals with pre-AIDS and less than 1% of hundreds of heterosexuals. A gp41 is identified as a major viral antigen (Sarngadharan, Popovic, Gallo and co-workers[35]). Later, it is demonstrated by Veronese, Sarngadharan and Gallo to be the HTLV-III viral transmembrane component of the envelope[36].

(4) Partial characterization of the immunologically reactive proteins by the Western blot technique. (Schupbach, Sarngadharan, Popovic, Gallo and co-workers[37]).

June 1984. Safai, Gallo, Popovic and Sarngadharan report 34 of 34 (100%) of AIDS patients positive for HTLV-III antibodies, 16 of 19 (84%) of LAS patients and 0 of 14 (0%) of controls (1984)[38].

Brun-Vezinet, Barre-Sinoussi, Montagnier, Chermann and co-workers (1984)[39] publish detection of antibodies against LAV proteins by ELISA in 74.5% of the patients presenting with lymphadenopathy syndrome, 37.5% of patients with frank AIDS, 18% of healthy homosexuals, 1% of blood donors.

July 1984. Kalyanaraman, Montagnier, Francis and co-workers (1984)[40] report the detection of anti-p25 (LAV) antibodies in 51 of 125 (41%) of AIDS patients, 81 of 113 (72%) of LAS patients, and 0 of 70 of healthy individuals; Montagnier and co-workers (1984)[41] report the growth of LAV in continuous B-cell lines, most of them transformed by Epstein-Barr virus.

Klatzmann, Gluckman, Chermann, Montagnier and co-workers (1984)[42] publish: (1) the selective isolation of LAV from CD4⁺ (T4⁺) lymphocytes of a healthy carrier of the virus; (2) the inhibition of CD4 cell growth at the same time of *in vitro* virus production; (3) the simultaneous disappearance of the CD4 antigen at the surface of the infected CD4 lymphocytes.

August 1984. A third group, Levy *et al.*, (1984)[43] isolate virus antigenically and structurally related to LAV from San Francisco AIDS patients.

September 1984. Cheinsong-Popov, Weiss and collaborators publish identical prevalence of antibodies against antigens of HTLV-III grown in H9 line and of LAV-1 grown in CEM line in UK patients with AIDS or at risk of AIDS (1984)[44].

Goedert, Gallo and co-workers (1984)[45] report that in a cohort of homosexual men at risk of AIDS, 53% were antibody-positive for HTLV-III. In HTLV-III antibody positive subjects, AIDS developed at 6.9% per year.

October 1984. Brun-Vezinet, Montagnier, Piot, Quinn and co-workers (1984)[46] publish the presence of antibody against LAV in 35 of 37 Zaïrean patients with AIDS.

Zagury, Gallo and co-workers (1984)[47] isolate HTLV-III from cells cultured from semen of two patients with AIDS.

November 1984. Hahn, Gallo and co-workers (1984)[48] report the molecular cloning of HTLV-III virus.

Kitchen, Allan, Essex and co-workers (1984)[49], (1985)[50] identify the viral external glycoprotein gp120, a finding confirmed by Montagnier and co-workers (1985)[51].

December 1984. Alizon, Barre-Sinoussi, Wain-Hobson, Montagnier and co-workers (1984)[52] report the molecular cloning of LAV-1.

Wong-Staal, Shaw, Gallo and co-workers (1984)[53] discover genomic heterogeneity of HTLV-III.

Dagleish, Weiss and co-workers (1984)[54] and independently Klatzmann, Gluckman, Montagnier and co-workers (1984)[55] show the CD4 molecule is involved in the receptor to the virus.

Popovic, Read-Connole and Gallo (1984)[56] publish a series of CD4-positive human neoplastic cell lines susceptible to and permissive for HTLV-III, including HUT78, Molt3 and CEM cell lines.

January 1985. The nucleotide sequence of the AIDS virus

genome is established independently at the Pasteur Institute (1985)[57], at the NCI/NIH (1985)[58], at Genentech, Inc. (1985)[59] and at Chiron (1985)[60], revealing the similarity of the various isolates.

Sodroski, Wong-Staal, Gallo, Haseltine and co-workers (1985)[61] demonstrate transactivation of transcription in HTLV-III infected cells.

Shaw, Gallo and co-workers (1985)[62] discover the presence of virus in the brain.

March 1985. Redfield, Gallo and co-workers (1985)[63] describe heterosexual transmission of HTLV-III.

We wish to acknowledge with gratitude the generous help of many of our colleagues in the preparation of this history. We cannot individually thank them all here, but would like to offer special thanks to Dr. Jonas Salk for his help and guidance in completing this project.

Notes

1. Temin, H.M. & Mizutani, S. *Nature* 226, 1211–1213 (1970).
2. Baltimore, D. *Nature* 226, 1209–1211 (1970).
3. Hill, M. & Hillova, J. *C.r. Acad. Sci. Paris* 272D, 3094 (1971).
4. Montagnier, L. & Vigier, P. *C.r. Acad. Sci. Paris* 274D, 1977–1980 (1972).
5. Svoboda, I, et al. *J. gen. Virol.* 21, 47–55 (1973).
6. Spiegelman, S, et al. *Nature* 237, 1029–1031 (1970).
7. Gallo, R.C. *Nature* 234, 194–198 (1971).
8. Sarngadharan, M.G., Sarin, P.S., Reitz, M.S. & Gallo, R.C. *Nature new Biol.* 240 67–72 (1972).
9. Gerwin, B.I. & Hilstein, J.B. *Proc. natn. Acad. Sci. U.S.A.* 69, 2599–2603 (1972).
10. Morgan, D.A., Ruscatti, F.W. & Gallo, R.C. *Science* 193, 1007–1008 (1976).
11. Barre-Sinoussi, F. et al. *Ann. Microbiol. (Inst. Pasteur)* 130B, 349–362 (1979).
12. Polesz, B.J. et al. *Proc. natn. Acad. Sci. U.S.A.* 77, 7415–7419 (1980).
13. Rbo, H.M. et al. *Virology* 112, 355–360 (1981); Reitz, M.S. Jr et al. *Proc. natn. Acad. Sci. U.S.A.* 78, 1887–1891. (1981); Kalyanaraman, V.S. et al. *Nature* 294, 271–273 (1981); Robert-Guroff, M. et al. *J. exp. Med.* 154, 1957–1964 (1981).
14. Hinuma, Y. et al. *Proc. natn. Acad. Sci. U.S.A.* 78, 6476–6480 (1981).
15. Yoshida, M., Miyoshi, I. & Hinuma, Y. *Proc. natn. Acad. Sci. U.S.A.* 79, 2031–2035 (1983).
16. Popovic, M. et al. *Nature* 306, 63–66 (1982).
17. Catovsky, D. et al. *Lancet* i, 639–642 (1982).
18. Blattner, W.A. et al. *Ins. J. Cancer* 30, 257–264 (1982).
19. Kalyanaraman, V.S. et al. *Science* 218, 571–575 (1982).
20. Gottlieb, M.S. et al. *Morbid. Mortal. weekly Rep.* 30, 250–252 (1981); Gottlieb, M.S. et al. *N. Engl. J. Med.* 305, 1423–1431 (1981).
21. Friedman-Kien, S.M. et al. *Morbid. Mortal. weekly Rep.* 30, 305–308 (1981).
22. Siegel, P.P. et al. *N. Engl J. Med.* 306, 1439–1444 (1981).
23. Masur, H. et al. *N. Engl. J. Med.* 305, 1431–1438 (1981).
24. Mildvan, D. et al. *Morbid. Mortal. weekly Rep.* 31, 249–251 (1982).

310   Appendix F

25. Centers for Disease Control Task Force on Kaposi's Sarcoma and Opportunistic Infections N. Engl. J. Med. 306, 1248–1252 (1982).
26. Barre-Sinoussi, F. et al. Science 220, 868–871 (1983).
27. Essex, M. et al. Science 220, 859–862 (1983).
28. Gelman, E.P. et al. Science 220, 862–865 (1983).
29. Montagnier, L. et al. in Human T-cell Leukaemia Lymphoma Viruses (eds Gallo, R.C., Essex, M.E. & Gross, L.) 363–379 (Cold Spring Harbor Laboratory, New York, 1984).
30. Robert-Guroff, M. et al. in Human T-Cell Leukaemia Lymphoma Viruses (eds Gallo, R.C., Essex, M.E. & Gross, L.) 363–379 (Cold Spring Harbor Laboratory, New York, 1984).
31. Montagnier, L. et al. Ann. Virol. (Inst Pasteur) 186E. 119–134 (1984).
32. Vilmer, E. et al. Lancet i 753–757 (1984).
33. Popovic, M., Sarngadharan, M.Q., Read, E. & Gallo, R.C. Science 224, 497–500 (1984).
34. Gallo, R.C. et al. Science 224, 500–503 (1984).
35. Sarngadharan, M.G., Popovic, M., Bruch, L., Schupbach, J. & Gallo, R.C. Science 224, 506–508 (1984).
36. Veronese, F. et al. Science 229, 1402–1405 (1985).
37. Schupbach, J. et al. Science 224, 503–505 (1984).
38. Safat, B. et al. Lancet i, 1435–1440 (1984).
39. Brun-Vezinet, F. et al. Lancet i 1253–1256 (1984).
40. Kalyanaraman, V.S. et al, Science 225, 321–323 (1984).
41. Montagnier, L. Science 226, 63–66 (1984).
42. Klatzmann, D. et al. Science 225, 59–69 (1984).
43. Levy, J.A. et al. Science 225, 840–842 (1984).
44. Cheinsong-Popov, R. et al. Lancet ii, 477–480 (1984).
45. Goedert, J.J. et al. Lancet ii, 711–716 (1984).
46. Brun-Vezinet, F. et al. Science 226, 453–456 (1984).
47. Zagury, D. et al. Science 226, 449–451 (1984).
48. Hahn, B.H. et al. Nature 312, 166–169 (1984).
49. Kitchen, L.W. et al. Nature 312, 367–369 (1984).
50. Allan, J. et al. Science 226, 1091–1094 (1985).
51. Montagnier, L. et al. Virology 144, 283–289 (1985).
52. Alizon, M. et al. Nature 312, 757–760 (1984).
53. Wong-Staal, F. et al. Science 227, 759–762, (1985).
54. Dagleish, A.G. et al. Nature 312, 763–767 (1984).
55. Klatzmann, D. et al. Nature 312, 767–768 (1984).
56. Popovic, M., Read-Connole, E. & Gallo, R.C. Lancet ii, 1472–1473 (1984).
57. Wain-Hobson, S., Sonigo, P., Danos, O., Cole, S. & Alizon, M. Cell 40, 9–17 (1985).
58. Ratner, L., Gallo, R.C. & Wong-Staal, F. Nature 313, 636–637 (1985).
59. Hausing, M.A. et al. Nature 313, 460–468 (1985).
60. Sanchez-Pescador, R. et al. Science 227, 484–492 (1985).
61. Sodroski, J. et al. Science 227, 171–173 (1985).
62. Shaw, G.M. et al. Science 227, 177–182 (1985).
63. Redfield, R.R. et al. J. Am. med. Ass. 253, 1571–1573 (1985).

Appendix G

Public Health Service Recommendations for the Education and Foster Care of Children Infected with HIV

The information and recommendations contained in this document were developed and compiled by CDC in consultation with individuals appointed by their organizations to represent the Conference of State and Territorial Epidemiologists, the Association of State and Territorial Health Officers, the National Association of County Health Officers, the Division of Maternal and Child Health (Health Resources and Services Administration), the National Association for Elementary School Principals, the National Association of State School Nurse Consultants, the National Congress of Parents and Teachers, and the Children's Aid Society. The consultants also included the mother of a child with acquired immunodeficiency syndrome (AIDS), a legal advisor to a state education department, and several pediatricians who are experts in the field of pediatric AIDS. This document is made available to assist state and local health and education departments in developing guidelines for their particular situations and locations.

These recommendations apply to all children known to be infected with human immunodeficiency virus (HIV). This includes children with AIDS as defined for reporting purposes [see Appendix B]; children who are diagnosed by their physicians as having an illness due to infection with HIV but who do not meet the case definition; and children who are asymptomatic but have virologic or serologic evidence of infection with HIV. These recommendations do not apply to siblings of infected children unless they are also infected.

Source: Reprinted in part from "PHS Recommendations: Education and Foster Care of Children Infected with HTLV-III/LAV," *Morbidity and Mortality Weekly Report,* 34 (August 30, 1985), 517–521.

★ The term *HIV* has been substituted throughout for the older term *HTLV-III/LAV.*

Background

Legal Issues Among the legal issues to be considered in forming guidelines for the education and foster care of HIV infected children are the civil rights aspects of public school attendance, the protections for handicapped children under 20 U.S.C. 1401 et seq. and 29 U.S.C. 794, the confidentiality of a student's school record under state laws and under 20 U.S.C. 1232g, and employee right-to-know statutes for public employees in some states.

Confidentiality Issues The diagnosis of AIDS or associated illnesses evokes much fear from others in contact with the patient and may evoke suspicion of life styles that may not be acceptable to some persons. Parents of HIV-infected children should be aware of the potential for social isolation should the child's condition become known to others in the care or educational setting. School, day-care, and social service personnel and others involved in educating and caring for these children should be sensitive to the need for confidentiality and the right to privacy in these cases.

Assessment of Risks

Risk Factors for Acquiring HIV Infection and Transmission In adults and adolescents, HIV is transmitted primarily through sexual contact (homosexual or heterosexual) and through parenteral exposure to infected blood or blood products. HIV has been isolated from blood, semen, saliva, and tears but transmission has not been documented from saliva and tears. Adults at increased risk for acquiring HIV include homosexual/bisexual men, intravenous drug abusers, persons transfused with contaminated blood or blood products, and sexual contacts of persons with HIV infection or in groups at increased risk for infection.

The majority of infected children acquire the virus from their infected mothers in the perinatal period (1–4). In utero or intrapartum transmission are likely, and one child reported from Australia apparently acquired the virus postnatally, possibly from ingestion of breast milk (5). Children may also become infected through transfusion of blood or blood products that contain the virus . . .

Risk of Transmission in the School, Day-Care or Foster-Care Setting None of the identified cases of HIV infection in the United States are known to have been transmitted in the school, day-care, or foster-care setting or through other casual person-to-person contact. Other than the sexual partners of HIV-infected patients and infants born to infected mothers, none of the family members of the over 12,000 AIDS patients reported to CDC have been reported to have AIDS. Six studies of family members of patients with HIV infection have failed to demonstrate HIV transmission to adults who were not sexual contacts of the infected patients or to older children who were not likely at risk from perinatal transmission (6–11).

Based on current evidence, casual person-to-person contact as would occur among schoolchildren appears to pose no risk. However, studies of the risk of transmission through contact between younger children and neurologically handicapped children who lack control of their body secretions are very limited. Based on experience with other communicable diseases, a theoretical potential for transmission would be greatest among these children. It should be emphasized that any theoretical transmission would most likely involve exposure of open skin lesions or mucous membranes to blood and possibly other body fluids of an infected person.

Risks to the Child with HIV Infection HIV infection may result in immunodeficiency. Such children may have a greater risk of encountering infectious agents in a school or day-care setting than at home. Foster homes with multiple children may also increase the risk. In addition, younger children and neurologically handicapped children who may display behaviors such as mouthing of toys would be expected to be at greater risk for acquiring infections. Immunodepressed children are also at greater risk of suffering severe complications from such infections as chickenpox, cytomegalovirus, tuberculosis, herpes simplex, and measles. Assessment of the risk to the immunodepressed child is best made by the child's physician who is aware of the child's immune status. The risk of acquiring some infections, such as chickenpox, may be reduced by prompt use of specific immune globulin following a known exposure.

Recommendations

1. Decisions regarding the type of educational and care setting for HIV-infected children should be based on the behavior, neurologic development, and physical condition of the child and the expected type of interaction with others in that setting. These decisions are best made using the team approach including the child's physician, public health personnel, the child's parent or guardian, and personnel associated with the proposed care or educational setting. In each case, risks and benefits to both the infected child and to others in the setting should be weighed.

2. For most infected school-aged children, the benefits of an

unrestricted setting would outweigh the risks of their acquiring potentially harmful infections in the setting and the apparent nonexistent risk of transmission of HIV. These children should be allowed to attend school and after-school day-care and to be placed in a foster home in an unrestricted setting.

3. For the infected preschool-aged child and for some neurologically handicapped children who lack control of their body secretions or who display behavior, such as biting, and those children who have uncoverable, oozing lesions, a more restricted environment is advisable until more is known about transmission in these settings. Children infected with HIV should be cared for and educated in settings that minimize exposure of other children to blood or body fluids.

4. Care involving exposure to the infected child's body fluids and excrement, such as feeding and diaper changing, should be performed by persons who are aware of the child's HIV infection and the modes of possible transmission. In any setting involving an HIV-infected person, good handwashing after exposure to blood and body fluids and before caring for another child should be observed, and gloves should be worn if open lesions are present on the caretaker's hands. Any open lesions on the infected person should also be covered.

5. Because other infections in addition to HIV can be present in blood or body fluids, all schools and day-care facilities, regardless of whether children with HIV infection are attending, should adopt routine procedures for handling blood or body fluids. Soiled surfaces should be promptly cleaned with disinfectants, such as household bleach (diluted 1 part bleach to 10 parts water). Disposable towels or tissues should be used whenever possible, and mops should be rinsed in the disinfectant. Those who are cleaning should avoid exposure of open skin lesions or mucous membranes to the blood or body fluids.

6. The hygienic practices of children with HIV infection may improve as the child matures. Alternatively, the hygienic practices may deteriorate if the child's condition worsens. Evaluation to assess the need for a restricted environment should be performed regularly.

7. Physicians caring for children born to mothers with AIDS or at increased risk of acquiring HIV infection should consider testing the children for evidence of HIV infection for medical reasons. For example, vaccination of infected children with live virus vaccines, such as the measles-mumps-rubella vaccine (MMR), may be hazardous. [For a discussion of the current recommendations on the immunization of children infected with HIV, see Chapter 3.] These children also need to be followed closely for problems with growth and development and given prompt and aggressive therapy for

infections and exposure to potentially lethal infections, such as varicella. In the event that an antiviral agent or other therapy for HIV infection becomes available, these children should be considered for such therapy. Knowledge that a child is infected will allow parents and other caretakers to take precautions when exposed to the blood and body fluids of the child.

8. Adoption and foster-care agencies should consider adding HIV screening to their routine medical evaluations of children at increased risk of infection before placement in the foster or adoptive home, since these parents must make decisions regarding the medical care of the child and must consider the possible social and psychological effects on their families.

9. Mandatory screening as a condition for school entry is not warranted based on available data.

10. Persons involved in the care and education of HIV-infected children should respect the child's right to privacy, including maintaining confidential records. The number of personnel who are aware of the child's condition should be kept at a minimum needed to assure proper care of the child and to detect situations where the potential for transmission may increase (e.g., bleeding injury).

11. All educational and public health departments, regardless of whether HIV-infected children are involved, are strongly encouraged to inform parents, children, and educators regarding HIV and its transmission. Such education would greatly assist efforts to provide the best care and education for infected children while minimizing the risk of transmission to others.

References

1. Scott GB, Buck BE, Leterman JG, Bloom FL, Parks WP. Acquired immunodeficiency syndrome in infants. N Engl J Med 1984;310:76–81.
2. Thomas PA, Jaffe HW, Spira TJ, Reiss R, Guerrero IC, Auerbach D. Unexplained immunodeficiency in children. A surveillance report. JAMA 1984;252;639–44.
3. Rubinstein A, Sicklick M, Gupta A, et al. Acquired immunodeficiency with reversed T4/T8 ratios in infants born to promiscuous and drug-addicted mothers. JAMA 1983;249:2350–6.
4. Oleske J, Minnefor A, Cooper R Jr, et al. Immune deficiency syndrome in children. JAMA 1983;249:2345–9.
5. Ziegler JB, Cooper DA, Johnson RO, Gold J. Postnatal transmission of AIDS-associated retrovirus from mother to infant. Lancet 1985;i;896–8.
6. CDC. Unpublished data.
7. Kaplan JE, Oleske JM, Getchell JP, et al. Evidence against transmission of HTLV-III/LAV in families of children with AIDS. Pediatric Infectious Disease (in press).
8. Lewin EB, Zack R, Ayodele A. Communicability of AIDS in a foster care setting. International Conference on Acquired Immunodeficiency Syndrome (AIDS), Atlanta, Georgia, April 1985.

9. Thomas PA, Lubin K, Enlow RW, Getchell J. Comparison of HTLV-III serology, T-cell levels, and general health status of children whose mothers have AIDS with children of healthy inner city mothers in New York. International Conference on Acquired Immunodeficiency Syndrome (AIDS), Atlanta, Georgia, April 1985.

10. Fischl MA, Dickinson G, Scott G, Klimas N, Fletcher M, Parks W. Evaluation of household contacts of adult patients with the acquired immunodeficiency syndrome. International Conference on Acquired Immunodeficiency Syndrome (AIDS), Atlanta, Georgia, April 1985.

11. Friedland GH, Saltzman BR, Rogers MF, et al. Lack of household transmission of HTLV-III infection. EIS Conference, Atlanta, Georgia, April 1985.

Appendix H
Public Health Service Recommendations for Preventing Transmission of HIV Infection in Non–Health Care Work Settings

Personal-Service Workers (PSWs)

PSWs are defined as individuals whose occupations involve close personal contact with clients (e.g., hairdressers, barbers, estheticians, cosmetologists, manicurists, pedicurists, massage therapists). PSWs whose services (tattooing, ear piercing, acupuncture, etc.) require needles or other instruments that penetrate the skin should follow precautions indicated for HCWs [health care workers]. Although there is no evidence of transmission of HIV* from clients to PSWs, from PSWs to clients, or between clients of PSWs, a risk of transmission would exist from PSWs to clients and vice versa in situations where there is both (1) trauma to one of the individuals that would provide a portal of entry for the virus and (2) access of blood or serous fluid from one infected person to the open tissue of the other, as could occur if either sustained a cut. A risk of transmission from client to client exists when instruments contaminated with blood are not sterilized or disinfected between clients. However, HBV [hepatitis B virus] transmission has been documented only rarely in acupuncture, ear piercing, and tattoo establishments and never in other personal-service settings, indicating that any risk for HIV transmission in personal-service settings must be extremely low.

All PSWs should be educated about transmission of bloodborne infections, including HIV and HBV. Such education should emphasize principles of good hygiene, antisepsis, and disinfection. This education can be accomplished by national or state professional organizations, with assistance from state and local health departments, using lectures at meetings or self-instructional materials. Licensure requirements should include evidence of such education.

Source: Reprinted in part from "PHS Recommendations for Preventing Transmission of Infection with HTLV-III/LAV in the Workplace," *Morbidity and Mortality Weekly Report,* 34 (November 15, 1985), 693–694.
 * The term *HIV* has been substituted throughout for the older term *HTLV-III/LAV.*

Instruments that are intended to penetrate the skin (e.g., tattooing and acupuncture needles, ear piercing devices) should be used once and disposed of or be thoroughly cleaned and sterilized after each use using procedures recommended for use in health-care institutions. Instruments not intended to penetrate the skin but which may become contaminated with blood (e.g., razors), should be used for only one client and be disposed of or thoroughly cleaned and disinfected after use using procedures recommended for use in health-care institutions. Any PSW with exudative lesions or weeping dermatitis, regardless of HIV infection status, should refrain from direct contact with clients until the condition resolves. PSWs known to be infected with HIV need not be restricted from work unless they have evidence of other infections or illnesses for which any PSW should also be restricted.

Routine serologic testing of PSWs for antibody to HIV is not recommended to prevent transmission from PSW to clients.

Food-Service Workers (FWSs)

FSWs are defined as individuals whose occupations involve the preparation or serving of food or beverages (e.g., cooks, caterers, servers, waiters, bartenders, airline attendants). All epidemiologic and laboratory evidence indicates that bloodborne and sexually transmitted infections are not transmitted during the preparation or serving of food or beverages, and no instances of HBV or HIV transmission have been documented in this setting.

All FSWs should follow recommended standards and practices of good personal hygiene and food sanitation [1]. All FSWs should exercise care to avoid injury to hands when preparing food. Should such an injury occur, both aesthetic and sanitary conditions would dictate that food contaminated with blood be discarded. FSWs known to be infected with HIV need not be restricted from work unless they have evidence of other infection or illness for which any FSW should also be restricted.

Routine serologic testing of FSWs for antibody to HIV is not recommended to prevent disease transmission from FSWs to consumers.

Other Workers Sharing the Same Work Environment

No known risk of transmission to co-workers, clients, or consumers exists from HIV-infected workers in other settings (e.g., offices, schools, factories, construction sites). This infection is spread by sexual contact with infected persons, injection of contaminated blood or blood products, and by perinatal transmission. Workers known to be infected with HIV should not be restricted from work solely based on this finding. Moreover, they should not be restricted from using telephones, office equipment, toilets, showers, eating facilities, and water fountains. Equipment contaminated with blood or other body fluids of any workers, regardless of HIV infection status, should be cleaned with soap and water or a detergent. A disinfectant solution or a fresh solution of sodium hypochlorite (household bleach [diluted 1 part bleach to 10 parts water]) should be used to wipe the area after cleaning.

Other Issues in the Workplace

The information and recommendations contained in this document do not address all the potential issues that may have to be considered when making specific employment decisions for persons with HIV infection. The diagnosis of HIV infection may evoke unwarranted fear and suspicion in some co-workers. Other issues that may be considered include the need for confidentiality, applicable federal, state, or local laws governing occupational safety and health, civil rights of employees, workers' compensation laws, provisions of collective bargaining agreements, confidentiality of medical records, informed consent, employee and patient privacy rights, and employee right-to-know statutes.

Reference

1. Food Service Sanitation Manual 1976. DHEW publication no. (FDA) 78-2081. First printing June 1978.

Glossary

Acquired immunodeficiency syndrome (AIDS). A severe manifestation of infection with human immunodeficiency virus (HIV).

ARC (AIDS-related complex). A term formerly used to describe a variety of chronic symptoms and physical findings found in HIV-infected people whose conditions did not meet the CDC case surveillance definition of AIDS. Symptoms included chronic swollen glands, recurrent fevers, unintentional weight loss, chronic diarrhea, lethargy, minor alterations of the immune system, and oral thrush. The term is now considered to be obsolete.

Antibody. A protein in the blood produced in response to exposure to specific foreign molecules. Antibodies neutralize toxins and interact with other components of the immune system to eliminate infectious microorganisms from the body.

Antigen. A substance that stimulates the production of antibodies.

ARV (AIDS-associated retrovirus). Name given by researchers at the University of California at San Francisco to isolates of the retrovirus that causes AIDS.

Autologous transfusion. A blood transfusion in which the patient receives his or her own blood, donated several weeks before elective surgery.

B lymphocyte or B cell. A type of white blood cell that produces antibody in response to stimulation by an antigen.

Candida albicans. A yeastlike fungus that causes whitish sores in the mouth. The infection is called candidiasis or, more commonly, thrush. In AIDS patients, candidiasis often extends into the esophagus.

Casual contact. Day-to-day interactions between HIV-infected individuals and others in the home, at school, or in the workplace. It does not include intimate contact, such as sexual or drug use interactions, and it implies closer contact than chance passing on a street or sharing a subway car.

CD4 lymphocyte or CD4 T cell. A T lymphocyte that expresses the cell surface marker molecule CD4. The majority of these cells are thought to consist of helper/inducer lymphocytes, which play important regulatory roles in the human immune system. These cells appear to be a primary target for infection by HIV.

CD8 lymphocyte or CD8 T cell. A T lymphocyte that expresses the cell surface marker molecule CD8. The majority of these cells are thought to consist of suppressor/cytotoxic lymphocytes, which play important regulatory and functional roles in the human immune system.

Cell-mediated immunity. A defense mechanism involving the coordinated activity of 2 subpopulations of T lymphocytes, helper T cells and killer T cells. Helper T cells produce a variety of substances that stimulate and regulate other participants in the immune response. Killer T lymphocytes destroy cells in the body that bear foreign antigens (for example, cells that are infected with viruses or other microorganisms).

Cofactor. A factor other than the basic causative agent of a disease that increases the likelihood of developing that disease. Cofactors may include the presence of other microorganisms or psychosocial factors, such as stress.

Cryptosporidium. A protozoan parasite that causes severe, protracted diarrhea. In persons with a normal immune system, the diarrhea is self-limited and lasts one to two weeks. In AIDS patients, the diarrhea often becomes chronic and may lead to severe malnutrition.

Cytomegalovirus (CMV). A virus that belongs to the herpesvirus group. Before the appearance of AIDS, it was most commonly associated with a severe congenital infection of infants and with life-threatening infections in patients who had undergone bone marrow transplants and other procedures requiring suppression of the immune system. It rarely causes disease in healthy adults. In AIDS patients, CMV may produce pneumonia, as well as inflammation of the retina, liver, kidneys, and colon.

DNA (deoxyribonucleic acid). A nucleic acid found chiefly in the nucleus of living cells that is responsible for transmitting hereditary characteristics.

ELISA (enzyme-linked immunosorbent assay). A test used to detect antibodies against HIV in blood samples.

Encephalitis. Inflammation of the brain.

Encephalopathy. Any degenerative disease of the brain.

Epstein-Barr virus. A member of the herpes group of viruses and the principal cause of infectious mononucleosis in young adults. It also has been implicated as a causal factor in the development of Burkitt's lymphoma in Africa.

False negative. A negative test result for a condition that in fact is present.

False positive. A positive test result for a condition that in fact is not present.

Genome. The genetic endowment of an organism.

Hemophilia. A rare, hereditary bleeding disorder of males, inherited through the mother, caused by a deficiency in the ability to make one or more blood-clotting proteins.

Herpes simplex. An acute disease caused by herpes simplex viruses types 1 and 2. Groups of watery blisters, often painful, form on the skin and mucous membranes, especially the borders of the lips (cold sores) or the mucous surface of the genitals.

Herpesvirus group. A group of viruses that includes the herpes simplex viruses, the varicella–zoster virus (the cause of chicken pox and shingles), cytomegalovirus, and Epstein–Barr virus.

HIV (human immunodeficiency virus). The widely accepted name for the causative agent of AIDS. It was first proposed by a subcommittee of the International Committee on the Taxonomy of Viruses. (*See also* ARV, HTLV-III, and LAV.)

HTLV-III (human T-cell lymphotropic virus type III). The name given by researchers at the National Cancer Institute to isolates of the retrovirus that causes AIDS.

Humoral immunity. The human defense mechanism that involves the production of antibodies and associated molecules present in body fluids such as serum and lymph.

Immune system. The natural system of defense mechanisms, in which specialized cells and proteins in the blood and other body fluids work together to eliminate disease-producing microorganisms and other foreign substances.

Incidence. The number of new cases of a specific disease occurring over a certain period.

Interferons. A class of proteins important in immune function and known to inhibit certain viral infections.

Interleukin-2. A substance produced by T lymphocytes that stimulates activated T lymphocytes and some activated B lymphocytes to proliferate. Also known as T-cell growth factor.

In vitro. Literally, within glass. The term refers to experiments conducted in tissue culture or another artificial environment.

In vivo. Literally, within a living body. The term refers to experiments conducted in animals or humans.

Interstitial pneumonitis. Localized acute inflammation of the lung. A definite diagnosis of interstitial pneumonitis in a child under 13 years of age is indicative of AIDS unless another cause is identified or tests for HIV are negative.

Intravenous. Injected into or delivered through a needle in a vein.

Kaposi's sarcoma. A cancer or tumor of the blood and/or lymphatic vessel walls. It usually appears as blue-violet to brownish skin blotches or bumps. Before the appearance of AIDS, it was rare in the United States and Europe, where it occurred primarily in men over age 50 or 60, usually of Mediterranean origin. AIDS-associated Kaposi's sarcoma is much more aggressive than the earlier form of the disease.

LAV (lymphadenopathy-associated virus). The name given by French researchers to the first reported isolate of the retrovirus now known to cause AIDS. This retrovirus was recovered from a person with lymphadenopathy (enlarged lymph nodes) who also was in a group at high risk for AIDS.

Lentiviruses. A subfamily of retroviruses that until recently included only the visna viruses of sheep, the equine infectious anemia virus of horses, and the caprine arthritis-encephalitis virus of goats. Newly recognized members of the family include the human immunodeficiency viruses (HIVs—the viruses that cause AIDS), the simian immunodeficiency virus (SIV), the feline immunodeficiency virus (FIV), and the bovine immunodeficiency virus (BIV). The original ungulate lentiviruses produce diverse chronic diseases in their natural hosts, but all cause encephalitis. The diseases are characterized by erratic relapses and remissions. The visna viruses cause a chronic interstitial pneumonitis similar to that seen in AIDS in young children. Lentiviruses persist in the body by evading natural defense mechanisms; the chronic carrier state—in which infected animals do not get sick themselves but can transmit the virus to other animals—is common.

Macrophage. A cell derived from the circulating monocyte. It has the capacity to ingest or phagocytize foreign particulate matter, such as bacteria.

Monocyte. A phagocytic white blood cell that engulfs and destroys bacteria and other disease-producing microorganisms. It produces interleukin-1, a substance that activates T lymphocytes in the presence of antigen.

Oncoviruses. A subfamily of retroviruses that includes tumor-causing agents such as the Rous sarcoma virus and the bovine leukemia virus.

Opportunistic infection. An infection caused by a microorganism that rarely causes disease in persons with normal defense mechanisms.

Parenteral. Involving introduction into the bloodstream.

Persistent generalized lymphadenopathy (PGL). A condition characterized by persistent, generalized swollen glands in the absence of any current illness or drug use known to cause such symptoms.

Phagocyte. A cell in blood or tissues that binds to, engulfs, and destroys microorganisms, damaged cells, and foreign particles.

Pneumocystis carinii *pneumonia.* The most common life-threatening opportunistic infection diagnosed in AIDS patients. It is caused by the parasite *Pneumocystis carinii.*

Prevalence. The total number of cases of a disease in existence at a particular time in a specified area.

Provirus. A copy of the genetic information of an animal virus that is integrated into the DNA of an infected cell. Copies of the provirus are passed on to each of the infected cell's daughter cells.

Retrovirus. A class of viruses that contain the genetic material RNA and have the capability to copy this RNA into DNA inside an infected cell. The resulting DNA is incorporated into the genetic structure of the cell in the form of a provirus.

Reverse transcriptase. An enzyme produced by retroviruses that allows them to produce a DNA copy of their RNA. This is the first step in the virus's natural cycle of reproduction.

RNA (ribonucleic acid). A nucleic acid associated with the control of chemical activities inside a cell. One type of RNA transfers information from the cell's DNA to the protein-forming system of a cell outside the nucleus. Some viruses carry RNA instead of the more familiar genetic material DNA.

Sensitivity. In serologic testing, the percentage of people who test positive who in fact do have the condition being tested for. (*See also* Specificity.)

Seroconversion. The initial development of antibodies specific to a particular antigen.

Serologic study. A study that compares the characteristics of the serum of individuals, especially those markers in blood that indicate exposure to a particular agent of disease.

Seropositive. In the context of HIV, the condition in which antibodies to the virus are found in the blood.

Specificity. In serologic testing, the percentage of people who test negative who in fact do not have the condition being tested for. (*See also* Sensitivity.)

Subunit vaccine. A vaccine that contains only portions of a surface molecule of a disease-producing microorganism.

T lymphocyte or T cell. A cell that matures in the thymus gland. T lymphocytes are found primarily in the blood, lymph, and lymphoid organs. Subsets of T cells have a variety of specialized functions within the immune system.

T4 lymphocyte or T4 cell. A synonym for CD4 T cell.

T8 lymphocyte or T8 cell. A synonym for CD8 T cell.

Toxoplasma gondii. A protozoan parasite that is one of the most common causes of inflammation of the brain in AIDS patients. The infection is called toxoplasmosis.

Virion. A complete viral particle.

Western blot technique. A test that involves the identification of antibodies against specific protein molecules. This test is believed to be more specific than the ELISA test in detecting antibodies to HIV in blood samples; it is also more difficult to perform and considerably more expensive. Western blot analysis is used by some laboratories as a confirmatory test on samples found to be repeatedly reactive on ELISA tests.

Notes

Periodicals cited frequently in the Notes are abbreviated as follows:

AIM   *Annals of Internal Medicine*
BMJ   *British Medical Journal*
JAMA   *Journal of the American Medical Association*
MMWR   *Morbidity and Mortality Weekly Report*
NEJM   *New England Journal of Medicine*

1. The Scope of AIDS

1. Institute of Medicine, *Confronting AIDS: Update 1988* (Washington, D.C.: National Academy Press, 1988).
2. Don C. Des Jarlais, Samuel R. Friedman, and Rand L. Stoneburner, "HIV Infection and Intravenous Drug Use: Critical Issues in Transmission Dynamics, Infection Outcomes, and Prevention," *Reviews of Infectious Diseases* 10 (1988):151–158.
3. Richard Rothenberg, Mary Woelfel, Rand Stoneburner, John Milberg, Robert Parker, and Benedict Truman, "Survival with the Acquired Immunodeficiency Syndrome," *NEJM* 317 (1987): 1297–1302.
4. U.S. Congress, Office of Technology Assessment, *AIDS and Health Insurance: An OTA Survey* (Washington, D.C., 1988).

2. Tracking the Epidemic

1. Preliminary evidence suggests that an AIDS-related death may have occurred in 1969 in St. Louis, but this has not been confirmed. See Chapter 4.
2. James W. Curran, Harold W. Jaffe, Ann M. Hardy, W. Meade Morgan, Richard M. Selik, and Timothy J. Dondero, "Epidemiology of HIV Infection and AIDS in the United States," *Science* 239 (1988):610–616.

328 Notes to Pages 17–20

3. Kung-Jong Lui of the Centers for Disease Control and his coworkers recently reported that the maximum likelihood estimate for the mean incubation period for AIDS in homosexual men is 7.8 years; Kung-Jong Lui, William W. Darrow, and George W. Rutherford III, "A Model-Based Estimate of the Mean Incubation Period for AIDS in Homosexual Men," *Science* 240 (1988):1333–1335.

4. Andrew R. Moss, Peter Bacchetti, Dennis Osmond, Walter Krampf, Richard E. Chaisson, Daniel Stites, Judith Wilber, Jeanne-Pierre Allain, and James Carlson, "Seropositivity for HIV and the Development of AIDS or AIDS Related Condition: Three-Year Follow-up of the San Francisco General Hospital Cohort," *BMJ* 296 (1988):745–750.

5. The OOI category included pneumonia, meningitis, and encephalitis caused by 9 different viruses, bacteria, fungi, and protozoa; esophagitis (inflammation of the esophagus) caused by candidiasis, cytomegalovirus, or herpes simplex; progressive brain disease with multiple lesions; chronic inflammation of the intestine caused by protozoan parasites of the genus *Cryptosporidium* (lasting more than 4 weeks); and unusually extensive herpes simplex infections of the mouth or rectum (lasting more than 5 weeks); Centers for Disease Control, "Update on Acquired Immune Deficiency Syndrome (AIDS)—United States," *MMWR* 31 (1982):507–514.

6. See "The Case Definition of AIDS Used by CDC for National Reporting (CDC-reportable AIDS)," Document no. 0312S Centers for Disease Control (Atlanta: August 1, 1985).

7. Centers for Disease Control, "Quarterly Report to the Domestic Policy Council on the Prevalence and Rate of Spread of HIV and AIDS in the United States," *MMWR* 37 (1988):223–226.

8. Curran et al., "Epidemiology," p. 611.

9. Centers for Disease Control, "Acquired Immunodeficiency Syndrome (AIDS) among Blacks and Hispanics—United States," *MMWR* 35 (1986):655–658, 663–666.

10. Donald R. Hopkins, "AIDS in the Minority Population," *Public Health Reports* 102 (1987):677–681.

11. Vickie Mays and Susan D. Cochran, "Acquired Immunodeficiency Syndrome and Black Americans: Special Psychosocial Issues," *Public Health Reports* 102 (1987):224–231.

12. Hopkins, "AIDS in the Minority Population," p. 679.

13. Bruce Lambert, "One in 61 Babies in New York City Has AIDS Antibodies, Study Says," *New York Times,* January 13, 1988, p. 1.

14. Curran et al., "Epidemiology," p. 611.

15. Kim Painter, "How AIDS May Change Society," *USA Today,* June 2, 1988, p. 1D.

16. Centers for Disease Control, "Human Immunodeficiency Virus Infection in the United States: A Review of Current Knowledge," *MMWR* 36, supp. 6 (1987):1–48.

17. A. C. Kinsey, W. B. Pomeroy, and C. E. Martin, *Sexual Behavior in the Human Male* (Philadelphia: Saunders, 1948).

18. Charles F. Turner, Heather Miller, and Lewellys Barker, "AIDS Research and the Behavioral and Social Sciences," in *AIDS 1988: AAAS Symposia Papers,* ed. Ruth Kulstad (Washington, D.C.: American Association for the Advancement of Science, 1988), pp. 253–254.

19. Rodney Hoff, Victor P. Berardi, Barbara J. Weiblen, Laurene Mahoney-Trout, Marvin L. Mitchell, and George F. Grady, "Seroprevalence of Human Immunodeficiency Virus among Childbearing Women," *NEJM* 318 (1988):525–530.

20. Hoff and his coworkers found evidence of infection in 1 of every 476 women (2.1 per 1,000) giving birth in Massachusetts. In testing of military recruits from October 1985 to March 1987, 2 of 2,029 (.99 per 1,000) Massachusetts women were found to be seropositive; between 1986 and mid-1987, the rate of seropositivity in female blood donors was about 1 per 25,000 (.04 per 1,000).

21. Centers for Disease Control, "Quarterly Report" (1988).

22. Centers for Disease Control, "HIV Infection in the United States: A Review of Current Knowledge."

23. Warren Winkelstein, Jr., Michael Samuel, Nancy S. Padian, James A. Wiley, William Lang, Robert E. Anderson, and Jay A. Levy, "The San Francisco Men's Health Study: III. Reduction in Human Immunodeficiency Virus Transmission among Homosexual/Bisexual Men, 1982–1986," *American Journal of Public Health* 77 (1987): 685–689.

24. Lawrence K. Altman, "Spread of AIDS Virus Found Slowing among Drug Users in 3 Cities," *New York Times,* June 16, 1988, p. A25.

25. Ibid.

26. CDC researchers explain that "stable observed prevalence levels do not imply absence of new infection. On the contrary, in the age-specific data from military applicants, for example, 20-year-olds in early 1987 had higher rates than 19-year-olds in early 1986; this suggests that new infection continues to occur. Preliminary analysis by birth-year cohort for applicants 17–25 years of age suggests incidence rates for new infection of 0.5 per 1,000 per year for men and 0.1 for women"; Centers for Disease Control, "HIV Infection in the United States: A Review of Current Knowledge," p. 13.

27. Judy Foreman, "U.S. Study: AIDS Virus in 1M," *Boston Globe,* June 14, 1988, p. 1.

28. Curran et al., "Epidemiology." According to Winkelstein et al., "San Francisco Men's Health Study," measures of seroprevalence in a city may differ by as much as 20 percent, depending on the source of the study population. Homosexual men recruited from sexually transmitted disease clinics have a higher rate of HIV seroprevalence than homosexual men recruited by random sampling of target neighborhoods. For example, the San Francisco City Clinic Cohort (obtained by sampling from a population recruited from STD clinics) showed an HIV seroprevalence rate of 69 percent by the first half of 1985; during the same period, the San Francisco Men's Health Study (a population-based sample from a 6-square-kilometer area of San Francisco) showed an HIV seroprevalence rate of 49 percent.

29. Centers for Disease Control, "HIV Infection in the United States: A Review of Current Knowledge."

30. Joan S. Chmiel, Roger Detels, Richard A. Kaslow, Mark Van Raden, Lawrence A. Kingsley, Ron Brookmeyer, and the Multicenter AIDS Cohort Study Group, "Factors Associated with Prevalent Human Immunodeficiency Virus (HIV) Infection in the Multicenter AIDS Cohort Study," *American Journal of Epidemiology* 126 (1987):568–575.

31. William W. Darrow, Dean F. Echenberg, Harold W. Jaffe, Paul M. O'Malley, Robert H. Byers, Jane P. Getchell, and James W. Curran, "Risk Factors for Human Immunodeficiency Virus (HIV) Infections in Homosexual Men," *American Journal of Public Health* 77 (1987):482.

32. Gerald H. Friedland and Robert S. Klein, "Transmission of the Human Immunodeficiency Virus," *NEJM* 317 (1987):1125–1135.

33. W. Meade Morgan and James W. Curran, "Acquired Immunodeficiency Syndrome: Current and Future Trends," *Public Health Reports* 101 (1986):459–465.

34. Friedland and Klein, "Transmission."

35. Mary E. Guinan and Ann Hardy, "Epidemiology of AIDS in Women in the United States: 1981 through 1986," *JAMA* 257 (1987):2041.

36. Don C. Des Jarlais, Samuel R. Friedman, and Rand L. Stoneburner, "HIV Infection and Intravenous Drug Use: Critical Issues in Transmission Dynamics, Infection Outcomes, and Prevention," *Reviews of Infectious Diseases* 10 (1988):151–158.

37. Thomas A. Peterman, Rand L. Stoneburner, James R. Allen, Harold W. Jaffe, and James W. Curran, "Risk of Human Immunodeficiency Virus Transmission from Heterosexual Adults with Transfusion-Associated Infections," *JAMA* 259 (1988):55–58.

38. One explanation for the association between infection and anal intercourse in the Padian study is that her sample included 55 women whose partners were bisexual men. Bisexual men may be more likely than men in other risk groups to practice anal intercourse with their female partners. See Nancy Padian, Linda Marquis, Donald P. Francis, Robert E. Anderson, George W. Rutherford, Paul M. O'Malley, and Warren Winkelstein, Jr., "Male-to-Female Transmission of Human Immunodeficiency Virus," *JAMA* 258 (1987):788–790.

39. Peter Piot, Francis A. Plummer, Fred S. Mhalu, Jean-Louis Lamboray, James Chin, and Jonathan M. Mann, "AIDS: An International Perspective," *Science* 239 (1988):575.

40. Norman Hearst and Stephen B. Hulley, "Preventing the Heterosexual Spread of AIDS: Are We Giving Our Patients the Best Advice?" *JAMA* 259 (1988):2428–2432.

41. They define high-risk groups to include anyone who, within the past 10 years, has engaged in male homosexual activity or intravenous drug use, has resided in Haiti or central Africa, has a history of multiple blood transfusions, or is a hemophiliac. Anyone who has had a regular sexual partner belonging to one of these groups is also included.

42. Experts estimate that the risk of receptive anal intercourse with an infected partner is about 10 times that of vaginal intercourse; Philip M. Boffey, "Researchers List Odds of Getting AIDS in Heterosexual Intercourse," *New York Times,* April 21, pp. 1, A18.

43. Ibid.

44. W. Robert Lange, Frederick R. Snyder, David Lozovsky, Vivek Kaistha, Mary A. Kaczaniuk, Jerome H. Jaffe, and the ARC Epidemiology Collaborating Group, "Geographic Distribution of HIV Markers in Parenteral Drug Abusers," *American Journal of Public Health* 78 (1988):443–446.

45. D. M. Novick, M. J. Kreek, D. C. Des Jarlais, T. J. Spira, E. T. Khuri, J. Ragunath, V. S. Kalyarnaraman, A. M. Gelb, and A. Miescher, 1986. "LAV among Parenteral Drug Users: Therapeutic, Historical, and Ethical Aspects," in *Problems of Drug Dependence 1985: Proceedings of the 47th Annual Scientific Meeting, the Committee on Problems of Drug Dependence, Inc.* ed. L. J. Harris, NIDA Research Monograph 67 (Washington, D.C.: U.S. Government Printing Office, 1986).

46. J. R. Robertson, A. B. V. Bucknall, P. D. Welsby, J. J. K. Roberts, J. M. Inglis, J. F. Peutherer, and R. P. Brettle, "Epidemic of AIDS Related Virus (HTLV-III/LAV) Infection among Intravenous Drug Abusers," *BMJ* 292 (1986):527–529.

47. Stephen C. Joseph, "Public Health Problems at the Local

Level: The New York City Experience with AIDS" (Paper prepared for the Committee for the Oversight of AIDS Activities, Institute of Medicine, National Academy of Sciences, 1987).

48. Des Jarlais, Friedman, and Stoneburner, "HIV Infection and Intravenous Drug Use."

49. Martha F. Rogers, "Transmission of Human Immunodeficiency Virus Infection in the United States," in *Report of the Surgeon General's Workshop on Children with HIV Infection and Their Families,* DHHS Publication no. HRS-D-MC 87-1 (Washington, D.C.: U.S. Department of Health and Human Services, 1987), pp. 17–19.

50. Institute of Medicine, *Confronting AIDS: Update 1988* (Washington, D.C.: National Academy Press, 1988).

51. John W. Ward, Deborah A. Deppe, Susan Samson, Herbert Perkins, Paul Holland, Leonor Fernando, Paul M. Feorino, Paul Thompson, Steven Kleinman, and James R. Allen, "Risk of Human Immunodeficiency Virus Infection from Blood Donors Who Later Developed the Acquired Immunodeficiency Syndrome," *AIM* 106 (1987):61–62.

52. Centers for Disease Control, "Human Immunodeficiency Virus Infection in Transfusion Recipients and Their Family Members," *MMWR* 36 (1987):137–140.

53. Ibid.

54. G. F. Medley, R. M. Anderson, D. R. Cox, and L. Billard, "Incubation Period of AIDS in Patients Infected via Blood Transfusion," *Nature* 328 (1987):719.

55. Gina Kolata, "AIDS Babies' Prospects," *New York Times,* May 24, 1988, p. C3.

56. Some uncertainty exists about the length of time an infected person may test seronegative. The 6-to-14 week figure is based on studies in transfusion recipients. Other routes of transmission, in which the initial dose of virus is smaller, may be associated with longer periods between infection and seroconversion. See the discussion on timing of the antibody response in Chapter 5.

57. John W. Ward, Scott D. Holmberg, James R. Allen, David L. Cohn, Sara E. Critchley, Steven H. Kleinman, Bruce A. Lenes, Otto Ravenholt, Jacqualyn R. Davis, M. Gerald Quinn, and Harold W. Jaffe, "Transmission of Human Immunodeficiency Virus (HIV) by Blood Transfusions Screened as Negative for HIV Antibody," *NEJM* 318 (1988):473–478.

58. Another form of autologous transfusion involves intraoperative blood salvage. Blood is recovered from the operative wound during surgery, purified, and reinfused into the patient.

59. In the future, recombinant DNA technology may eliminate the need for factor VIII concentrate made from human plasma. Both

factor VIII and factor IX have been produced in the laboratory by bacteria containing copies of the human genes. Researchers began clinical trials of recombinant factor VIII in 1987.

60. Centers for Disease Control, "HIV Infection in the United States."

61. M. Elaine Eyster, Mitchell H. Gail, James O. Ballard, Hamid Al-Mondhiry, and James J. Goedert, "Natural History of Human Immunodeficiency Virus (HIV) Infections in Hemophiliacs: Effects of T-cell Subsets, Platelet Counts, and Age," *AIM* 107 (1987):1–6. See also Gina Kolata, "AIDS Symptoms Found Slowed in Teen-Agers," *New York Times,* March 3, 1988, p. 18.

62. Centers for Disease Control, "Update: Acquired Immunodeficiency Syndrome and Human Immunodeficiency Virus Infection among Health-Care Workers," *MMWR* 37 (1988):231–234, 239.

63. Centers for Disease Control, "Occupationally Acquired Human Immunodeficiency Virus Infections in Laboratories Producing Virus Concentrates in Large Quantities," *MMWR* 37, supp. 4 (1988):19–22.

64. Curran et al., "Epidemiology."

65. Stephen Chanock and Kenneth McIntosh, "Human Immunodeficiency Virus Infections," in *Hematologic Contributions to Fetal Health,* ed. Murray Bern and Frederic Frigoletto (New York: Alan R. Liss, forthcoming).

66. Philippe Lepage, Philippe Van de Perre, Michel Caraël, Francois Nsengumuremyi, Jean Nkurunziza, Jean-Paul Butzler, and Suzanne Sprecher, "Postnatal Transmission of HIV from Mother to Child," *Lancet* (1987) ii:400–402.

67. Howard L. Minkoff, "Care of Pregnant Women Infected with Human Immunodeficiency Virus," *JAMA* 258 (1987):2714–2717.

68. Kenneth Castro, Alan R. Lifson, Carol R. White, Timothy J. Bush, Mary E. Chamberland, Anastasia Lekatsas, and Harold W. Jaffe, "Investigations of AIDS Patients with No Previously Identified Risk Factors," *JAMA* 259 (1988):1338–1342.

69. Curran et al., "Epidemiology."

70. Friedland and Klein, "Transmission."

71. Alan R. Lifson, "Do Alternate Modes for Transmission of Human Immunodeficiency Virus Exist? A Review," *JAMA* 259 (1988):1355.

72. Ibid., pp. 1353–1356.

73. Ibid., p. 1353.

74. Centers for Disease Control, "Acquired Immunodeficiency Syndrome (AIDS) in Western Palm Beach County, Florida," *MMWR* 35 (1986):609–612.

75. U.S. Congress, Office of Technology Assessment, *Do Insects Transmit AIDS?* (Washington, D.C.: U.S. Government Printing Office, 1987), pp. 23, iii.

76. Researchers estimate that reporting systems capture about 80 percent of AIDS cases in the United States. Reporting of AIDS cases from Africa has been much less complete. One indication of this is that more than 70 percent of all cases from Africa were reported in 1987. African nations are working hard to improve their diagnostic and surveillance systems.

77. Piot et al., "AIDS: An International Perspective."

78. Centers for Disease Control, "Update: Acquired Immunodeficiency Syndrome (AIDS)—Worldwide," *MMWR* 37 (1988): 286–288, 293–295.

79. Ibid., pp. 294–295.

80. "Study Traces AIDS in Africa Children," *New York Times,* January 22, 1988, p. A6.

81. Thomas C. Quinn, "AIDS in Africa: An Epidemiologic Paradigm," *Science* 234 (1986):955–963.

82. Thomas C. Quinn, Peter Piot, Joseph B. McCormick, Fred M. Feinsod, Henry Taelman, Bela Kapita, Wim Stevens, and Anthony S. Fauci, "Serologic and Immunologic Studies in Patients with AIDS in North America and Africa: The Potential Role of Infectious Agents as Cofactors in Human Immunodeficiency Virus Infection," *JAMA* 257 (1987):2617.

83. Centers for Disease Control, "Update—Worldwide." Zimbabwe officially retracted its report of 380 cases in April 1988 pending a national review of the accuracy of its reporting system.

84. Lawrence K. Altman, "AIDS Hits Drug Users in Thailand, Panel Told," *New York Times,* April 19, 1988, p. C12.

85. Piot et al., "AIDS: An International Perspective."

3. The Spectrum of Disease

1. Ronald L. Burkes, Anthony A. Gal, Mary L. Stewart, Parkash S. Gill, Wataru Abo, and Alexandra M. Levine, "Simultaneous Occurrence of *Pneumocystis carinii* Pneumonia, Cytomegalovirus Infection, Kaposi's Sarcoma, and B-Immunoblastic Sarcoma in a Homosexual Man," *JAMA* 253 (1985):3425–3428; and Margaret A. Fischl, Arthur E. Pitchenik, and Thomas J. Spira, "Tuberculous Brain Abscess and *Toxoplasma* Encephalitis in a Patient with the Acquired Immunodeficiency Syndrome," ibid., pp. 3428–3430.

2. David A. Cooper, Prudence MacLean, Robert Finlayson, Harry M. Michelmore, Julian Gold, Basil Donovan, Timothy G.

Barnes, Peter Brooke, and Ronald Penny, "Acute AIDS Retrovirus Infection: Definition of a Clinical Illness Associated with Seroconversion," *Lancet* (1985) i:537–540.

3. Dana H. Gabuzda and Martin S. Hirsch, "Neurologic Manifestations of Infection with Human Immunodeficiency Virus," *AIM* 107 (1987):383–391.

4. Richard A. Kaslow, John P. Phair, Heidi B. Friedman, David Lyter, Rachel E. Solomon, Jan Dudley, B. Frank Polk, and William Blackwelder, "Infection with the Human Immunodeficiency Virus: Clinical Manifestations and Their Relationship to Immune Deficiency," *AIM* 107 (1987):474–480.

5. Ronald L. Burkes of the Los Angeles County–University of Southern California Medical Center and his coworkers say that the elevation of beta$_2$-microglobulin in patients with AIDS suggests "an increased turnover of a certain subpopulation of lymphocytes in these patients." Serum levels of the molecule also are elevated in patients with rheumatoid arthritis, kidney disease, and some forms of cancer; Ronald L. Burkes, Andy E. Sherrod, Mary L. Stewart, Parkash S. Gill, Scott Aguilar, Clive R. Taylor, Mark D. Krailo, and Alexandra M. Levine, "Serum Beta-2 Microglobulin Levels in Homosexual Men with AIDS and with Persistent, Generalized Lymphadenopathy," *Cancer* 57 (1986): 2190–2192.

6. Centers for Disease Control, "Revision of the CDC Surveillance Case Definition of Acquired Immunodeficiency Syndrome," *MMWR* 36, supp. 1 (1987):3–15.

7. Jay A. Nelson, Catherine Reynolds-Kohler, William Margaretten, Clayton A. Wiley, Charles E. Reese, and Jay A. Levy, "Human Immunodeficiency Virus Detected in Bowel Epithelium from Patients with Gastrointestinal Symptoms," *Lancet* (1988) i:259–262.

8. Robert Pear, "Key Jobs in Military Off Limits for AIDS-Infected," *New York Times*, December 19, 1987, p. 1.

9. Igor Grant, J. Hampton Atkinson, John R. Hesselink, Caroline J. Kennedy, Douglas D. Richman, Stephen A. Spector, and J. Allen McCutchan, "Evidence for Early Central Nervous System Involvement in the Acquired Immunodeficiency Syndrome (AIDS) and Other Human Immunodeficiency Virus (HIV) Infections," *AIM* 107 (1987):828–836.

10. Steve Eisenberg, "Early HIV Effects on Nervous System Found," *Science News* 133 (1988):6.

11. "WHO Statement on Neuropsychological Aspects of HIV Infection" (Geneva: World Health Organization, Division of Mental Health, Global Programme on AIDS, March 18, 1988).

12. Michael R. Spence and Elias Abrutyn, "Syphilis and Infec-

tion with the Human Immunodeficiency Virus," Editorial, *AIM* 107 (1987):587.

13. K. P. Goldman, "AIDS and Tuberculosis," *BMJ* 295 (1987):511–512.

14. Carmen J. Allegra, Bruce A. Chabner, Carmelita U. Tuazon, Debra Ogata-Arakaki, Barbara Baird, James C. Drake, J. Thayer Simmons, Ernest E. Lack, James H. Shelhamer, Frank Balis, Robert Walker, Joseph A. Kovacs, H. Clifford Lane, and Henry Masur, "Trimetrexate for the Treatment of *Pneumocystis Carinii* Pneumonia in Patients with the Acquired Immunodeficiency Syndrome," *NEJM* 317 (1987):978–985.

15. A. Bruce Montgomery, John M. Luce, Joan Turner, Emil T. Lin, Robert J. Debs, Kevin J. Corkery, Elisa N. Brunette, Philip C. Hopewell, "Aerosolised Pentamidine as Sole Therapy for *Pneumocystis carinii* Pneumonia in Patients with Acquired Immunodeficiency Syndrome," *Lancet* (1987) ii:480–483.

16. John E. Conte, Jr., Harry Hollander, and Jeffrey A. Golden, "Inhaled or Reduced-Dose Intravenous Pentamidine for *Pneumocystis carinii* Pneumonia," *AIM* 107 (1987):495–498.

17. Margaret A. Fischl, Gordon M. Dickinson, and Lawrence La Voie, "Safety and Efficacy of Sulfamethoxazole and Trimethoprim Chemoprophylaxis for *Pneumocystis carinii* Pneumonia in AIDS," *JAMA* 259 (1988):1185–1189.

18. See *IV International Conference on AIDS: Book 1* (Stockholm, June 12–16, 1988), abstracts 7164–7172, pp. 418–420.

19. Mads Melbye, James J. Goedert, Ronald J. Grossman, M. Elaine Eyster, and Robert J. Biggar, "Risk of AIDS after Herpes Zoster," *Lancet* (1987) i:728–730.

20. Edmund C. Tramont, "Syphilis in the AIDS Era," *NEJM* 316 (1987): 1600–1601.

21. Centers for Disease Control, "Diagnosis and Management of Mycobacterial Infection and Disease in Persons with Human T-lymphotropic Virus Type III/Lymphadenopathy-Associated Virus Infection," *MMWR* 35 (1986):448–452.

22. James J. Goedert, Robert J. Biggar, Mads Melbye, Dean L. Mann, Susan Wilson, Mitchell H. Gail, Ronald J. Grossman, Richard A. DiGioia, William C. Sanchez, Stanley H. Weiss, and William A. Blattner, "Effect of T4 Count and Cofactors on the Incidence of AIDS in Homosexual Men Infected with Human Immunodeficiency Virus," *JAMA* 257 (1987):331–334.

23. Richard Knox, "Caution Urged on Some Ways to Treat AIDS," *Boston Globe,* June 13, 1988, p. 1.

24. Personal communication.

25. Robert J. Biggar, John Horm, James J. Goedert, and Mads

Melbye, "Cancer in a Group at Risk of Acquired Immunodeficiency Syndrome (AIDS) through 1984," *American Journal of Epidemiology* 126 (1987):578–586.

26. Joan A. Phelan and Paul D. Freedman, "Oral Manifestations of Acquired Immunodeficiency Syndrome (AIDS) and HTLV-III/LAV Infection," *New York Journal of Dentistry* 56 (1986): 176–178.

27. Centers for Disease Control, "Oral Viral Lesion (Hairy Leukoplakia) Associated with Acquired Immunodeficiency Syndrome," *MMWR* 34 (1985):549–550.

28. H. Hollander, D. Greenspan, S. Stringari, J. Greenspan, and M. Schiodt, "Hairy Leukoplakia and the Acquired Immunodeficiency Syndrome," *AIM* 104 (1986):892.

29. Gina Kolata, "AIDS Overturns Theories on Two Medical Mysteries," *New York Times,* October 27, 1987, p. C1.

30. "AIDS Development Is Tracked in Babies Born with the Virus," *New York Times,* June 15, 1988, p. A21. See also Catherine Peckham and the European Collaborative Study, "Consequences of HIV Infection in Pregnancy: Results from the European Collaborative Study," in *IV International Conference on AIDS,* abstract 4027, p. 266.

31. Andrew R. Moss, Peter Bacchetti, Dennis Osmond, Walter Krampf, Richard E. Chaisson, Daniel Stites, Judith Wilber, Jean-Pierre Allain, and James Carlson, "Seropositivity for HIV and the Development of AIDS or AIDS Related Condition: Three-Year Follow-up of the San Francisco General Hospital Cohort," *BMJ* 296 (1988):745–750.

32. Stephen Chanock and Kenneth McIntosh, "Human Immunodeficiency Virus Infections," in *Hematologic Contributions to Fetal Health,* ed. Murray Bern and Frederic Frigoletto (New York: Alan R. Liss, forthcoming).

33. Robert W. Marion, Andrew A. Wiznia, Gordon Hutcheon, and Ayre Rubinstein, 1986. "Human T-Cell Lymphotropic Virus Type III (HTLV-III) Embryopathy," *American Journal of Diseases of Children* 140 (1986):638–640.

34. Silvia Iosub, Mahrukh Bamji, Richard K. Stone, Donald S. Gromisch, and Edward Wasserman, "More on Human Immunodeficiency Virus Embryopathy," *Pediatrics* 80 (1987):512–516.

35. Gwendolyn B. Scott, "Natural History of HIV Infection in Children," in *Report of the Surgeon General's Workshop on Children with HIV Infection and Their Families,* DHHS Publication no. HRS-D-MC 87-1 (Washington, D.C.: U.S. Department of Health and Human Services, 1987), pp.22–23.

36. Immunization Practices Advisory Committee, "Immunization of Children Infected with Human T-Lymphotropic Virus

Type III/Lymphadenopathy-Associated Virus," *MMWR* 35 (1986): 595–598, 603–606.

37. U.S. Public Health Service, Immunization Practices Advisory Committee, "Immunization of Children Infected with Human Immunodeficiency Virus—Supplementary ACIP Statement," *MMWR* 37 (1988):181–183.

4. Discovery of the Virus

1. Robert C. Gallo, "The First Human Retrovirus," *Scientific American* 255 (1986): 88–98.

2. Recent evidence indicates that HTLV-I has begun spreading rapidly among intravenous drug abusers in some major U.S. cities. Although HTLV-I causes disease in only about 1 percent of those infected and the incubation period may be as long as 30 years, some scientists expect an increase in the prevalence of adult T-cell leukemia.

3. F. Barré-Sinoussi, J.-C. Chermann, F. Rey, M. T. Nugeyre, S. Chamaret, J. Gruest, C. Dauguet, C. Axler-Blin, F. Vézinet-Brun, C. Rouzioux, W. Rozenbaum, and L. Montagnier, "Isolation of a T-lymphotropic Retrovirus from a Patient at Risk for Acquired Immune Deficiency Syndrome (AIDS)," *Science* 220 (1983):868–871.

4. Mikulas Popovic, M. G. Sarngadharan, Elizabeth Read, and Robert C. Gallo, "Detection, Isolation, and Continuous Production of Cytopathic Retroviruses (HTLV-III) from Patients with AIDS and Pre-AIDS," *Science* 224 (1984):497–500.

5. Robert C. Gallo, Syed Z. Salahuddin, Mikulas Popovic, Gene M. Shearer, Mark Kaplan, Barton F. Haynes, Thomas J. Palker, Robert Redfield, James Oleske, Bijan Safai, Gilbert White, Paul Foster, and Phillip D. Markham, "Frequent Detection and Isolation of Cytopathic Retroviruses (HTLV-III) from Patients with AIDS and at Risk for AIDS," *Science* 224 (1984):500–503.

6. Jay A. Levy, Anthony D. Hoffman, Susan M. Kramer, Jill A. Landis, Joni M. Shimabukuro, and Lyndon S. Oshiro, "Isolation of Lymphocytopathic Retroviruses from San Francisco Patients with AIDS," *Science* 225 (1984):840–842.

7. "The Chronology of AIDS Research," *Nature* 326 (1987): 435–436.

8. Efforts to understand the relationship between HTLV-IV and LAV-2 were hampered by a serious technical problem in the Essex laboratory. At some point the cell cultures used by the researchers to study the new human virus were contaminated with a particular strain of STLV-III. This created confusion when Essex and

his associates tried to isolate and sequence the new human virus. See Harry W. Kestler III, Yen Li, Yathirajalu M. Naidu, Carole V. Butler, Michael F. Ochs, Gerlinde Jaenel, Norval W. King, Muthiah D. Daniel, and Ronald C. Desrosiers, "Comparison of Simian Immunodeficiency Virus Isolates," *Nature* 331 (1988):619–622.

9. John Coffin, Ashley Haase, Jay A. Levy, Luc Montagnier, Steven Oroszlan, Natalie Teich, Howard Temin, Kumao Toyoshima, Harold Varmus, Peter Vogt, and Robin Weiss, "Human Immunodeficiency Viruses," *Science* 232 (1986):697.

10. Mireille Guyader, Michael Emerman, Pierre Sonigo, François Clavel, Luc Montagnier, and Marc Alizon, "Genome Organization and Transactivation of the Human Immunodeficiency Virus Type 2," *Nature* 326 (1987):662–669.

11. Temple F. Smith, A. Srinivasan, Gerald Schochetman, Mira Marcus, and Gerald Myers, "The Phylogenetic History of AIDS," *Nature* 333 (1988):573–575.

12. The first documented case of AIDS caused by HIV-2 in the United States was diagnosed in December 1987. The patient had come to the United States from West Africa. After reviewing the patient's history, CDC epidemiologists concluded that the case "undoubtedly represents infection acquired in West Africa since illness began before the patient's arrival in the United States"; Centers for Disease Control, "AIDS Due to HIV-2 Infection—New Jersey," *MMWR* 37 (1987):33–35.

5. HIV and Its Effects on the Body

1. Anthony S. Fauci, "The Human Immunodeficiency Virus: Infectivity and Mechanisms of Pathogenesis," *Science* 239 (1988): 617–622.

2. Judy Foreman, "Problem Cited with Promising AIDS Drug," *Boston Globe,* June 15, 1988, p. 3.

3. Regine Leonard, Daniel Zagury, Isabelle Desportes, Jacky Bernard, Jean-François Zagury, and Robert C. Gallo, "Cytopathic Effect of Human Immunodeficiency Virus in T4 Cells Is Linked to the Last Stage of Virus Infection," *Proceedings of the National Academy of Sciences* 85 (1988):3570–3574.

4. S. Zaki Salahuddin, Dharam V. Ablashi, Phillip D. Markham, Steven F. Josephs, Susi Sturzenegger, Mark Kaplan, Gregory Halligan, Peter Biberfeld, Flossie Wong-Staal, Bernhard Kramarsky, and Robert C. Gallo, "Isolation of a New Virus, HBLV, in Patients with Lymphoproliferative Disorders," *Science* 234 (1986):596–601.

5. D. V. Ablashi, S. Z. Salahuddin, H. Z. Streicher, M.

Kaplan, G. R. F. Krueger, G. M. Shearer, and R. C. Gallo, "Elevated HBLV (Human Herpesvirus-6) Antibody in HIV-1 Antibody-Positive Symptomatic and Asymptomatic Individuals," in *IV International Conference on AIDS: Book 1* (Stockholm, June 12–16, 1988), abstract 1134, p. 146.

6. Robert Gallo, Flossie Wong-Staal, Luc Montagnier, William A. Haseltine, and Mitsuaki Yoshida, "HIV/HTLV Gene Nomenclature," *Science* 333 (1988):504.

7. Institute of Medicine, *Confronting AIDS: Update 1988* (Washington, D.C.: National Academy Press, 1988).

8. A. S. Fauci, "AIDS: Immunopathogenic Mechanisms and Research Strategies" *Clinical Research* 35 (1987):503–510.

9. Howard E. Gendelman, J. M. Orenstein, M. A. Martin, Carol Ferrua, Rita Mitra, Terri Phipps, L. A. Wahl, H. C. Lane, A. S. Fauci, D. S. Burke, Donald Skillman, and M. S. Meltzer, "Efficient Isolation and Propagation of Human Immunodeficiency Virus on Recombinant Colony-Stimulating Factor 1–Treated Monocytes," *Journal of Experimental Medicine* 167 (1988):1428–1441.

10. Scott Koenig, Howard E. Gendelman, Jan M. Orenstein, Mauro C. Dal Canto, Gholam H. Pezeshkpour, Margaret Yungbluth, Frank Janotta, Allen Aksamit, Malcolm A. Martin, and Anthony S. Fauci, "Detection of AIDS Virus in Macrophages in Brain Tissue from AIDS Patients with Encephalopathy," *Science* 233 (1986):1089–1093.

11. Gina Kolata, "AIDS Virus Found to Hide in Cells, Eluding Detection by Normal Tests," *New York Times,* June 5, 1988, pp. 1, 28.

12. S. Crowe, J. Mills, J. Kirihara, P. Lekas, and M. McGrath, "Splenic and Peritoneal Macrophages Provide a Major Reservoir of HIV *In Vivo,*" in *IV International Conference on AIDS, Book 1* (Stockholm, June 12–16, 1988), abstract 2062, p. 179.

13. Gina Kolata, "The Evolving Biology of AIDS: Scavenger Cell Looms Large," *New York Times,* June 7, 1988, p. C1.

14. H. Clifford Lane, Henry Masur, Lynn C. Edgar, Gail Whalen, Alain H. Rook, and Anthony S. Fauci, "Abnormalities of B-Cell Activation and Immunoregulation in Patients with the Acquired Immune Deficiency Syndrome," *NEJM* 309 (1983):453–458.

15. Mario Stevenson of the University of Nebraska Medical Center, Xinhua Zhang, and David J. Volsky report that HIV causes multiple abnormalities in the surface receptors of infected T cells; "Downregulation of Cell Surface Molecules during Noncytopathic Infection of T Cells with Human Immunodeficiency Virus," *Journal of Virology* 61 (1987):3741–3748.

16. Folks and his coworkers also have shown that substances produced by activated lymphocytes can lead to increased virus production in chronically infected monocytes; Thomas M. Folks, Jesse Justement, Audrey Kinter, Charles A. Dinarello, and Anthony S. Fauci, "Cytokine-Induced Expression of HIV-1 in a Chronically Infected Promoncyte Cell Line," *Science* 238 (1987):800–802.

17. Howard E. Gendelman, William Phelps, Lionel Feigenbaum, Jeffrey Ostrove, Aiko Adachi, Peter M. Howley, George Khoury, Harold S. Ginsberg, and Malcolm A. Martin, "Transactivation of the Human Immunodeficiency Virus Terminal Repeat Sequence by DNA Viruses," *Proceedings of the National Academy of Sciences* 83 (1986):9759–9763.

18. Annamari Ranki, Minerva Krohn, Jean-Pierre Allain, Genoveffa Franchini, Sirkka-Liisa Valle, Jaakko Antonen, Michael Leuther, and Kai Krohn, "Long Latency Precedes Overt Seroconversion in Sexually Transmitted Human Immunodeficiency Virus Infection," *Lancet* (1987) ii:589–593.

19. Gina Kolata, "Study of 18 Men with AIDS Virus Finds Delay in Antibody Production," *New York Times,* June 14, 1988, p. C7.

20. Homayoon Farzadegan, Michael A. Polis, Steven M. Wolinsky, Charles R. Rinaldo, Jr., John J. Sninsky, Shirley Kwok, Robert L. Giffith, Richard A. Kaslow, John P. Phair, B. Frank Polk, and Alfred J Saah, "Loss of Human Immunodeficiency Virus Type 1 (HIV-1) Antibodies with Evidence of Viral Infection in Asymptomatic Homosexual Men," *AIM* 108 (1988):785–790.

21. Thomas F. Zuck, "Silent Sequences and the Safety of Blood Transfusions," *AIM* 108 (1988):895–897. Gina Kolata, "Halt in AIDS Virus Growth Is Discovered in 4 Patients," *New York Times,* June 1, 1988, p. A18.

22. David D. Ho, M. G. Sarngadharan, Martin S. Hirsch, Robert T. Schooley, Teresa R. Rota, Ronald C. Kennedy, Tran C. Chanh, and Vicki L. Sato, "Human Immunodeficiency Virus Neutralizing Antibodies Recognize Several Conserved Domains on the Envelope Glycoproteins," *Journal of Virology* 61 (1987): 2024–2028. (David Ho is now in the Infectious Diseases Division at Cedars-Sinai Medical Center, Los Angeles, California.)

23. Bruce D. Walker, Sekhar Chakrabarti, Bernard Moss, Timothy J. Paradis, Theresa Flynn, Amy G. Durno, Richard S. Blumberg, Joan C. Kaplan, Martin S. Hirsch, and Robert T. Schooley, "HIV-specific Cytotoxic T Lymphocytes in Seropositive Individuals," *Nature* 328 (1987):345–348; Fernando Plata, Brigitte Autran, Livia Pedroza Martins, Simon Wain-Hobson, Martine Raphael, Charles Mayaud, Michel Denis, Jean-Marc Guillon, and

Patrice Debré, "AIDS Virus-specific Cytotoxic T Lymphocytes in Lung Disorders," ibid., pp. 348–351.

24. Stephen Dewhurst, Koji Sakai, Joel Bresser, Mario Stevenson, Mary Jean Evinger-Hodges, and David J. Volsky, "Persistent Productive Infection of Human Glial Cells by Human Immunodeficiency Virus (HIV) and by Infectious Molecular Clones of HIV," *Journal of Virology* 61 (1987):3774–3782.

25. Deborah M. Barnes, "Brain Function Decline in Children with AIDS," *Science* 232 (1986):1196.

26. Susan Squire, "New Clues to the Immune System," *New York Times Magazine,* January 29, 1987, p. 32.

27. Gina Kolata, "Where Is the AIDS Virus Harbored?" *Science* 232 (1986): 1197.

28. Robert E. Donahue, Margaret M. Johnson, Leonard I. Zon, Steven C. Clark, and Jerome E. Groopman, "Suppression of In Vitro Haematopoiesis Following Human Immunodeficiency Virus Infection," *Nature* 326 (1987):200–203.

29. Thomas M. Folks, S. Kessler, M. Cottler-Fox, J. Justement, J. Orenstein, and A. S. Fauci, "Infection and Replication of Human Immunodeficiency Virus-1 (HIV-1) in Purified CD4 Negative Precursor Cells from Normal Human Bone Marrow," in *IV International Conference on AIDS,* abstract 2067, p. 180

30. J. Orenstein, quoted in Timothy F. Kirn, "Immunodeficiency Virus Slowly Yields Secrets," *JAMA* 259 (1988):3378–3379.

31. Jay A. Nelson, Catherine Reynolds-Kohler, William Margaretten, Clayton A. Wiley, Charles E. Reese, and Jay A. Levy, "Human Immunodeficiency Virus Detected in Bowel Epithelium from Patients with Gastrointestinal Symptoms," *Lancet* (1988) i:259–262.

32. Roger J. Pomerantz, Suzanne M. de la Monte, S. Patrick Donegan, Teresa R. Rota, Markus W. Vogt, Donald E. Craven, and Martin S. Hirsch, "Human Immunodeficiency Virus Infection of the Human Uterine Cervix," *AIM* 108 (1988):321–327.

6. Prevention

1. Harvey V. Fineberg, "Education to Prevent AIDS: Prospects and Obstacles," *Science* 239 (1988):592–596.

2. Ellen Goodman, "When the 'Experts' Start Dueling on AIDS," *Boston Globe,* March 10, 1988, p. 21.

3. Quoted in *Newsweek,* March 14, 1988, p. 42. The sex therapists base their statement on a study of 800 heterosexuals recruited from churches, colleges, and singles bars in 4 cities. Six percent of those who reported at least 6 sexual partners a year were

infected with HIV, a figure much higher than that found in other studies. Critics point out that the authors did not reinterview those who tested positive. Other studies have shown that people who are faced with a positive result will often admit that they have not been truthful about risk factors such as homosexuality or drug abuse; Christine Gorman, "An Outbreak of Sensationalism," *Time,* March 21, 1988, p. 59.

4. "AIDS Risk Articles Criticized," *New York Times,* February 20, 1988. p. 10.

5. "Koop Blasts AIDS Book's 'Scare Tactics,' " *Boston Globe,* March 10, 1988, p. 84.

6. Goodman, "When the 'Experts' Start Dueling."

7. One of the ads showed a woman slipping a condom into her purse as she prepared for a date. The other began with a young couple embracing in a doorway; the girl left when the young man balked at the idea of using a condom.

8. James Barron, "Media Executives Hesitant to Run Explicit AIDS Ads," *New York Times,* May 12, 1987, p. B3.

9. C. Everett Koop, "Physician Leadership in Preventing AIDS," *JAMA* 258 (1987):2111.

10. William W. Darrow, "Condom Use and Use-Effectiveness in High-Risk Population" (Paper presented at a meeting of the CDC, Atlanta, February 20, 1987).

11. Koop, "Physician Leadership." For additional information see Centers for Disease Control, "Condoms for Prevention of Sexually Transmitted Diseases," *MMWR* 37 (1988):133–137.

12. Jonathan Mann, Thomas C. Quinn, Peter Piot, Ngaly Bosenge, Nzila Nzilambi, Mpunga Kalala, Henry Francis, Robert L. Colebunders, Robert Byers, Pangu Kasa Azila, Ngandu Kabeya, and James W. Curran, "Condom Use and HIV Infection among Prostitutes in Zaire," *NEJM* 316 (1987):345.

13. Koop, "Physician Leadership," p. 2111.

14. Thomas J. Coates, Stephen Morin, and Leon McKusick, "Behavioral Consequences of AIDS Antibody Testing among Gay Men," *JAMA* 258 (1987): 1988; also Thomas J. Coates, Stephen Morin, Leon McKusick, Colleen Hoff, Joseph A. Catania, Susan M. Kegeles, and Lance Pollock, "Long-Term Consequences of AIDS Antibody Testing on Gay and Bisexual Men," in *IV International Conference on Aids: Book 1* (Stockholm, June 12–16, 1988), abstract 8101, p. 474.

15. Organizations that discouraged homosexual men from obtaining HIV testing generally recommended that all homosexual men assume that they were antibody positive regardless of test results and behave accordingly—follow safer-sex guidelines and

refrain from donating blood, semen, or organs for transplantation. See Thomas J. Coates, Ronald D. Stall, Susan M. Kegeles, Bernard Lo, Stephen F. Morin, and Leon McKusick, "AIDS Antibody Testing: Will It Stop the AIDS Epidemic? Will It Help People Infected with HIV?" *American Psychologist,* 43 (November 1988).

16. Council on Ethical and Judicial Affairs, "Ethical Issues Involved in the Growing AIDS Crisis," *JAMA* 259 (1988):1360–1361.

17. Ronald Sullivan, "New Attack on AIDS Is Planned: Patients to Be Urged to Name Partners," *New York Times,* December 5, 1987, p. 29.

18. Dean F. Echenberg, "Education and Contact Notification for AIDS Prevention," *New York State Journal of Medicine,* May 1987, pp. 296–297.

19. Thomas M. Vernon, letter to Committee for the Oversight of AIDS Activities, Institute of Medicine, National Academy of Sciences, December 8, 1987.

20. Bernard M. Dickens, "Legal Rights and Duties in the AIDS Epidemic," *Science* 239 (1988):580–586.

21. Mark A. Rothstein, "Screening Workers for AIDS," in *AIDS and the Law: A Guide for the Public,* ed. Harlon L. Dalton, Scott Burris, and the Yale AIDS Law Project (New Haven: Yale University Press, 1987), pp. 126–141.

22. U.S. Congress, House, 100th Cong., 1st sess., H.R. 3071 (Mr. Waxman and cosponsors).

23. Thomas J. Coates, Ron D. Stall, and Colleen C. Hoff, "Changes in Sexual Behavior among Gay and Bisexual Men Since the Beginning of the AIDS Epidemic" (Paper prepared for U.S. Congress, Office of Technology Assessment, Washington, D.C., 1988). See also John L. Martin, "The Impact of AIDS on Gay Male Sexual Behavior Patterns in New York City," *American Journal of Public Health* 77 (1987):578–581.

24. Fineberg, "Education to Prevent AIDS."

25. Maria L. Ekstrand and Thomas J. Coates, "Predictors of AIDS High-Risk Behavior among a Probability Sample of Gay and Bisexual Men: The San Francisco Men's Health Study," in *IV International Conference on Aids,* abstract 9078, p. 495.

26. Leonard H. Calabrese, Buck Harris, Kirk A. Easley, and Max R. Proffitt, "Persistence of High Risk Sexual Activity among Homosexual Men in an Area of Low Incidence for Acquired Immunodeficiency Syndrome," *AIDS Research* 2 (1986):357–361.

27. Clifton C. Jones, Hetty Waskin, Brigid Gerety, Betty J. Skipper, Harry F. Hull, and Gregory J. Mertz, "Persistence of High-Risk Sexual Activity among Homosexual Men in an Area of

Low Incidence of the Acquired Immunodeficiency Syndrome," *Sexually Transmitted Diseases* 14 (1987):79–82.

28. Coates, Stall, and Hoff, "Changes in Sexual Behavior."

29. Sandra G. Boodman, "Despite AIDS, Many Gays Snub 'Safe Sex' Warnings," *Washington Post,* November 26, 1987, p. A27.

30. Gina Kolata, "Erotic Films in AIDS Study Cut Risky Behavior," *New York Times,* November 3, 1987, p. C3.

31. Ronald O. Valdiserri, David W. Lyter, Lawrence A. Kingsley, Laura C. Leviton, Janet W. Schofield, James Huggins, Monto Ho, and Charles R. Rinaldo, "The Effect of Group Education on Improving Attitudes about AIDS Risk Reduction," *New York State Journal of Medicine,* May 1987, pp. 272–278.

32. Presidential Commission on the Human Immunodeficiency Virus Epidemic, "Interim Report" (Washington, D.C., March 15, 1988), p. 6.

33. Peter Kerr, "Drug Treatment Shortage Imperils AIDS Control," *New York Times,* October 4, 1987, p. 32.

34. Don C. Des Jarlais, Samuel R. Friedman, and Rand L. Stoneburner, "HIV Infection and Intravenous Drug Use: Critical Issues in Transmission Dynamics, Infection Outcomes, and Prevention," *Reviews of Infectious Diseases* 10 (1988):151–158.

35. Ibid., p. 155.

36. Ibid., p. 156.

37. Don C. Des Jarlais, Samuel R. Friedman, and William Hopkins, "Risk Reduction for the Acquired Immunodeficiency Syndrome among Intravenous Drug Abusers," *AIM* 103 (1985): 755–759.

38. Chris Anne Raymond, "First Needle-Exchange Program Approved: Other Cities Await Results," *JAMA* 259 (1988): 1289–1290.

39. In June 1988 the American Foundation for AIDS Research in New York announced that it would sponsor the nation's first authorized needle-exchange program in Portland, Oregon. At the time, the New York plan still faced several obstacles. The *New York Times* reported: "A long-pending proposed experiment to distribute needles to 200 New York City addicts is hinging on the efforts of local health officials to persuade law enforcement officials to refrain from arresting and prosecuting participants"; Bruce Lambert, "Addicts in Portland, Ore., Will Get Free Hypodermic Needles," June 10, 1988, p. A13.

40. Des Jarlais, Friedman, and Stoneburner, "HIV Infection and Intravenous Drug Use," p. 156.

41. Mary Chamberland, L. Conley, and T. Dondero. "Epide-

miology and Evolution of Heterosexually Acquired AIDS—United States," in *IV International Conference on Aids,* abstract 4017, p. 264.
42. Robert Pear, "Sharp Rise Found in Syphilis in U.S.," *New York Times,* October 4, 1987, p. 1.
43. "AIDS Effort for High-Risk Women Set for Boston," *Boston Globe,* December 16, 1987, p. 29.
44. Centers for Disease Control, "Antibody to Human Immunodeficiency Virus in Female Prostitutes," *MMWR* 36 (1987): 157–161.
45. John F. Decker, "Prostitution as a Public Health Issue," in Dalton, Burris, and Yale AIDS Law Project, *AIDS and the Law,* p. 86. Decker says that blood testing generally is not considered an unreasonable method of search, as long as it has been demonstrated that there is probable cause to search for infection (for example, if a high proportion of prostitutes in a given area are infected) and the search has been authorized by a judicial warrant; ibid., p. 87.
46. Quoted in Harold Schmeck, Jr., "Hemophiliacs' Mates Shun AIDS Tests," *New York Times,* September 12, 1987, p. 6. See also Centers for Disease Control, "HIV Infection and Pregnancies in Sexual Partners of HIV-Seropositive Hemophilic Men—United States," *MMWR* 36 (1987):593–595.
47. Keith Krasinski, William Borkowsky, Donna Bebenroth, and Tiina Moore, "Failure of Voluntary Testing for Human Immunodeficiency Virus to Identify Infected Parturient Women in High-Risk Population," *NEJM* 318 (1988):185; also Sheldon Landesman, Howard Minkoff, Susan Holman, Sandra McCalla, and Odalis Sijin, "Serosurvey of Human Immunodeficiency Virus Infection in Parturients: Implications for Human Immunodeficiency Virus Testing Programs of Pregnant Women," *JAMA* 258 (1987):2701–2703.
48. In several states the prevalence of HIV infection among childbearing women has been determined by anonymous testing of blood samples from newborn babies (see Chapter 2). The presence of HIV antibodies in the blood of a newborn indicates that the mother is infected with the virus.
49. Howard L. Minkoff, "Care of Pregnant Women Infected with Human Immunodeficiency Virus," *JAMA* 258 (1987):2714–2717.
50. Ibid.
51. Ibid.
52. In view of the tenuousness of these few case reports, it is not clear that the risks of breastfeeding outweigh the benefits in all settings. Many public health experts continue to recommend breastfeeding in developing countries with a high prevalence of HIV

infection; they believe that the hazards of bottle-feeding, associated with contaminated water, are probably greater than the chance of transmitting HIV through breast milk.

53. James L. Baker, Gabor D. Kelen, Keith T. Sivertson, and Thomas C. Quinn, "Unsuspected Human Immunodeficiency Virus in Critically Ill Emergency Patients," *JAMA* 257 (1987):2609–2611.

54. Centers for Disease Control, "Update: Human Immunodeficiency Virus Infections in Health-Care Workers Exposed to Blood of Infected Patients," *MMWR* 36 (1987):285–289.

55. James W. Curran, Harold W. Jaffe, Ann M. Hardy, W. Meade Morgan, Richard M. Selik, and Timothy J. Dondero, "Epidemiology of HIV Infection and AIDS in the United States," *Science* 239 (1988):610–616.

56. Robert Pear, "Health Workers to Get AIDS Protection," *New York Times*, July 24, 1987, p. A16.

57. "Hospitals Grapple with HIV Testing Issue," *Medical World News*, February 8, 1988, pp. 54–55.

58. Michael D. Hagen, Klemens B. Meyer, and Stephen G. Pauker, "Routine Preoperative Screening for HIV: Does the Risk to the Surgeon Outweigh the Risk to the Patient?" *JAMA* 259 (1988): 1357–1359.

59. Council on Ethical and Judicial Affairs, "Ethical Issues," p. 1361.

60. H. Hunter Handsfield, M. Jeanne Cummings, and Paul D. Swenson, "Prevalence of Antibody to Human Immunodeficiency Virus and Hepatitis B Surface Antigen in Blood Samples Submitted to a Hospital Laboratory: Implications for Handling Specimens," *JAMA* 258 (1987):3395–3397.

61. Stanley H. Weiss, James J. Goedert, Suzanne Gartner, Mikulas Popovic, David Waters, Philip Markham, Fulvia di Marzo Veronese, Mitchell H. Gail, W. Emmett Barkley, Joseph Gibbons, Fred A. Gill, Michael Leuther, George M. Shaw, Robert C. Gallo, and William A. Blattner, "Risk of Human Immunodeficiency Virus (HIV-1) Infection among Laboratory Workers," *Science* 239 (1988): 68–71.

62. Deborah Barnes, "AIDS Virus Creates Lab Risk," *Science* 239 (1988):348–349.

63. Ibid., p. 349.

64. Weiss et al., "Risk of HIV-1 Infection," p. 71.

65. "School Boards Favor AIDS Mandate," *New York Times*, February 27, 1988, p. 10.

66. Centers for Disease Control, "Guidelines for Effective School Health Education to Prevent the Spread of AIDS," *MMWR* 37, supp. 2 (1988):2.

67. "School Boards Favor AIDS Mandate."

68. Lee Strunin and Ralph Hingson, "Acquired Immunodeficiency Syndrome and Adolescents: Knowledge, Beliefs, Attitudes, and Behaviors," *Pediatrics* 79 (1987):825–828.

69. Susan M. Kegeles, Nancy E. Adler, and Charles E. Irwin, Jr., "Sexually Active Adolescents and Condoms: Changes over One Year in Knowledge, Attitudes, and Use," *American Journal of Public Health* 78 (1988):460–461.

70. Barbara Ann Caruso and John R. Haig, "AIDS on Campus: A Survey of College Health Service Priorities and Policies," *Journal of American College Health* 36 (1987):35.

71. David W. Fraser, "AIDS Education in Colleges: Recent Issues" (Paper prepared for the Committee for the Oversight of AIDS Activities, Institute of Medicine, National Academy of Sciences, 1987).

72. Centers for Disease Control, "Additional Recommendations to Reduce Sexual and Drug Abuse–Related Transmission of Human T-Lymphotropic Virus Type III/Lymphadenopathy-Associated Virus," *MMWR* 35 (1986):152–155.

73. Philip M. Boffey, "Reagan Urges Wide AIDS Testing but Does Not Call for Compulsion," *New York Times*, June 1, 1987, p. 1.

74. Institute of Medicine, *Confronting AIDS* (Washington, D.C.: National Academy Press, 1986), pp. 14–15.

75. Paul D. Cleary, Michael J. Barry, Kenneth H. Mayer, Allan M. Brandt, Larry Gostin, and Harvey V. Fineberg, "Compulsory Premarital Screening for the Human Immunodeficiency Virus," *JAMA* 258 (1987):1757–1762.

76. Isabel Wilkerson, "Illinoisans Fault Prenuptial AIDS Tests," *New York Times*, April 16, 1988, p. 6.

77. On December 18, 1987, the military services announced that military personnel infected with HIV would be "removed from sensitive, stressful jobs because of new evidence that the virus could impair mental function, even in people who show no overt symptoms of the disease"; Robert Pear, "Key Jobs in Military Off Limits for AIDS-Infected," *New York Times*, December 19, 1987, p. 1. Several months later, a WHO panel of experts convened to review scientific data on the neurological effects of HIV infection concluded that "otherwise healthy HIV-infected individuals are no more likely to be functionally impaired than uninfected persons"; "WHO Statement on Neuropsychological Aspects of HIV Infection" (Geneva: World Health Organization, Division of Mental Health, Global Programme on AIDS, March 18, 1988).

78. Presidential Commission on the Human Immunodeficiency

Virus Epidemic, *Preliminary Report: December 2, 1987* (Washington, D.C., 1987), app. C-1.

79. Decker, "Prostitution as a Public Health Issue."

7. Drugs and Vaccines

1. In an interview with the *Boston Globe* in December 1987, a spokesman for Burroughs Wellcome Company explained that AZT was licensed before the company had had time to develop full-scale production facilities. Expansion of the firm's manufacturing capabilities resulted in increased efficiency, which allowed a decrease in the price of the drug; Judy Foreman "Cost of Anti-AIDS Drug AZT to Be Reduced by 20 Percent," December 15, 1987, p. 3.

2. Some of the ACTUs were originally funded as AIDS Treatment Evaluation Units (ATEUs) and others were funded as AIDS Clinical Study Groups (CSGs).

3. Philip M. Boffey, "Trial of AIDS Drug in U.S. Lags as Too Few Participants Enroll," *New York Times,* December 28, 1987, p. 1.

4. Patricia Fultz, "Conspectus on Primate Models for AIDS" (Paper prepared for the Committee for the Oversight of AIDS Activities, Institute of Medicine, National Academy of Sciences, 1987).

5. Ruth M. Ruprecht, "Development and *In Vivo* Analysis of Antiretroviral Therapy," in *Biotechnology and Clinical Medicine,* ed. A. Albertini, C. Lenfant, and R. Paoletti (New York: Raven Press, 1987), pp. 227–234.

6. Richard A. Knox, "Symptoms of AIDS," *Boston Globe,* June 15, 1988, p. 21. See also J. M. Leonard, J. Abramczuk, D. Pezen, J. S. Khillan, H. E. Gendelman, H. Westphal, M. S. Meltzer, and M. A. Martin, "Expressions of an Infectious HIV Provirus in Transgenic Mice," in *IV International Conference on AIDS: Book 1* (Stockholm, June 12–16, 1988), abstract 3107, p. 246.

7. W. A. Carter, Isadore Brodsky, M. G. Pellegrino, H. F. Henriques, D. M. Parenti, R. S. Schulof, W. E. Robinson, D. J. Volsky, Helene Paxton, Katalin Karikó, R. J. Suhadolnik, D. R. Strayer, Mark Lewin, Leo Einck, G. L. Simon, R. G. Scheib, D. C. Montefiori, W. M. Mitchell, Deborah Paul, W. A. Meyer III, Nancy Reichenbach, and D. H. Gillespie, "Clinical, Immunological, and Virological Effects of Ampligen, a Mismatched Double-Stranded RNA, in Patients with AIDS or AIDS-Related Complex," *Lancet* (1987) i:1286–1292.

8. Gina Kolata, "Poor Results Bring End to Anti-AIDS Drug Study," *New York Times*, October 14, 1988, p. A17.

9. Martin Hirsch, "AIDS Update Commentary: Azidothymidine," *Journal of Infectious Diseases* 157 (1988):429.

10. Philip A. Pizzo, Janie Eddie, Judy Falloon, Frank M. Balis, Robert F. Murphy, Howard Moss, Pam Wolters, Pim Brouwers, et al., "Effect of Continuous Intravenous Infusion of Zidovadine (AZT) in Children with Symptomatic HIV Infection," *NEJM* 319 (1988): 889–896.

11. Martin S. Hirsch and Joan C. Kaplan, "Treatment of Human Immunodeficiency Virus Infections," *Antimicrobial Agents and Chemotherapy* 31 (1987):841.

12. Robert Yarchoan, R. V. Thomas, J.-P. Allain, Nanette McAtee, Richard Dubinsky, H. I. Mitsuya, T. J. Lawley, Bijan Safai, C. E. Myers, C. F. Perno, R. W. Klacker, R. J. Wills, M. A. Fischl, M. C. McNeely, J. M. Pluda, Michael Leuther, J. M. Collins, and Samuel Broder, "Phase 1 Studies of 2', 3'-Dideoxycytidine in Severe Human Immunodeficiency Virus Infection as a Single Agent and Alternating with Zidovudine (AZT)," *Lancet* (1988) i:76–81.

13. Other stimuli, including pieces of RNA, fragments of bacterial membranes, and certain chemicals, also can elicit secretion of interferons.

14. The neutrophil is the most numerous of the 3 types of white blood cells in the granulocytic series. The other 2 types are the eosinophil and the basophil.

15. Laboratory studies indicate that in some cases GM-CSF alone may actually stimulate HIV production. When recombinant GM-CSF was added to a model system consisting of chronically infected, cloned monocyte precursors, virus expression increased significantly; Thomas M. Folks, Jesse Justement, Audrey Kinter, Charles A. Dinarello, and Anthony S. Fauci, "Cytokine-Induced Expression of HIV-1 in a Chronically Infected Promonocyte Cell Line," *Science* 238 (1988):800–802.

16. Rob A. Gruters, Jacques J. Neefjes, Matthijs Tersmette, Ruud E. Y. de Goede, Abraham Tulp, Han G. Huisman, Frank Miedema, and Hidde L. Ploegh, "Interference with HIV-Induced Syncytium Formation and Viral Infectivity by Inhibitors of Trimming Glucosidase," *Nature* 330 (1987):74–77.

17. Institute of Medicine, *Confronting AIDS* (Washington, D.C.: National Academy Press, 1986), p. 26.

18. The concern over protecting people against different isolates of HIV actually has diminished somewhat. Researchers at the National Cancer Institute have reported that the use of booster shots after an initial immunization can broaden the immune response to a

vaccine. Chimpanzees that received several booster shots with a subunit vaccine developed an antibody response capable of recognizing multiple strains of HIV.

19. Some policymakers have expressed concern that the notarized documents could be counterfeited. NIAID is working with the Bureau of Engraving to develop a counterfeit-proof document that could be used when vaccine trials expand beyond the small studies now under way.

20. Axel Ellrodt and Phillipe Le Bras, "The Hidden Dangers of AIDS Vaccination," *Nature* 325 (1987):765.

21. If the recombinant vaccinia virus were transmissible, contacts of the vaccinee who had eczema or another severe skin disorder also might be at risk of developing disseminated vaccinia.

22. The goals of vaccine trials differ from the goals established for trials of therapeutic drugs. Researchers begin to assess the efficacy of a drug in phase 2 trials; vaccine efficacy is not addressed until phase 3.

23. Jonas Salk, "Prospects for the Control of AIDS by Immunizing Seropositive Individuals," *Nature* 327 (1987):473–476.

8. Individual and Societal Stress

1. Peter M. Marzuk, Helen Tierney, Kenneth Tardiff, Elliot M. Gross, Edward B. Morgan, Ming-Ann Hsu, and J. John Mann, "Increased Risk of Suicide in Persons with AIDS," *JAMA* 259 (1988):1333–1337.

2. Vickie M. Mays and Susan D. Cochran, "Acquired Immunodeficiency Syndrome and Black Americans: Special Psychosocial Issues," *Public Health Reports* 102 (1987):227.

3. Constance B. Wofsy, "Human Immunodeficiency Virus Infection in Women," Editorial *JAMA* 257 (1987):2074–2076.

4. Charles Lawrence, P. Thomas, D. Morse, B. Truman, I. Auger, R. Williams, and V. DeGruttola, "Incubation Periods for Maternally Transmitted Pediatric AIDS Cases," in *IV International Conference on AIDS: Book 1* (Stockholm, June 12–16, 1988), abstract 7268, p. 444.

5. Jane Gross, "Children with AIDS," *New York Times,* July 17, 1987, pp. 1, B4.

6. Samuel Perry and Paul Jacobsen, "Neuropsychiatric Manifestations of AIDS-Spectrum Disorders," *Hospital and Community Psychiatry* 37 (1986):135–142.

7. Michael Helquist, ed., *Working with AIDS: A Resource Guide for Mental Health Professionals* (San Francisco: AIDS Health Project, University of California at San Francisco, June 1987).

8. Mays and Cochran, "AIDS and Black Americans," p. 228.

9. Robert Steinbrook, Bernard Lo, Jeffrey Moulton, Glenn Saika, Harry Hollander, and Paul A. Volberding, "Preferences of Homosexual Men with AIDS for Life-Sustaining Treatment," *NEJM* 314 (1986):457–460. See also James A. Roberston, *The Rights of the Critically Ill* (New York: Bantam, 1983).

10. At the time, ARC referred to a variety of chronic symptoms and physical findings occurring in HIV-infected patients whose conditions did not meet the CDC definition of AIDS. The symptoms included chronic swollen glands, recurrent fevers, unintentional weight loss, chronic diarrhea, lethargy, minor alterations of the immune system, and oral thrush. The revision of the CDC surveillance case definition for AIDS in August 1987 (see Appendix B) made the term *ARC* obsolete. See Chapters 2 and 3 for more information.

11. David G. Ostrow, "Psychiatric Consequences of AIDS: An Overview," *International Journal of Neuroscience* 32 (1987):649.

12. Eric Lichtblau, "Rise in Antigay Violence Linked to AIDS in Study," *Boston Globe,* June 8, 1988, p. 5.

13. Caroline H. Sparks, "Report of the AIDS Prevention Forum for Women" (Report for the National Institute of Mental Health, Rockville, Md., 1986). See also idem, "Psychosocial Impact of AIDS on Women" (Report for the National Institute of Mental Health, Office of Prevention and Special Projects, Rockville, Md., 1987).

14. Wofsy, "HIV Infection in Women."

15. David Agle, Henry Gluck, and Glenn F. Pierce, "The Risk of AIDS: Psychologic Impact on the Hemophilic Population," *General Hospital Psychiatry* 9 (1987):11–17.

16. Ibid., p. 15.

17. Steven Steiber, "AIDS: Explosive Growth in Public Awareness," *Hospitals,* January 5, 1988, p. 96. Also "Public Supports AIDS Education, Research," ibid., January 5, 1988, p. 67.

18. Quoted in "81% Found to Support U.S. on Backing AIDS Research," *New York Times,* January 8, 1987, p. B6.

19. Personal communication.

20. John Ellement, "Robertson Says AIDS Spreads Easily," *Boston Globe,* December 17, 1987, p. 37; idem, "Tracking Robertson on AIDS: Briton Is Source of Disputed Views," *Boston Globe,* December 26, 1987, p. 3.

21. Ellement reported in the December 26 article that Seale "also believes homosexual men are part of a 'secret society,' some members of which are intent on 'destroying the rest of society.' "

22. Ronald Bayer, "AIDS, Power, and Reason," *Milbank Quarterly* 64, supp. 1 (1986):169.

23. Philip M. Boffey, "Doctors Who Shun AIDS Patients Are Assailed by Surgeon General," *New York Times*, September 10, 1987, p. 1.

24. Lindsey Gruson, "AIDS Fear Spawns Ethics Debate as Some Doctors Withhold Care," *New York Times*, July 11, 1987, pp. 1, 12.

25. Council on Ethical and Judicial Affairs," "Ethical Issues Involved in the Growing AIDS Crisis," *JAMA* 259 (1988):1360.

26. Charles E. Lewis, Howard E. Freeman, and Christopher C. Corey, "AIDS-Related Competence of California's Primary Care Physicians," *American Journal of Public Health* 77 (1987):795–799.

27. Jeffrey A. Kelly, Janet S. St. Lawrence, Steve Smith, Jr., Harold V. Hood, and Donna J. Cook, "Stigmatization of AIDS Patients by Physicians," ibid., p. 791.

28. Michael Specter, "Medical Profession Confronts New Generation's AIDS Fear," *Washington Post*, January 20, 1988, p. A1.

9. The Impact of AIDS on the Health Care System

1. Lydia Chavez, "Emergency Rooms: The New Wards," *New York Times*, January 15, 1988, p. B1.

2. Stacey Okun, "Lack of Nurses Impedes New York AIDS Care," *New York Times*, February 23, 1988, pp. 1, D30.

3. Bruce D. Lambert, "Outlook Dim for Expanding Health Care," *New York Times*, April 5, 1988, p. 1.

4. Deborah Barnes, "AIDS Stresses Health Care in San Francisco," *Science* 235 (1987):964.

5. Institute of Medicine, *Confronting AIDS: Update 1988* (Washington, D.C.: National Academy Press, 1988), p. 93.

6. Jane Gross, "New York City AIDS Patients Find Few Places to Ease Their Last Days," *New York Times*, June 12, 1987, pp. B1, B4.

7. Institute of Medicine, *Confronting AIDS: Update 1988*, p. 96.

8. Institute of Medicine, *Confronting AIDS* (Washington, D.C.: National Academy Press, 1986), p. 146.

9. Gina Kolata, "New York Shelters, a Last Stop for Hundreds of AIDS Patients," *New York Times*, April 4, 1988, pp. B1, B4.

10. Suzanne Daley, "Foster Care and AIDS: Joy and Pain," *New York Times*, May 7, 1988, pp. 29–30.

11. Institute of Medicine, *Confronting AIDS: Update 1988*, p. 96.

12. Daley, "Foster Care."

13. Joe Mahoney, "A Loving Home for Babies with AIDS," *Boston Globe,* May 29, 1988, p. 2.

14. David E. Bloom and Geoffrey Carliner, "The Economic Impact of AIDS in the United States," *Science* 239 (1988):604–609.

15. Ann M. Hardy, Kathryn Rauch, Dean Echenberg, W. Meade Morgan, and James W. Curran, "The Economic Impact of the First 10,000 Cases of Acquired Immunodeficiency Syndrome in the United States, *JAMA* 255 (1986):209–211.

16. Bloom and Carliner, "Economic Impact of AIDS," p. 604.

17. Anne A. Scitovsky, "Review of Current State of Knowledge Regarding the Personal Medical Care Costs of Persons with AIDS (PWA)" (Paper prepared for the Institute of Medicine, Washington, D.C., 1988).

18. Dennis P. Andrulis, Virginia S. Beers, James D. Bentley, and Larry S. Gage, "The Provision and Financing of Medical Care for AIDS Patients in U.S. Public and Private Teaching Hospitals," *JAMA* 258 (1987):1343–1346.

19. Bloom and Carliner, "Economic Impact of AIDS."

20. George R. Seage III, Stewart Landers, M. Anita Barry, Jerome Groopman, George A. Lamb, and Arnold M. Epstein, "Medical Care Costs of AIDS in Massachusetts," *JAMA* 256 (1986):3107–3109.

21. Fred J. Hellinger, "Forecasting the Personal Medical Care Costs of AIDS from 1988 through 1991," *Public Health Reports* 103 (1988):309–319.

22. Ibid.

23. Michael Specter, "450,000 AIDS Cases Seen by '93," *Washington Post,* June 5, 1988, p. A1.

24. Anne A. Scitovsky and Dorothy P. Rice, "Estimates of the Direct and Indirect Costs of Acquired Immunodeficiency Syndrome in the United States, 1985, 1986, and 1991," *Public Health Reports* 102 (1987):5–17.

25. Presidential Commission on the Human Immunodeficiency Virus Epidemic, "Interim Report" (Washington, D.C., March 15, 1988).

26. Hardy et al., "Economic Impact of First 10,000 Cases."

27. Bloom and Carliner, "Economic Impact of AIDS"; figures are based on extrapolation of Scitovsky and Rice's estimates.

28. For males aged 35 to 44, lifetime per-patient medical costs (in 1986 dollars) are $67,000 for heart attack, $47,500 for cancer of the digestive tract, and $28,600 for leukemia; ibid.

29. Ibid., p. 607.

30. Scitovsky and Rice, "Estimates of Costs."

31. Institute of Medicine, *Confronting AIDS: Update 1988.*

32. Bloom and Carliner, "Economic Impact of AIDS."

33. Andrulis et al., "Provision and Financing of Medical Care."

34. U.S. Congress, Office of Technology Assessment, *The Costs of AIDS and Other HIV Infections: Review of the Estimates,* Staff paper (Washington, D.C., 1987).

35. Institute of Medicine, *Confronting AIDS: Update 1988.*

36. U.S. Congress, Office of Technology Assessment, *AIDS and Health Insurance: An OTA Survey,* Staff paper (Washington, D.C., 1988).

37. Institute of Medicine, *Confronting AIDS: Update 1988,* p. 118.

Acknowledgments

The support and contributions of many people were indispensable to the writing of both editions of *Mobilizing against AIDS*. The first edition was based on the 1985 annual meeting of the Institute of Medicine. Chaired by Philip Leder, John Emory Andrus Professor and chairman, Department of Genetics, Harvard Medical School, the meeting was planned and carried out under the skillful direction of Enriqueta C. Bond, director of IOM's Division of Health Promotion and Disease Prevention. Speakers who addressed the meeting also graciously cooperated throughout the preparation of the book: Lewellys F. Barker, American Red Cross, Washington, D.C.; Ronald Bayer, Columbia University School of Public Health, New York City; Brett J. Cassens, Association of Physicians for Human Rights, Philadelphia; James W. Curran, Centers for Disease Control, Atlanta; Anthony S. Fauci, National Institute of Allergy and Infectious Diseases, NIH, Bethesda, Md.; Shervert Frazier, Harvard Medical School and McLean Hospital, Belmont, Mass.; Robert C. Gallo, National Cancer Institute, NIH, Bethesda; Richard T. Johnson, Johns Hopkins Medical Institutions, Baltimore; Philip R. Lee, University of California, San Francisco; Luc Montagnier, Institut Pasteur, Paris; June E. Osborn, University of Michigan School of Public Health, Ann Arbor; Frederick C. Robbins, former president, Institute of Medicine; and Mervyn F. Silverman, American Foundation for AIDS Research, New York City.

Guidance for the revised and enlarged edition was generously provided by the Committee for the Oversight of AIDS Activities at the Institute of Medicine/National Academy of Sciences, and by Robin Weiss, director of AIDS Activities at IOM. Committee members include: Theodore Cooper (chair), Upjohn Company, Kalamazoo, Mich.; Stuart Altman, Brandeis University, Waltham, Mass.; David Baltimore, Whitehead Institute for Biomedical Research and Massachusetts Institute of Technology, Cambridge, Mass.; Kristine Gebbie, Oregon Health Division, Portland; Donald R. Hopkins, Carter Presidential Center, Atlanta; Kenneth Prewitt, The Rockefeller Foundation, New York City; Howard M. Temin, University of Wisconsin School of Medicine, Madison; and Paul Volberding, San Francisco General Hospital.

I also would like to thank the following: Stephen Chanock, Children's Hospital, Boston; Fran Chevarley, National Center for Health Statistics; Thomas J. Coates, University of California, San Francisco; John Coffin, Tufts University School of Medicine; Deborah Cotton, Beth Israel Hospital, Boston; Emily DeVoto, Harvard University Press; D. Peter Drotman, AIDS Program, Centers for Disease Control; Walter Dzik, New England Deaconess Hospital; Max Essex, Harvard School of Public Health; Mark Feinberg, Whitehead Institute for Biomedical Research; Jerome E. Groopman, New England Deaconess Hospital; Cherie Haitz, Mount Auburn Hospital, Cambridge, Mass.; Leslie Hardy, Institute of Medicine; William Haseltine, Dana-Farber Cancer Institute; Martin Hirsch, Massachusetts General Hospital; Colleen C. Hoff, University of California, San Francisco; Rodney Hoff, Massachusetts Department of Public Health; Frank Landry, Mount Auburn Hospital; Norman L. Letvin, New England Regional Primate Research Center; Lynn I. Levin, Institute of Medicine; Gayle Lloyd, Centers for Disease Control; Ann C. London, National Institute of Allergy and Infectious Diseases; Heather Miller, National Research Council/National Academy of Sciences; Lata Nerurkar, National Cancer Institute; Mary Jane Potash, Institute of Medicine; Juan Ramos, National Institute of Mental Health; Zeda Rosenberg, National Institute of Allergy and Infectious Diseases; Ruth Ruprecht, Dana-Farber Cancer Institute; Temple Smith, Dana-Farber Cancer Institute; Gail Spears, Institute of Medicine; Dale R. Spriggs, National Institute of Allergy and Infectious Diseases; Jeff Stryker, University of Michigan School of Public Health; Xiao-Hong Sun, Whitehead Institute for Biomedical Research; Charles F. Turner, National Research Council/National Academy of Sciences; and Roy Widdus, Global Programme on AIDS, World Health Organization.

Special thanks to Timothy Pace, now a student at George Washington University School of Medicine, who spent many hours in the library tracking down references for this book; and to Wallace K. Waterfall, senior editor at the Institute of Medicine, who improved the clarity of early drafts and provided encouragement when the task seemed most daunting. I also have benefited from the excellent advice and support of Howard Boyer and the editorial expertise of Ann Hawthorne at Harvard University Press. The writing of the manuscript was funded in large part by a grant from Hoffmann–La Roche, Inc.

Finally, I would like to thank three people whose patience and support made this book possible: my husband, Nick, and my children, Matthew and Elizabeth.

Index

Homosexual men (*cont.*)
Kinsey 1948 data on, 21
lymphomas in, 74, 77
macrophages in, 129
mandatory reporting with, 156
military personnel, 186
opportunistic infections in, 65
partner notification, 302
pneumocystis carinii pneumonia in, 93–94
promiscuity as risk factor in, 27, 51, 94, 157, 158
psychosocial effects on, 239, 246–247
risk factors, 94, 111
sexual behavior of, 14
shingles in, 70
teenagers, 182
testing for, 15, 151
transmission in, 26–27, 140
in vaccine safety trials, 228, 232
Homosexual women
incidence in, 27
venereal disease in, 27
Hopkins, Donald, 20
Hormones, and HIV infection, 41
Hospice care, 236, 260, 261, 262
Hospital patients
counseling for, 175
incidence in, 25
testing of, 174–175, 301–302
Hospital workers. *See* Health care workers
Hotlines, 160, 277
Housing discrimination, 156, 239
Houston, 27
HTLV-I, 97, 100, 104
HTLV-II, 100, 104
HTLV-III, 101, 104. *See also* HIV-1
HTLV-III/LAV, 104
HTLV-IV, 105
Hulley, Stephen, 32
Human B-lymphotropic virus. *See* Herpes virus; HHV-6

Human immunodeficiency viruses (HIVs). *See* HIV-1; HIV-2
Human T-cell leukemia/lymphoma virus (HTLV), 97, 100, 101. *See also* Human T-cell lymphotropic virus (HTLV)
Human T-cell lymphotropic virus (HTLV), 101, 104, 105. *See also* HIV-1; Human T-cell leukemia/lymphoma virus (HTLV)
Hypergammaglobulinemia, 86–87
Hypogammaglobulinemia, 86, 88

IDAV, 104
Illinois, 184, 185
Immigrants, testing of, 183, 186
Immune modulators, 191, 217–220
Immune system
cell fusion process and, 117
in children and adults, 81, 86
defects in and susceptibility to AIDS, 112
envelope proteins and, 118–119, 134, 135–136, 213
HTLV-I and HTLV-II and, 100
infection process and, 93–94, 121, 126–136
and infectivity, 31, 52
lymphomas and, 77, 78
normal function of, 121–126
regulatory genes and, 119–121
response to HIV, 132–136
and sexual behavior, 94
Immunization. *See* Vaccines
Immunization Practices Advisory Committee, 89
Immunodeficiency-associated virus (IDAV), 104
Immunoenhancement, 229
Immunosuppression
and AIDS-related symptoms, 80
and lymphomas, 78
Imreg-1, 219–220